MINDFULNESS-ORIENTED INTERVENTIONS FOR TRAUMA

Also Available

Cognitive-Behavioral Therapies for Trauma,
Second Edition
Edited by Victoria M. Follette and Josef I. Ruzek

Mindfulness and Acceptance:
Expanding the Cognitive-Behavioral Tradition
*Edited by Steven C. Hayes, Victoria M. Follette,
and Marsha M. Linehan*

Mindfulness-Oriented Interventions for Trauma

Integrating Contemplative Practices

edited by
Victoria M. Follette, John Briere, Deborah Rozelle,
James W. Hopper, and David I. Rome

THE GUILFORD PRESS
New York   London

To D. H. who helps me on the path—VMF

*To Cheryl Lanktree, for her support
with this book and in all other things*—JB

*To Gelek Rimpoche, whose guidance, life,
and work are an inspiration and model*—DR

*To DaRa Williams, former Director of the Women's
Wellness Project at the Garrison Institute*—DIR

© 2015 The Guilford Press
A Division of Guilford Publications, Inc.
370 Seventh Avenue, Suite 1200, New York, NY 10001
www.guilford.com

Paperback edition 2018

Printed in the United States of America

This book is printed on acid-free paper.

Last digit is print number: 9 8 7 6 5 4 3

The authors have checked with sources believed to be reliable in their efforts to provide
information that is complete and generally in accord with the standards of practice that
are accepted at the time of publication. However, in view of the possibility of human error
or changes in behavioral, mental health, or medical sciences, neither the authors, nor the
editors and publisher, nor any other party who has been involved in the preparation or
publication of this work warrants that the information contained herein is in every respect
accurate or complete, and they are not responsible for any errors or omissions or the
results obtained from the use of such information. Readers are encouraged to confirm the
information contained in this book with other sources.

Library of Congress Cataloging-in-Publication Data

Mindfulness-oriented interventions for trauma : integrating contemplative practices / edited
by Victoria M. Follette, John Briere, Deborah Rozelle, James W. Hopper, David I. Rome.
     p. ; cm.
Includes bibliographical references and index.
ISBN 978-1-4625-1858-6 (hardcover : alk. paper)
ISBN 978-1-4625-3384-8 (paperback : alk. paper)
  I. Follette, Victoria M., editor. II. Briere, John, editor. III. Rozelle, Deborah, 1954– ,
editor. IV. Hopper, James W., editor. V. Rome, David I., editor.
  [DNLM: 1. Stress Disorders, Traumatic—therapy. 2. Mindfulness—methods.
3. Spiritual Therapies—methods. WM 172.5]
  RD93
  617.1′0652—dc23
                                                                        2015044240

About the Editors

Victoria M. Follette, PhD, is Foundation Professor in the Department of Psychology at the University of Nevada, Reno. Her work has focused on treating complex trauma using acceptance and commitment therapy. A Fellow and a past president of the Western Psychological Association, Dr. Follette is coeditor of *Cognitive-Behavioral Therapies for Trauma, Second Edition,* and *Mindfulness and Acceptance: Expanding the Cognitive-Behavioral Tradition.*

John Briere, PhD, is Associate Professor in the Departments of Psychiatry and Psychology at the Keck School of Medicine, University of Southern California (USC), and Director of the USC Adolescent Trauma Training Center, National Child Traumatic Stress Network. He is a recipient of the Robert S. Laufer Memorial Award for Scientific Achievement from the International Society for Traumatic Stress Studies and the Award for Outstanding Contributions to the Science of Trauma Psychology from Division 56 of the American Psychological Association. Designated a "Highly Cited Researcher" by the Institute of Scientific Information, Dr. Briere has published widely in the areas of trauma, child abuse, and interpersonal violence, as well as the application of mindfulness to trauma therapy.

Deborah Rozelle, PsyD, is a certified therapist and Approved Consultant in eye movement desensitization and reprocessing (EMDR). She trains and consults widely on psychological trauma, trauma therapy, and their relation to contemplative practice. Dr. Rozelle is on the faculties of the Institute for Meditation and Psychotherapy in Cambridge, Massachusetts, and the Nalanda Institute for Contemplative Science in New York City. She is a long-time practicing Buddhist and has a clinical practice in Lexington, Massachusetts.

James W. Hopper, PhD, is Clinical Instructor in Psychology in the Department of Psychiatry at Harvard Medical School. His work as a consultant, clinician, and researcher has focused on the effects of child abuse and sexual assault, the nature of traumatic memories, the psychology and biology of trauma, and the brain bases of meditation and other spiritual practices. Dr. Hopper trains and consults with a wide range of organizations and professionals.

David I. Rome, BA, is a teacher, writer, and editor focusing on applications of contemplative methods in personal and social change. He has directed the development of the Garrison Institute's Transforming Trauma Initiative as well as programs applying contemplative methods in K–12 education and environmental change work. Mr. Rome is the developer of mindful focusing, a contemplative technique integrating focusing and Buddhist mindfulness-awareness practices, and is a senior trainer with the Focusing Institute and Shambhala International.

Contributors

Thorsten Barnhofer, PhD, Charité Clinic, Freie Universitaet Berlin, Berlin, Germany

Tara Brach, PhD, private practice, Great Falls, Virginia

John Briere, PhD, Departments of Psychiatry and Psychology, Keck School of Medicine, University of Southern California, and USC Adolescent Trauma Training Center, National Child Traumatic Stress Network, Los Angeles, California

Brooke Dodson-Lavelle, MA, Emory–Tibet Partnership, Emory University, Atlanta, Georgia

Mary Ann Dutton, PhD, Center for Trauma and the Community, Department of Psychiatry, Georgetown University Medical Center, Washington, DC

David Emerson, E-RYT, The Trauma Center at Justice Resource Institute, Brookline, Massachusetts

Jessica L. Engle, BA, Department of Psychology, University of Nevada, Reno, Reno, Nevada

Devika R. Fiorillo, PhD, Department of Psychiatry and Behavioral Sciences, Emory University School of Medicine, Atlanta, Georgia

Victoria M. Follette, PhD, Department of Psychology, University of Nevada, Reno, Reno, Nevada

Alan E. Fruzzetti, PhD, Department of Psychology, University of Nevada, Reno, Reno, Nevada

Christopher K. Germer, PhD, Department of Psychology, Harvard Medical School, Boston, Massachusetts

Moriah Gottman, BA, College of Natural Sciences, University of Texas at Austin, Austin, Texas

Doralee Grindler Katonah, PsyD, MDiv, Department of Psychology, Sofia University, Palo Alto, California, and private practice, Woodland, California

Elizabeth K. Hopper, PhD, The Trauma Center at Justice Resource Institute, Brookline, Massachusetts

James W. Hopper, PhD, Department of Psychiatry, Harvard Medical School, Boston, Massachusetts

David J. Kearney, MD, Department of Medicine, VA Puget Sound Health Care System, Seattle, Washington

David J. Lewis, PhD, private practice, Brighton, Massachusetts

Laila A. Madni, BA, Department of Psychology, California School of Professional Psychology, Alliant International University, San Diego, California

Trish Magyari, MS, private practice and Department of Health, Behavior and Society, Johns Hopkins Bloomberg School of Public Health, Baltimore, Maryland

Kristin D. Neff, PhD, Department of Educational Psychology, University of Texas at Austin, Austin, Texas

Geshe Lobsang Tenzin Negi, PhD, Department of Religion, Emory University, Atlanta, Georgia

Pat Ogden, PhD, Sensorimotor Psychotherapy Institute, Boulder, Colorado

Brendan Ozawa-de Silva, PhD, Emory–Tibet Partnership, Emory University, Atlanta, Georgia

Robert A. Parker, PhD, private practice, White Plains, New York

Jenny Phillips, PhD, private practice, Concord, Massachusetts

Charles L. Raison, MD, Department of Psychiatry, University of Arizona, Tucson, Arizona

David I. Rome, BA, writer, Garrison, New York

Deborah Rozelle, PsyD, Institute for Meditation and Psychotherapy, Cambridge, Massachusetts, and Nalanda Institute for Contemplative Science, New York, New York

Richard C. Schwartz, PhD, Department of Psychiatry, Harvard Medical School, Boston, Massachusetts

Randye J. Semple, PhD, Department of Psychiatry and Behavioral Sciences, Keck School of Medicine, University of Southern California, Los Angeles, California

Daniel J. Siegel, MD, Department of Psychiatry, School of Medicine, University of California, Los Angeles, Los Angeles, California

Ronald D. Siegel, PsyD, Department of Psychology, Harvard Medical School, Boston, Massachusetts

Flint Sparks, PhD, private practice, Austin, Texas

Lynn C. Waelde, PhD, Pacific Graduate School of Psychology, Palo Alto University, Palo Alto, California

J. Mark G. Williams, DPhil, Oxford Mindfulness Centre, Department of Psychiatry, University of Oxford, Prince of Wales International Centre, Warneford Hospital, Oxford, United Kingdom

Contents

Introduction   1

Victoria M. Follette, John Briere, Deborah Rozelle,
James W. Hopper, and David I. Rome

PART I. FOUNDATIONS

1. Pain and Suffering: A Synthesis of Buddhist   11
   and Western Approaches to Trauma

   John Briere

2. Healing Traumatic Fear: The Wings of Mindfulness and Love   31

   Tara Brach

3. Cultivating Self-Compassion in Trauma Survivors   43

   Christopher K. Germer and Kristin D. Neff

PART II. ADAPTING CONTEMPLATIVE APPROACHES

4. Mindfulness and Valued Action: An Acceptance   61
   and Commitment Therapy Approach to Working
   with Trauma Survivors

   Jessica L. Engle and Victoria M. Follette

5. Dialectical Behavior Therapy for Trauma Survivors   75

   Devika R. Fiorillo and Alan E. Fruzzetti

 6. Mindfulness-Based Cognitive Therapy for Chronic   91
    Depression and Trauma
    J. Mark G. Williams and Thorsten Barnhofer

 7. Eye Movement Desensitization and Reprocessing   102
    and Buddhist Practice: A New Model of Posttraumatic
    Stress Disorder Treatment
    Deborah Rozelle and David J. Lewis

 8. The Internal Family Systems Model in Trauma Treatment: 125
    Parallels with Mahayana Buddhist Theory and Practice
    Richard C. Schwartz and Flint Sparks

 9. Teaching Mindfulness-Based Stress Reduction   140
    and Mindfulness to Women with Complex Trauma
    Trish Magyari

10. Focusing-Oriented Psychotherapy: A Contemplative   157
    Approach to Healing Trauma
    Doralee Grindler Katonah

11. Yoga for Complex Trauma   170
    David Emerson and Elizabeth K. Hopper

PART III. NEUROBIOLOGICAL/SOMATIC ISSUES AND APPROACHES

12. Harnessing the Seeking, Satisfaction, and Embodiment   185
    Circuitries in Contemplative Approaches to Trauma
    James W. Hopper

13. An Interpersonal Neurobiology Approach   210
    to Developmental Trauma: The Possible Role
    of Mindful Awareness in Treatment
    Daniel J. Siegel and Moriah Gottman

14. Embedded Relational Mindfulness: 227
    A Sensorimotor Psychotherapy Perspective
    on the Treatment of Trauma
    Pat Ogden

PART IV. SPECIAL APPLICATIONS AND POPULATIONS

15. Mindfulness-Based Stress Reduction for Underserved 243
Trauma Populations
Mary Ann Dutton

16. Mindfulness in the Treatment of Trauma-Related 257
Chronic Pain
Ronald D. Siegel

17. Mindfulness-Based Stress Reduction and Loving-Kindness 273
Meditation for Traumatized Veterans
David J. Kearney

18. Treating Childhood Trauma with Mindfulness 284
Randye J. Semple and Laila A. Madni

19. Mindfulness and Meditation for Trauma-Related 301
Dissociation
Lynn C. Waelde

20. Focusing-Oriented Therapy with an Adolescent 314
Sex Offender
Robert A. Parker

21. Intensive Vipassana Meditation Practice 329
for Traumatized Prisoners
Jenny Phillips and James W. Hopper

22. Cognitively Based Compassion Training for Adolescents 343
*Brooke Dodson-Lavelle, Brendan Ozawa-de Silva,
Geshe Lobsang Tenzin Negi, and Charles L. Raison*

Conclusion 359
*John Briere, Victoria M. Follette, Deborah Rozelle,
James W. Hopper, and David I. Rome*

Index 363

Introduction

Victoria M. Follette, John Briere, Deborah Rozelle,
James W. Hopper, and David I. Rome

The past several decades have witnessed a major increase in our understanding of psychological trauma and its effects and a burgeoning of empirically based therapies for treating posttraumatic stress. Many of these treatments are cognitive-behavioral, although others involve relational or psychodynamic perspectives, and some combine multiple approaches. Accumulated data and clinical experience suggest that these various interventions can be quite helpful in ameliorating posttraumatic stress disorder (PTSD; American Psychiatric Association, 2013) and related outcomes.

At the same time, two additional developments have caught the attention of trauma-focused clinicians. The first is the growing scientific realization that the effects of trauma are widespread, often involving far more symptoms, difficulties, and problems than those subsumed under the umbrella of PTSD, anxiety, or depression. These include interpersonal difficulties, impaired self-awareness, negative relational schemas, bodily preoccupations, dissociation, and attempts to cope with painful internal states through substance abuse, self-harm, dysfunctional sexual behaviors, and aggression (Briere & Scott, 2014). Further, many survivors struggle with existential concerns such as demoralization, loss of meaning, and alienation, as well as insufficient self-acceptance and happiness (Nader, 2006; Thompson & Walsh, 2010; Shay, 1995). These issues are less likely to respond to traditional, empirically validated interventions, which are typically more concerned with the classic symptoms of posttraumatic stress and dysphoria. As a result, some of the most pressing effects of traumatic events

1

and losses may not be fully addressed by commonly available psychological therapies.

The second development involves the application of mindfulness-based and contemplative interventions to address psychological suffering. These approaches, especially those derived from Buddhist psychology but including other traditions as well, often appear more immediately relevant to the existential effects of trauma. They also potentially provide new options for the treatment of trauma-related distress and disorders.

Primary among these contemplative methodologies is the development of *mindfulness*, often described as "paying attention in a particular way: on purpose, in the present moment, and non-judgmentally" (Kabat-Zinn, 1994, p. 4). As discussed by several authors in this book, those who develop a greater capacity for mindfulness appear to experience reductions in anxiety, depression, illness-related pain and distress, and a host of other emotional and physical difficulties. Importantly, as also described, newer research indicates that mindfulness also may specifically assist trauma survivors struggling with PTSD.

At the same time, it is becoming increasingly clear that other mindfulness-related approaches, such as yoga, loving-kindness meditation, or compassion practices, also can be helpful for those suffering from psychological or emotional issues, perhaps especially those associated with trauma. Yet these approaches have appeared less frequently in mainstream journals or books. Part of the difficulty in studying and applying these latter approaches is their (until recently) less robust empirical validation, as well as possible conflicts between their underlying assumptions and those of current scientific theories of trauma and its effects. Further, such approaches may be attached to religious or spiritual traditions that are not as widely held by trauma survivors and clinicians.

In this regard, we wish to clarify here the notion of *contemplative practice*, used in the subtitle of this volume and in various chapters. The online Oxford dictionary (*www.oxforddictionaries.com/us/definition/american_english*) defines this term as follows: (1) deep reflective thought; (2) the state of being thought about or planned; (3) religious meditation; and (4) (in Christian spirituality) a form of prayer or meditation in which a person seeks to pass beyond mental images and concepts to a direct experience of the divine. In this volume, we refer primarily to the first usage, which implies inwardly focused attention, observation, and inquiry rather than more religiously oriented notions, which may include devotional attention to a deity. This focus is not intended to dismiss religious or spiritual perspectives, only to highlight the idea that contemplation, most broadly, reflects the often repetitive act of turning inward, of examining one's thoughts, feelings, and other internal experiences in order to reach deepened conceptual and nonconceptual understandings. Although such practices typically engender some form of mindfulness, additional out-comes, psychotherapeutic, spiritual, or otherwise, also may pertain.

In response to these various issues, we, as the editors of this volume, sought to examine ways in which mindfulness and related contemplative methodologies have been, or could be, applied to the complex psychological and existential suffering associated with trauma. One inspiration was a groundbreaking conference held in June 2009 at The Garrison Institute in Garrison, New York. This eclectic forum—"Transforming Trauma: Integrating Contemplative Practices, Neuroscience, and Cross-Cultural Perspectives"—was convened to explore the potential benefits of a wide range of contemplative practices in assisting those exposed to traumatic events. The attendees represented a wide range of different contemplative traditions, ranging from different schools of Buddhism to hatha yoga. Others were neurobiologists, trauma researchers, and/or widely respected clinicians, some of whom were involved in some form of contemplative practice and others who were not. The only requirements for their attendance were that they were thought leaders in their respective domains, that they focused on trauma resolution, and that they endorsed some form of empiricism regarding their methodologies.

Importantly, the Garrison meeting suggested that a broader, transdisciplinary focus on trauma and its treatment could, in some ways, "open up" our discussions and approaches to trauma and its resolution. Among the questions that this meeting encouraged us to ask were the following:

- Do mindfulness-oriented traditions contain elements that might be helpful in the remediation of posttraumatic difficulties?
- How might these elements be safely applied?
- What evidence can be marshaled for their efficacy?
- How might the more existential effects of trauma be addressed by such interventions?
- Is it possible to combine Western, empirical treatments for trauma with more contemplative approaches to create new, especially efficacious trauma treatments?

This edited volume represents an initial step in exploring these questions. It includes the thinking of more than 30 clinicians, researchers, and/or spiritual practitioners, all of whom share the same goal: to articulate the potential roles of various forms of contemplative practice in the modern treatment of trauma. They all are writers, teachers, and/or researchers, and most are not new to book chapters. But bringing them together in a single volume was an ambitious task; they represent a variety of perspectives, traditions, and professions—inside and outside of academia, clinically focused or largely theoretical—and not all of their views are entirely complementary. However, our intention was not to achieve harmony. Rather, we sought to highlight the tremendous potential inherent in a wide range of mindfulness-oriented approaches to trauma treatment—a diversity that is intended to stimulate thought and, we hope, new syntheses and cross-collaborations. For this reason, it is likely that the reader will find much to agree and, perhaps, disagree with in this book. Although we held all contributors to relatively high standards of exposition, we invited them to be free to offer new ideas and modes of expression.

Organization of the Volume

This volume is divided into four sections that examine the foundations of mindfulness-oriented treatment for trauma, treatments that include contemplative practices and have some empirical support, neurobiological and somatic perspectives and therapies related to trauma, and applications for special populations.

In Part I, three chapters provide the background and premises that support using mindfulness-oriented approaches in trauma treatment. In Chapter 1, John Briere offers an overview of the issue of pain versus suffering in relation to trauma, integrating Buddhist and Western approaches to address the myriad outcomes that can be associated with exposure to traumatic events. He argues for a multimodal approach that can be considered a hybrid of Eastern and Western philosophies of dealing with painful life experiences. In Chapter 2, Tara Brach goes to the core of contemplatively grounded Buddhist psychology to describe how survivors of trauma suffer and lose the ability to identify with their true and whole self. Through description and transcripts, she provides guidance on helping clients to reconnect to their intrinsic resources, while strengthening their sense of safety and connection to life. In Chapter 3, Christopher K. Germer and Kristin D. Neff discuss empirical findings suggesting that contemplative therapies can have a direct impact on self-compassion, which is considered a key factor in healing for trauma survivors. They provide one method of directly working with self-compassion but note the linkages, both direct and indirect, to other treatment modalities presented here.

Part II focuses on those treatments that include contemplative activities or perspectives in their approach to trauma therapy. Jessica Engle and Victoria M. Follette, in Chapter 4, provide an overview of acceptance and commitment therapy (ACT; Hayes, Wilson, Gifford, Follette, & Strosahl, 1996) as it relates to working with trauma survivors. While ACT for the treatment of trauma has been the subject of books and articles, this chapter emphasizes the importance of using mindfulness practices to assist the client in connecting to core values. This connection is thought to lead to greater engagement in life and to be associated with remaining in the present, with kindness and compassion. Chapter 5, by Devika R. Fiorillo and Alan E. Fruzzetti, describes how dialectical behavior therapy (DBT; Linehan, 1993)—originally developed to address a range of emotional difficulties typically associated with borderline personality disorder—is particularly well suited to the treatment of trauma survivors. The authors speak to the ways in which DBT supports the client in developing mindfulness, remaining in the present moment, and moving forward with effective skills for managing trauma-related symptoms.

Depression is a common outcome of trauma and adversity. In Chapter 6, J. Mark G. Williams and Thorsten Barnhofer discuss how mindfulness-based cognitive therapy (MBCT; Segal, Williams, & Teasdale, 2013), originally developed for the prevention of relapse in chronic depression, is quite relevant to the treatment of trauma survivors. Presenting theoretical issues, especially overgeneralized memory, as well as empirical findings and suggestions for adapting MBCT, the authors provide an overview of the current state of the art in working with trauma and depression. Deborah Rozelle and David J. Lewis, in Chapter 7, discuss eye movement desensitization and reprocessing (EMDR; Shapiro, 2001), a therapy for PTSD that is not usually considered contemplative. Expanding beyond the typical views of EMDR, they describe a significant correspondence with Buddhism, linking empirically based practice with contemplative methods and suggesting new insights into PTSD and its treatment. In Chapter 8, Richard C. Schwartz and Flint Sparks describe the internal family systems (IFS; Schwartz, 1994) model as it pertains to the treatment of trauma effects, in particular in facilitating healthy functioning of the hypothesized internal components of the self. They relate their treatment approach to elements of Mahayana Buddhism, highlighting the trauma sufferer's innate capacities for mindfulness, loving-kindness, and compassion in the treatment process.

Trish Magyari, in Chapter 9, writes on the utility of mindfulness-based stress reduction (MBSR; Kabat-Zinn, 1982) in the treatment of women sexually abused as children. MBSR involves didactic presentations, meditation practice, and a stance of mindful inquiry that encourages acceptance of internal experience. Magyari describes special adaptations of MBSR to more complex forms of posttraumatic symptomatology. Doralee Grindler Katonah, in Chapter 10, presents contemplative aspects of focusing-oriented psychotherapy (Gendlin, 1998), a treatment that has been used for a variety of psychological difficulties, and makes the case for the relevance of this work to trauma survivors, especially with its intentional focus on "bodily knowing" and on the wholeness of the person. This approach encourages the client to integrate traumatic experiences and begin the process of growth that can lead to a more meaningful life. Finally, in Chapter 11, David Emerson and Elizabeth K. Hopper provide a clinically rich discussion of their distinctive use of "trauma-sensitive" hatha yoga, described as a complementary intervention that facilitates healing and can help the client to become more centered and to move through life in a more embodied and intentional way. Moreover, as with other chapters in this section, they provide empirical findings that support the adaptation of their approach to trauma survivors.

There has been increasing interest in the neurobiological foundations of contemplative work. Kabat-Zinn and Davidson's writings with the Dalai Lama (e.g., Kabat-Zinn, Davidson, & Houshmand, 2011) have strengthened the linkage between mindfulness and compassion practices and the more secular "hard sciences." Part III describes fundamental physiological processes as they relate to trauma and recovery. James W. Hopper (Chapter 12) begins with an overview of brain dynamics, with an emphasis on the impact of posttraumatic fear and depression on psychological functioning. Interweaving the impact of contemplative practices on brain circuitries, he offers a framework for linking scientific, clinical, and contemplative knowledge that can serve as a basis for advancing our understanding of trauma and healing. Daniel J. Siegel and Moriah Gottman (Chapter 13) expand on biological foundations with a discussion of the developmental impact of trauma using an interpersonal neurobiology approach. They discuss the role of disorganized attachment and decreased neural integration in leading to a number of less adaptive psychological processes and suggest the utility of mindfulness in addressing these long-term difficulties. In the final chapter of Part III, Pat Ogden (Chapter 14) describes sensorimotor psychotherapy, which involves implicit processing of cognition, emotion, sense perception, movement, and interoception. She describes how client–therapist interactions involving "relational mindfulness" can lead to growth and healing by facilitating the client's processing of "here and now" experiences.

In Part IV, we consider special applications of mindfulness-oriented practice with particular populations or unique presentations. Mary Ann Dutton (Chapter 15) begins Part IV by addressing the use of MBSR with low-income minority women who have had repeated trauma exposures. The clients she serves are unique in that they were not seeking treatment but rather assumed that they had to live with trauma-related symptoms. Empirical evaluation of this application of MBSR demonstrated improvement in a range of symptoms, including increased self-compassion. Ronald D. Siegel's chapter (Chapter 16) on mindfulness approaches to physical pain describes studies indicating that specific interventions can decrease the experience of pain and pain-related suffering on both psychological and neurological levels. His treatment approach focuses on processing and "letting go of" or accepting pain. David J. Kearney addresses the special needs of combat veterans in Chapter 17, on the utility of MBSR and loving-kindness meditation (LKM; Kearney et al., 2013). Veterans who are treated in the Veterans Administration (VA) system are generally offered medications and therapies with a specific focus on PTSD, such as prolonged exposure or cognitive processing therapy. However, not all clients benefit from these approaches, and Kearney makes a strong case for the use of mindfulness-based interventions for treating the range of issues faced by returning veterans. In Chapter 18, Randye J. Semple and Laila A. Madni provide a clear rationale and data for the application of mindfulness-based cognitive therapy to children with trauma histories. Their 12-week group program, adapted from adult treatments to include various activities that help to sustain children's involvement in the therapy, has been successfully utilized in children ages 8–12. Lynn C. Waelde notes, in Chapter 19, that dissociation can take a number of forms and serve a range of functions. She presents clear directions for implementing a program of treatment that involves mindfulness and meditation, as well as providing special considerations and cautions related to clients with significant dissociative symptoms.

Although this volume primarily addresses treating survivors of trauma and abuse, Robert A. Parker (Chapter 20) discusses focusing-oriented therapy as a form of guided mindfulness for treating an adolescent sex offender. Mindfulness is used to connect to the "implicit knowing" that the body is thought to possess with movement toward behaving in a more compassionate way in relation to others. In Chapter 21, Jenny Phillips and James W. Hopper write about the use of contemplative practices with another underserved group, traumatized prisoners. They describe an intensive vipassana meditation program that has been offered in a maximum security prison and discuss how intensive vipassana practice may address prisoners' suffering and deficits in compassion for themselves and others. In the final chapter of Part IV (Chapter 22), Brooke Dodson-Lavelle, Brendan Ozawa-de Silva, Geshe Lobsang Tenzin Negi, and Charles L. Raison describe a contemplative treatment for adolescents in foster care, cognitively based compassion training, which has been implemented and evaluated with a range of populations. After describing the treatment in detail, the authors present a case for using this approach with children in foster care, who have trauma-related symptoms at a rate similar to that of combat veterans.

Taken together, the chapters in this book offer support for what we believe to be an exciting development in the field: that is, that although traditional clinical approaches to trauma effects have proven to be helpful for many traumatized people, there are important insights, theoretical perspectives, and methodologies now available to us that come from an entirely different domain. As these chapters reveal, many of these "new" methods can be tested and empirically validated and often can be combined with more traditional psychological therapies. This synthesis may constitute an important advancement in trauma treatment, which may both sharpen the effectiveness of existing trauma therapies and promote outcomes that extend beyond symptom reduction to encompass general psychological well-being.

References

American Psychiatric Association. (2013). *Diagnostic and statistical manual of mental disorders* (5th ed.). Arlington, VA: Author.

Briere, J., & Scott, C. (2014). *Principles of trauma therapy: A guide to symptoms, evaluation, and treatment* (2nd ed., DSM-5 update). Thousand Oaks, CA: Sage.

Gendlin, E. T. (1998). *Focusing-oriented psychotherapy: A manual of the experiential method.* New York: Guilford Press.

Hayes, S. C., Wilson, K. W., Gifford, E. V., Follette, V. M., & Strosahl, K. (1996). Experiential avoidance and behavioral disorders: A functional dimensional approach to diagnosis and treatment. *Journal of Consulting and Clinical Psychology, 64*(6), 1152–1168.

Kabat-Zinn, J. (1982). An outpatient program in behavioral medicine for chronic pain patients based on the practice of mindfulness meditation: Theoretical considerations and preliminary results. *General Hospital Psychiatry, 4,* 33–47.

Kabat-Zinn, J. (1994). *Wherever you go there you are: Mindfulness meditation for everyday life.* New York: Hyperion.

Kabat-Zinn, J., Davidson, R. J., & Houshmand, Z. (Eds.). (2012). *The mind's own physician: A scientific dialogue with the Dalai Lama on the healing power of meditation.* Oakland, CA: New Harbinger.

Kearney, D. J., Malte, C. A., McManus, C., Martinez, M., Felleman, B., & Simpson, T. L. (2013). Loving-kindness meditation for posttraumatic stress disorder: A pilot study. *Journal of Traumatic Stress, 26*(4), 426–434.

Linehan, M. M. (1993). *Cognitive-behavioral treatment of borderline personality disorder.* New York: Guilford Press.

Nader, K. (2006). Childhood trauma: The deeper wound. In J. P. Wilson (Ed.), *The posttraumatic self: Restoring meaning and wholeness to personality* (pp. 117–156). London: Routledge.

Schwartz, R. C. (1994). *Internal family systems therapy.* New York: Guilford Press.

Segal, Z. V., Williams, J. M. G., & Teasdale, J. D. (2013). *Mindfulness-based cognitive therapy for depression* (2nd ed.). New York: Guilford Press.

Shapiro, F. (2001). *Eye movement desensitization and reprocessing (EMDR): Basic principles, protocols, and procedures* (2nd ed.). New York: Guilford Press.

Shay, J. (1995). *Achilles in Vietnam: Combat trauma and the undoing of character.* New York: Touchstone.

Thompson, N., & Walsh, M. (2010). The existential basis of trauma. *Journal of Social Work Practice: Psychotherapeutic Approaches to Health, Welfare and the Community, 24,* 377–389.

Part I

FOUNDATIONS

Pain and Suffering

A Synthesis of Buddhist and Western Approaches to Trauma

John Briere

Adversity, pain, and loss are inevitable aspects of life, whether they involve the death of a loved one, an automobile accident, a grave diagnosis, or the unexpected end of a long-term relationship. In this chapter, we examine events that are especially overwhelming, generally referred to as *psychological trauma*, and explore similarities and differences between Western and Buddhist approaches to such phenomena. Along the way, we will consider what it means to have been hurt, how this relates to subsequent emotional suffering, and how much one necessarily has to result in the other. Ultimately, we will explore ways in which Buddhist psychology, especially mindfulness training, can uniquely inform the trauma recovery/integration process. Before we do so, we will review what trauma actually represents, what its effects often are, and the interventions that Western psychology typically marshals to address trauma-related difficulties.

Trauma and Posttraumatic Outcomes

Trauma is defined in Western psychology as an event that involves actual or threatened death, injury, or other threat to physical integrity, commonly resulting in great emotional distress (American Psychiatric Association, 2013). Memories of trauma, which may have sensory, cognitive, and emotional aspects, can be triggered and relived at later points in time as flashbacks, painful emotional states, and intrusive thoughts. These phenomena, in turn, can motivate avoidance responses that are themselves problematic. Traumatic events also may hypersensitize the "fight or flight" (noradrenergic) component of the autonomic nervous system, resulting in long-standing tension, anxiety, jumpiness, hypervigilance, sleeplessness, and irritability (Hopper, Chapter 12, this volume; Yehuda, 1998). When they are sufficient in number and intensity, these various symptoms are considered evidence of posttraumatic stress disorder (PTSD; American Psychiatric Association, 2013).

Trauma can have additional effects, including depression, anxiety, interpersonal disturbance, and difficulties in tolerating and regulating emotional states, the latter of which can motivate distress-reducing behaviors such as substance abuse, dissociation, self-injury, suicidality, aggression, and impulsive behavior (Briere, 2004; Courtois & Ford, 2012; van der Kolk et al., 1996). Other impacts of trauma are more obviously existential in nature, for example, feeling that one's life has little or no meaning or purpose, fears about death, loss of spiritual beliefs, and alienation from others or society (Nader, 2006; Thompson & Walsh, 2010; Shay, 1995).

Given these disparate outcomes, no single psychological intervention or approach is likely to address all instances or types of trauma-related distress or disturbance. For example, although cognitive-behavioral therapies have been shown to reduce or resolve PTSD in some individuals (Cahill, Rothbaum, Resick, & Follette, 2009; Hembree & Foa, 2003), they do not appear to be especially helpful for others (Dutton, Chapter 15, this volume; Belleville, Guay, & Marchand, 2011; Bradley, Greene, Russ, Dutra, & Westen, 2005; Kar, 2011; Schottenbauer, Glass, Arnkoff, Tendick, & Gray, 2008). Similarly, classical psychoanalysis may not be immediately useful for flashbacks or autonomic hyperarousal, and psychiatric medications, although sometimes helpful, have not been shown to remediate all aspects of PTSD, let alone outcomes such as trauma-related affect dysregulation, relational problems, or identity disturbance (Scott, Jones, & Briere, 2014). Beyond the incomplete efficacy of Western treatment techniques for individual psychological symptoms, more complex trauma effects (e.g., borderline personality disorder [American Psychiatric Association, 2013] or developmental trauma disorder [van der Kolk et al., 2005]) may be especially resistant to traditional psychological interventions (Courtois & Ford, 2012; Dutton, Chapter 15, this volume), and the existential effects of adverse experiences are unlikely to be fully addressed by current empirically informed treatments (Schneider, Bugental, & Fraser Pierson, 2002).

Because no one treatment approach is likely to be helpful for all clients, recent research and clinical practice have focused more on multimodal therapies, in which different treatment components are applied for different problems, symptoms, or difficulties. Especially of interest in the trauma field are methodologies that increase trauma survivors' affect regulation skills, facilitate emotional processing, and address posttraumatic cognitions (e.g., Cloitre, Stovall-McClough, Miranda, & Chemtob, 2004; Follette & Vijay, 2009; Wagner & Linehan, 1998). Notable among these more recent approaches are interventions that include the development or amplification of *mindfulness*—described later in this chapter and covered in depth throughout this volume. Before we can consider mindfulness in the context of trauma treatment, however, we should examine its antithesis, which is one of the most problematic aspects of trauma.

The Pain Paradox

In the face of emotional pain, a common human response is to withdraw, numb, distract, deny, or otherwise suppress awareness. Yet psychological avoidance may actually prolong or intensify psychological distress. Those who abuse drugs or alcohol, dissociate, externalize through dysfunctional behavior, or suppress upsetting thoughts and memories, for example, are more likely than others to develop intrusive and chronic problems and symptoms (e.g., Briere, Scott, & Weathers, 2005; Cioffi & Holloway, 1993; Gold & Wegner, 1995; Morina, 2007; Pietrzak, Harpaz-Rotem, & Southwick, 2011; Siegel, Chapter 16, this volume), seemingly because avoided material cannot be engaged and thereby psychologically metabolized.

Being involved in distress-sustaining behaviors while trying to, in fact, avoid painful or upsetting internal states can be referred to as a *pain paradox* (Briere & Scott, 2014). In an effort to reduce distress, we may do things that ultimately increase, not decrease, unwanted thoughts and feelings and make them more enduring. As well, by narrowing our attention and deadening our awareness, we may miss out on important aspects of life that are associated with well-being. This numbing of experience, in turn, may further reinforce avoidance by eliminating from consciousness any evidence that more positive options and feelings are possible.

A common reason for avoidance is the need to maintain psychological homeostasis: When an individual's emotional distress exceeds his or her affect regulation/tolerance capacities, he or she is motivated to avoid (or at least reduce) awareness of that distress so that it no longer challenges his or her emotional equilibrium (Briere & Scott, 2014; van der Kolk et al., 1996). A homeless person may abuse alcohol or methamphetamine as a way to temporarily escape the emotional pain associated with his or her situation, especially when the privations and cruelties of his or her life exceed his or her already limited affect regulation capacities. Similarly, a survivor of childhood abuse may engage in dissociation or dysfunctional sexual behavior in an attempt to reduce or distract from overwhelming anxiety or shame associated with painful memories.

Beyond its psychological functions, avoidance is broadly supported in our culture, generally reflecting social training to deal with uncomfortable states through denial, distraction, or suppression. For example, a person who remains depressed, anxious, or angry for more than a few weeks or months after a major loss or trauma may be told by others to "just get over it," "let go of the past," or "move on." Advertisements on television and other media promote drugs or remedies to eliminate unhappiness or simple discomfort and encourage the acquisition of things as a way to feel better or, in many cases, to address self-perceived inadequacies or dissatisfaction. The message is often that distress and discomfort are bad and should be removed, masked, or medicated—after which one will, by definition, feel good.

Unfortunately, as previously described, avoidance rarely works in the long term. In contrast, however, those who are able to more directly experience distress—whether through what we will refer to as mindfulness or in response to psychodynamic psychotherapy, therapeutic exposure, or other ways of accessing and "sitting with" traumatic material—are more likely to experience reduced distress over time than those who avoid or deny (e.g., Hayes, Strosahl, & Wilson, 2011; Foa, Huppert, & Cahill, 2006; Kimbrough, Magyari, Langenberg, Chesney, & Berman, 2010; Thompson & Waltz, 2007). In this regard, various theoretical perspectives suggest that directly engaging nonoverwhelming psychological pain allows the individual to process, and cognitively accommodate traumatic or upsetting mental material until it no longer is a source of distress or intrusive experience (Briere & Scott, 2014; Chödrön, 2002; Horowitz, 1986; Rothbaum & Davis, 2003).

Thus the pain paradox ultimately counsels us to directly feel painful states and/or to think painful thoughts and to avoid, in effect, avoidance. This notion of "inviting your fear to tea" (unknown early Zen teacher) or "leaning into pain" (Brach, 2004) is central to Buddhist and some Western approaches to trauma processing. To the extent that the trauma survivor can learn to apply consistent, full attention to the contents of his or her consciousness, regardless of their emotional valence, he or she seemingly engages the antithesis of avoidance. In Buddhist psychology, the ability to focus direct, nonevaluative attention on one's internal experience is considered a major component of *mindfulness.*

Mindfulness

Mindfulness refers to the capacity to maintain awareness of, and openness to, immediate experience—including internal mental states, thoughts, feelings, memories, and impinging elements of the external world—without judgment and with acceptance (for a range of definitions, see Bishop et al., 2004; Germer, 2013; Kabat-Zinn, 2003; Siegel, 2007). Mindfulness is often learned through meditation but is not equivalent to it. Whereas the former can be thought of as a mind capacity, meditation refers to practices ranging from sustained attention to one's breath or thoughts to specific types of movement (e.g., walking or dancing) or vocalizations (e.g., chanting or praying) in order to change or enhance consciousness. To the extent that they foster internally directed awareness, meditational activities teach mindful attention to the present moment, thereby reducing preoccupation with the past or worry about the future. Increased mindfulness, in turn, is associated with a range of psychological benefits, as described subsequently.[1]

As mindfulness has gained popularity, a growing number of clinicians have integrated it into their therapies, both cognitive-behavioral (e.g., Hayes, Follette, & Linehan, 2004; Segal, Williams, & Teasdale, 2002) and psychodynamic (e.g., Bobrow, 2010; Epstein, 2008). In many cases (e.g., Germer & Neff, Chapter 3, this volume; Dodson-Lavelle, Ozawa-de Silva, Negi, & Raison, Chapter 22, this volume; Gilbert, 2009), clinicians have incorporated additional aspects of Buddhist psychology—for example, compassion, metacognitive awareness, and appreciation of dependent origination, each described later in this chapter.

In addition to integrating mindfulness training or practices into established therapeutic approaches, researcher-clinicians have developed a number of mindfulness-specific interventions. These include *acceptance and commitment therapy* (ACT; Hayes et al., 2011; Engle & Follette, Chapter 4, this volume), *dialectical behavior therapy* (DBT; Linehan, 1993; Fiorillo & Fruzzetti, Chapter 5, this volume), *mindfulness-based cognitive therapy* (MBCT; Segal et al., 2002; Williams & Barnhofer, Chapter 6, this volume), *mindfulness-based relapse prevention* (MBRP; Bowen, Chawla, & Marlatt, 2011; Marlatt & Gordon, 1985), and *mindfulness-based stress reduction* (MBSR; Kabat-Zinn, 1982, and various chapters, this volume). A burgeoning literature supports the efficacy of these interventions in preventing or reducing various symptoms or problems associated with trauma, including anxiety, panic, depression, substance abuse, eating disorders, suicidality, self-injurious behavior, dissociation, low self-esteem, aggression, chronic pain, and what is described as borderline personality disorder (see meta-analyses by Baer, 2003; Coelho, Canter, & Ernst, 2007; Grossman, Neimann, Schmidt, & Walach, 2004; Hofmann, Sawyer, Witt, & Oh, 2010; Lynch, Trost, Salsman, & Linehan, 2007).

---

[1]Interestingly, the psychological impacts of mindfulness training, although prized by many in the West, may be relatively irrelevant (if not a distraction) for traditional Buddhists, who seek, instead, enlightenment, optimal rebirth, or other spiritual outcomes.

Especially relevant to this chapter, several studies indicate that MBSR and DBT have been specifically helpful for child abuse survivors (e.g., Kimbrough et al., 2010; Steil, Dyer, Priebe, Kleindienst, & Bohus, 2011; see also Fiorillo & Fruzzetti, Chapter 5, this volume, and Magyari, Chapter 9, this volume), veterans (Kearney, McDermott, Malte, Martinez, & Simpson, 2012), and victims of intimate partner violence (Dutton, Bermudez, Matas, Majid, & Myers, 2013). In addition, transcendental meditation, although not especially mindfulness-focused, also appears to reduce posttraumatic stress among those exposed to combat (Rosenthal, Grosswald, Ross, & Rosenthal, 2011).

Toward a Hybrid Approach

Given the benefits of both Western and mindfulness approaches, we suggest that they can be combined to provide an effective intervention for at least some survivors of psychological trauma. In some ways, this may be easier than it initially appears. Buddhist and Western psychology generally agree on a number of central points that facilitate their integration (Baer, 2003; Bruce, Shapiro, Constantino, & Manber, 2010; Hayes et al., 2011; Engle & Follette, Chapter 4, this volume). These include appreciation of the fact that cognitive variables (e.g., excessive need for control, inaccurate expectations, and negative attributions) can increase trauma effects and that avoidance of distress can prolong, and even intensify, psychological suffering. They also concur that greater awareness promotes processing and integration and that greater insight into the basis for subjective/distorted reactions to adversity may decrease those reactions.

At the same time, of course, there are significant differences between the two perspectives. Western interventions often rely on the notion of psychological disorder and its treatment, the goal of which is to return the client to his or her pretrauma level of functioning. In contrast, Buddhist approaches tend to focus on the development of sustained internal awareness, increased insight into—and acceptance of—the "true" nature of life's realities, and a perspective that focuses on developing new understanding, capacities, and skills rather than solely fixing injuries or pathology.

Why Not Mindfulness Training Alone?

Because mindfulness interventions have been helpful for a range of potentially trauma-related symptoms and problems and potentially address issues beyond those of the Western medical model, one might be tempted to simply teach mindfulness techniques to trauma survivors and forgo Western treatment approaches entirely. Yet, despite their usefulness, mindfulness-based interventions have a significant limitation for survivors of chronic and/or severe trauma: With the exception of ACT and, to some extent, DBT, they do not occur in the context of individual psychotherapy, which is seemingly an essential component in work with this cohort (Courtois & Ford, 2012). Instead, such interventions often take place in group settings and tend to be nonclinically oriented, focusing more on the acquisition of certain skills (e.g., mindfulness and the capacity to meditate) than on the specific resolution of psychological symptoms per se (Baer, 2003). Further, most mindfulness groups are relatively brief, typically involving eight weekly sessions of approximately 2½ hours and one day-long meeting. In contrast, the psychological impacts of severe and extended trauma may require considerably more time in treatment, given their complexity and breadth (Courtois & Ford, 2012). Finally, and perhaps most important, the treatment outcome literature described later in this chapter suggests that the therapeutic relationship—including the attuned, compassionate attention of the therapist toward the client—serves important functions in therapy, ones that are unlikely to be replicated in mindfulness groups or meditation alone (see an early paper by Buddhist teacher and psychologist Jack Kornfield [*www.buddhanet.net/psymed1.htm*] for a prescient discussion of the potential limits of meditation for those suffering major psychological distress).

Mindfulness-Augmented Trauma Therapy

Given these concerns, we (e.g., Briere & Scott, 2014) have suggested an algorithm for the application of Buddhist and Western psychology to trauma-related issues. This combination of Eastern and Western models, we suggest, may allow the clinician to offer the best of both worlds: the established benefits of empirically validated trauma therapy, including the healing power of the therapeutic relationship, and also the fruits of mindfulness and what we will call *existential insight*. This is just one perspective, of course, and the reader is referred to the many other chapters in this volume that describe other approaches.

1. *Screen for the appropriateness of meditation.* Clinical experience suggests that clients who are subject to especially intrusive thoughts, flashbacks, rumination, or easily triggered trauma memories are at greater risk of experiencing distress when meditating (Siegel, Chapter 16, this volume; Shapiro, 1992; Williams & Swales, 2004), probably because meditation and mindfulness reduce cognitive and emotional avoidance and thereby provide greater exposure to internal experience, including trauma memories and painful emotional states (Baer, 2003; Germer, 2013; Hayes et al., 2011; Treanor, 2011). As well, some survivors of severe trauma suffer from reduced affect regulation/tolerance capacities (Briere, Hodges, & Godbout, 2010; van der Kolk et al., 1996) and thus may be more easily overwhelmed

by the sensory and emotional material that can arise during meditation. More obviously, those experiencing psychosis, extreme depression, a dissociative disorder, mania/hypomania, substance addiction, suicidality, or susceptibility to significant relaxation-induced anxiety generally should avoid meditation-based mindfulness interventions until these symptoms or conditions are improved or resolved.

In instances in which mindfulness meditation is potentially problematic but not entirely contraindicated, other, related options may be potentially less activating. For example, although there are few research data on this to date, loving-kindness (*metta*) meditation (Salzberg, 1995) or yoga (Harvard Health Publications, 2009; Emerson & Hopper, Chapter 11, this volume) focus less directly on awareness of the mind—and thus on its potentially disturbing contents—and thereby may provide more titrated access to painful memories or dysregulating internal experience. The trade-off is that, while potentially providing greater safety, decreased access to painful mind states may mean less exposure to trauma-related material and thus less emotional processing.

2. Consider referral to a mindfulness group or a qualified meditation or yoga center. Specialized trauma-focused mindfulness groups (e.g., as described by Kimbrough et al., 2010; see also Magyari, Chapter 9, this volume) may be especially helpful when available. Although most discussions of mindfulness-based trauma treatment suggest that the therapist teach meditation to the client, this may not always be the most appropriate path (although see compelling presentations by Brach, 2013, and others). Extensive mindfulness training, especially during early sessions, can be relatively inefficient; the development of mindfulness requires a significant investment of time and effort, during which the survivor may have decreased access to much-needed trauma-focused interventions. As well, modern meditation teachers typically have devoted many years not only to the study and practice of meditation but also to how to teach such skills to others—a background that most clinicians may not have.

Even when the clinician is sufficiently trained and experienced in trauma therapy, mindfulness, and teaching meditation, he or she should carefully consider what the traumatized client needs most at any given moment in time. For example, is mindfulness training most appropriate, or does the client more immediately require grounding, support, other forms of affect regulation training, cognitive intervention, or titrated therapeutic exposure? This is not an all-or-none scenario, of course. The mindfulness-trained clinician may introduce simple meditation instruction or mindfulness exercises, yet not spend an inordinate amount of time doing so, or may respond to client inquiries or interactions with a therapeutic style that is informed by a mindful perspective, while not necessarily directly teaching mindfulness per se (Germer, 2013).

Importantly, although the clinician may not be the client's primary meditation instructor, his or her personal experience with meditation and mindfulness is a prerequisite for the conduct of mindfulness-inclusive therapies (Kabat-Zinn, 2003; Semple & Lee, 2011; Shapiro & Carlson, 2009). When the survivor is simultaneously involved in psychotherapy and mindfulness training, the meditation-experienced therapist can monitor and inform the process, helping the client to explore, understand, and integrate what he or she is learning and experiencing in each domain.

3. *As the client gains meditation and mindfulness skills, these capacities can be called upon during concurrent trauma-focused psychotherapy.* These may include the following:

• *The use of settling skills.* The client who is able to decrease his or her anxiety or posttraumatic hyperarousal through mindfulness practices—for example, by attending to the breath, consciously engaging in the here-and-now, and noticing, in a nonreactive manner, emotions and cognitions—can use these skills to regulate distress when encountering painful memories or triggers of upsetting emotions (Baer, 2003; Ogden, Minton, & Pain, 2006; Siegel, Chapter 16, and Waelde, Chapter 19, this volume). Similarly, mindfulness skills involving the ability to "let go" of intrusive or persistent mental content may be helpful for the client who is prone to repetitive or sustained negative cognitive-emotional states (Segal et al., 2002). As noted later about metacognitive awareness, settling skills represent a form of affect regulation and may be especially helpful for those easily overwhelmed by anxiety, depression, or anger (Linehan, 1993).

• *Intrinsic therapeutic exposure.* Various writers (e.g., Baer, 2003; Fulton & Siegel, 2013; Kabat-Zinn, 2003; Treanor, 2011) note that the decreased avoidance associated with mindfulness can expose the individual to emotionally laden memories in the context of a relatively settled state and a less involved, nonjudgmental cognitive perspective—a process that is likely to desensitize and countercondition such material and decrease its power to produce distress (Briere & Scott, 2014). In the therapy session, this process may be encouraged by asking the client to describe traumatic events in relative detail and to feel the attendant emotions while at the same time engaging in as mindful a perspective as possible.

When the client can experience traumatic memories with less judgment and with more acceptance, their effects are less likely to be exacerbated or compounded by shaming or guilt-related cognitions. In fact, increased acceptance of trauma memories, by definition, makes them less "negative"—thereby potentially requiring less avoidance and allowing more exposure and psychological processing.

• *Metacognitive awareness.* During therapy, the client may be invited to consider his or her trauma-related thoughts and perceptions from a mindful, specifically *metacognitive* (Segal et al., 2002), perspective wherein they are viewed as "just" memories or products of the mind, as opposed to necessarily accurate information about self, others, or the environment. For example, in *trigger identification* (Briere & Lanktree, 2014), the client learns to apply a metacognitive perspective to symptoms of posttraumatic stress or when in the grips of especially shaming or self-blaming cognitions. As he or she becomes conversant with his or her specific trauma-related triggers (e.g., rejection, criticism, certain facial expressions, or interaction with authority figures), the states they engender (e.g., contextually inappropriate emotional states, intrusive thoughts, dissociative episodes, or a desire to engage in substance abuse or self-harming behaviors), and ways to intervene (e.g., noting the intrusion without necessarily accepting its validity, delaying avoidance behavior until the need for it fades, reaching out to safe others for context or perspective, or self-talk such as "this is just my past talking"), the trauma survivor begins to discriminate triggered implicit memories from accurate perceptions of current events, seeing the former as transient trauma-related phenomena rather than data on the true state of reality.

This ability to observe one's internal experiences—without necessarily identifying with them—appears to increase the client's affect regulation capacity. As he or she reinterprets intrusive cognitions as historic phenomena stored in memory, for example, there may be less to be afraid of or angry about in the current, "real" world. And as the survivor comes to view triggered thoughts and memories as merely the mind's response to trauma, avoidance strategies such as self-injury, substance abuse, or aggression may be less necessary because they are now less contextually relevant (Briere & Lanktree, 2012).

Another metacognitive technique is *urge surfing* (Bowen et al., 2011), wherein the client learns to apply mindfulness skills when the need to engage in substance abuse or distress-reduction activities is triggered. The survivor is encouraged to view the urge to engage in such behaviors as similar to riding (rather than trying to stop) a wave. In this regard, he or she learns to accept—but not react to—triggered need states as they start small, build in size, peak, and then fall away. If the client can experience activated states and compulsions as time-limited intrusions of history, internally generated phenomena that can be "held" in a mindful way rather than being suppressed or acted upon, he or she may be able to avoid or decrease problematic behaviors, whether they be drug abuse or self-injury.

Supporting Existential Insight

As suggested earlier, it is not just through mindfulness that Buddhist psychology can assist traumatized people. Also helpful may be what Buddhists call *wisdom* (Brach, 2013; Germer & Siegel, 2012) or, from a more secular perspective, *existential insight*. Although such contributions are less obviously science-based, many mindfulness-oriented clinicians consider the existential aspects of Buddhism to be of great assistance to people who have sustained major losses, traumas, or dramatically changed circumstances. In other words, beyond mindfulness skills, it may be important to develop an overbridging perspective that determines how life—including pain—is interpreted and experienced.

When the Buddha first described the "Four Noble Truths" (Bhikkhu, 2010), he introduced several organizing propositions. One is that life inevitably involves pain and loss, because the world exists implacably beyond our desires: Bad things happen, people we love sometimes die or leave, and we are both fragile and mortal. This was especially apparent in the Buddha's time, when disease was endemic, wars and other forms of violence were a regular part of life, poverty was omnipresent, and many were oppressed by an inflexible caste system and extreme ethnic and gender inequality.

A second proposition is that pain and loss are not necessarily the only, or even the primary, reasons for lasting human distress. Although Buddhist texts do not speak of trauma per se, they suggest that suffering can arise when life experiences challenge one's investment in things that cannot last or never were true and motivate resistance (avoidance) when acceptance of experience would be more helpful.[2] Thus suffering can occur when people's inaccurate expectations, historically acquired needs, and emotional investments keep them from accepting the transient and ever-changing nature of things. For example, a heart attack typically involves great pain, but it also may powerfully challenge previously held beliefs and expectations about personal immortality, autonomy, life trajectory, and the assumption of a life without significant disability. These challenges, and the person's struggles against them, may be at least as devastating as the pain and terror associated with a physically damaged heart.

From this perspective, then, there are at least two sources of distress associated with any given traumatic experience: (1) the event itself and the emotional pain it produces, some of which may be lasting and intense, and (2) the suffering associated with attempts to avoid pain and the struggle to maintain previous models of self, others, and well-being in the face of intruding, unwanted reality.

It may be appropriately argued that some instances of long-term distress are due to the physiology of the human trauma response, as opposed to the effects of avoidance, challenged needs, or attachments. Even in such cases, however, nonbiological phenomena (e.g., cognitive factors or effortful avoidance) often play a part in sustaining posttraumatic stress over the

---

[2]This does not mean that the Buddha suggested passive acceptance of injustice or maltreatment, nor that modern, "engaged" Buddhists do not actively work to end oppression, violence, or social marginalization (Queen, 1995; Hanh, 2005).

long term (Foa et al., 2006; Rothbaum & Davis, 2003). Similarly, some memories of trauma (e.g., torture, rape, witnessing brutality against loved ones) are sufficiently anguishing that they never entirely depart from the survivor's ongoing awareness. Yet even these experiences may change in intensity and meaning with the metacognitive aspects of therapy or mindfulness-based acceptance (see, e.g., the perspective of a Cambodian torture survivor in Briere, 2012b).

In an example of the possible differences between the pain of trauma and the suffering that can arise from psychological factors, an early Buddhist teaching offers the parable of a person pierced by two arrows in rapid succession (Thanissaro, 1997). The first arrow is the objective pain and distress felt when encountering adversity, trauma, or loss. The second is the extent to which the pain challenges tightly held, albeit inaccurate, expectations, needs, and worldviews, resulting in resistance, avoidance, and the more complex state that Buddhists call suffering.

Buddhist psychology offers opportunities for the client to more directly address "second arrow" issues associated with his or her trauma. This generally occurs as the client explores his or her experiences, life assumptions, and aspects of the pain paradox in conversations with the clinician, as well as, in some cases, during meditation. Among the second-arrow aspects considered in this context are *attachment, impermanence,* and *dependent origination.*

Attachment can be defined as the need to hang on to, rely upon, obsess over, or overly invest in things that, ultimately, are impermanent. *Impermanence* refers to the fact that everything is in a state of flux and that no thing or event continues forever, including our lives and what we value. As a result, this perspective discourages preoccupation with possessions, social status, and rigid ideas or assumptions about oneself or others, because these things are inevitably unsustainable and unreliable, resulting in eventual crisis, loss, and unhappiness (Bodhi, 2005).

To the extent that Buddhist psychology can help the client access the implications of impermanence, at least two things may happen: He or she may feel initial distress and disillusionment associated with reduced expectations of immortality or sustained well-being, and yet eventually come to terms with such realities so that adverse events lose some of their associated qualities, including feelings of abandonment, betrayal, and crushing disappointment. Although observers of Buddhist cosmology sometimes remark on the seeming dismal nature of a perspective so concerned with suffering and its etiology, in actuality growing freedom from false beliefs and socially acquired or reinforced needs can lead to greater emotional stability, acceptance of life as it actually is, and appreciation of transient but special things in the moment.

The third existential aspect, *dependent origination,* holds that all things arise from concrete conditions and sustaining causes, which themselves occur in the context of a vast, mutually reciprocating array of other causes and conditions (Bodhi, 2005). It suggests that attributions of inherent badness, inadequacy, or even pathology of self or others may be due to insufficient information: If we could know the logic and history of a given person's (or our own) problematic behavior or sustained distress, we might be less likely to judge or blame him, her, or ourselves.

Importantly, bad acts committed by an individual also are influenced by antecedent causes and conditions, including socially based attitudes and beliefs, inadequate knowledge, psychological or physical distress or disorder, previous maltreatment or trauma, and exposure to oppressive or marginalizing social dynamics; they are unlikely to arise *de novo* from inherent evil (Briere, 2012b). The "free-will versus determinism" aspects of this view are exceedingly complex (see, e.g., Anderson & Huesmann, 2003; Baer, Kaufman, & Baumeister, 2008; and Gier & Kjellberg, 2004), whether they involve the issue of accountability for one's actions, the existence of an independent agent/self who can, in fact, be "free," or the traditional Buddhist notion of *karma*.

The fact that hurtful or abusive behavior is likely to arise from antecedent phenomena does not mean that the client should necessarily "forgive" his or her perpetrator—especially to the extent that doing so implies a lack of entitlement to negative feelings and thoughts, or signals pressure for premature closure. It is a very human response to hate, resent, or desire revenge against someone who has done one (or one's loved ones) serious harm. The pain paradox suggests that such feelings should not be suppressed or avoided if they are to be resolved. At the same time, it is likely that unprocessed anger is bad for people over the long term, whereas eventually reduced involvement in such states is associated with improved well-being (Dalai Lama & Goleman, 2003). As a result, we recommend that anger, even hatred, be experienced, accepted, and processed in the same manner as other trauma-related emotional phenomena, though obviously, not acted on in ways that harm others.

Working with the Second Arrow

In the context of the client's growing existential awareness, he or she can be encouraged to explore shattered or violated assumptions, hopes, and needs associated with previous traumas and can be provided with nondirective opportunities to consider at length the *what*s surrounding the worst of these events. As this largely cognitive process unfolds, themes of impermanence, attachment, dependent origination, and resistance may become more clear and may be addressed more directly. A few second-arrow questions that might be considered are:

- *What did the client believe about him- or herself, others, or life before the trauma that may not have been accurate?* Examples might be that life will go on forever that loved ones will never leave, that justice is a quality of the universe, and that positive experiences in the present should be sacrificed for the possibility of future well-being.

- *What social messages and acquired needs complicate and/or add to the client's current distress?* These may include notions that physical attractiveness is required in order to be loved or valued by others, that those who have been hurt or disabled are less or worse than others, that retribution provides "closure" and is a helpful thing, and that money, property, or status is critical to happiness.

- *What is the client resisting about the trauma and its implications? What might nonresistance lead to?* For example, although acceptance of things such as irrevocable loss, continuing pain or disability, or even impending death may seem like giving up or giving in, denying or fighting against negative states or realizations does not decrease their negativity and often exacerbates suffering. In contrast, because acceptance is less rooted in desperation or denial, "allowing" painful experiences may lead to more positive states, including greater peace and well-being.

Mindfulness and the Therapist

The therapist's own mindfulness also can contribute to the client's progress in treatment. A therapist who is able to focus his or her attention on the client in an alert, accepting, and compassionate way will almost inevitably increase the quality of the therapeutic relationship (Fulton, 2013; Siegel, 2007; Brach, Chapter 2, this volume). A positive client–therapist relationship, in turn, appears to be the most helpful general component of psychotherapy, often exceeding the effects of specific therapeutic interventions (Lambert & Barley, 2001; Lambert & Okishi, 1997; Martin, Garske, & Davis, 2000). This is certainly true for the trauma survivor, for whom a positive relationship can be both a minimal requirement and a powerful intervention (Cloitre et al., 2004; Courtois & Ford, 2012).

Because mindfulness involves the capacity to pay close, nondistracted, and nonjudgmental attention, it can assist the clinician in maintaining attunement to the client (Fulton, 2013; Morgan, Morgan, & Germer, 2013; Shapiro & Carlson, 2009). Not only does mindfulness increase the therapist's capacity to understand the client's ongoing experience, but it may also help the client to process negative interpersonal schema in the context of (antithetic) caring attention. When attunement is continuously experienced, especially if the clinician's compassion is evident, the client may enter a form of attachment activation, engaging psychological and neurobiological systems that encourage openness and connection, reduce expectations of danger (and therefore defensiveness), and increase well-being (Briere, 2012a; Gilbert, 2009; Schore, 1994). These positive feelings, elicited in an interpersonal context that otherwise might trigger fear, can countercondition relational distress, producing an increased likelihood of trust and interpersonal connection in the future.

Clinician mindfulness also can serve as a partial protection against countertransference (Bruce et al., 2010). As the therapist is more able to recognize the subjective and multidetermined nature of his or her own thoughts, feelings, and reactions, he or she can place triggered responses to the client in proper perspective before they result in nontherapeutic, or even harmful, behavior. As well, mindfulness may allow the therapist to be less reactive to, and become less identified with, the client's trauma history and disclosures, potentially reducing vicarious traumatization and "burnout."

Conclusion

Mindfulness-based interventions appear to be helpful for people suffering from a variety of problems and forms of distress, many of which are associated with exposure to traumatic events. In some cases, the processes underlying (or arising from) mindfulness-based activities parallel or reflect those well defined in modern trauma theory. In others, mindfulness and other aspects of Buddhist psychology (e.g., existential awareness) can provide skills and insights that are less easily accessed in Western therapies. For this reason, hybrid approaches that include both classic trauma therapy and mindfulness training may be especially useful. It is suggested in this chapter that mindfulness skills are often most efficiently acquired outside of therapy, after which they can be called on during psychotherapy sessions. This approach does not sacrifice the critically important aspects of trauma-focused psychotherapy—such as stabilization, relational processing, therapeutic exposure, and cognitive interventions—but augments them, to the extent possible, with mindfulness, existential awareness, and other helpful aspects of Buddhist psychology.

Acknowledgment

Portions of this chapter were adapted from Briere (2013). Copyright 2013 by The Guilford Press. Adapted by permission.

References

American Psychiatric Association. (2013). *Diagnostic and statistical manual of mental disorders* (5th ed.). Arlington, VA: Author.

Anderson, C. A., & Huesmann, L. R. (2003). Human aggression: A social-cognitive view. In M. A. Hogg & J. Cooper (Eds.), *The handbook of social psychology* (rev. ed., pp. 296–323). London: Sage.

Baer, J., Kaufman, J. C., & Baumeister, R. F. (2008). *Are we free?: Psychology and free will*. New York: Oxford University Press.

Baer, R. A. (2003). Mindfulness training as a clinical intervention: A conceptual and empirical review. *Clinical Psychology: Science and Practice, 10,* 125–143.

Belleville, G., Guay, S., & Marchand, A. (2011). Persistence of sleep disturbances following cognitive-behavior therapy for posttraumatic stress disorder. *Journal of Psychosomatic Research, 70,* 318–327.

Bhikkhu, A. (2010). *The earliest recorded discourses of the Buddha (from Lalitavistara, Mahākhandhaka & Mahāvastu)*. Kuala Lumpur, Malaysia: Sukhi Hotu.

Bishop, S. R., Lau, M., Shapiro, S., Carlson, L., Anderson, N. D., Carmody, J., et al. (2004). Mindfulness: A proposed operational definition. *Clinical Psychology: Science and Practice, 11,* 230–241.

Bobrow, J. (2010). *Zen and psychotherapy: Partners in liberation*. New York: Norton.

Bodhi, B. (2005). *In the Buddha's words: An anthology of discourses from the Pāli Canon*. Somerville, MA: Wisdom.

Bowen, S., Chawla, N., & Marlatt, G. A. (2011). *Mindfulness-based relapse prevention for addictive behaviors: A clinician's guide*. New York: Guilford Press.

Brach, T. (2004). *Radical acceptance: Embracing your life with the heart of a Buddha*. New York: Bantam.

Brach, T. (2013). *True refuge: Finding peace and freedom in your own awakened heart*. New York: Randon House.

Bradley, R., Green, J., Russ, E., Dutra, L., & Westen, D. (2005). A multidimensional meta-analysis of psychotherapy for PTSD. *American Journal of Psychiatry, 162,* 214–227.

Briere, J. (2004). *Psychological assessment of adult posttraumatic states: Phenomenology, diagnosis, and measurement* (2nd ed.). Washington, DC: American Psychological Association.

Briere, J. (2012a). Working with trauma: Mindfulness and compassion. In C. K. Germer & R. D. Siegel (Eds.), *Compassion and wisdom in psychotherapy* (pp. 265–279). New York: Guilford Press.

Briere, J. (2012b). When people do bad things: Evil, suffering, and dependent origination. In A. Bohart, E. Mendelowitz, B. Held, & K. Schneider (Eds.), *Humanity's dark side: Explorations in psychotherapy and beyond* (pp. 141–156). Washington, DC: American Psychological Association.

Briere, J. (2013). Mindfulness, insight, and trauma therapy. In C. K. Germer, R. D. Siegel, & P. R. Fulton (Eds.), *Mindfulness and psychotherapy* (2nd ed., pp. 208–224). New York: Guilford Press.

Briere, J., Hodges, M., & Godbout, N. (2010). Traumatic stress, affect dysregulation, and dysfunctional avoidance: A structural equation model. *Journal of Traumatic Stress, 23,* 767–774.

Briere, J., & Lanktree, C. B. (2012). *Treating complex trauma in adolescents and young adults*. Thousand Oaks, CA: Sage.

Briere, J., & Scott, C. (2014). *Principles of trauma therapy: A guide to symptoms, evaluation, and treatment* (2nd ed., DSM-5 update). Thousand Oaks, CA: Sage.

Briere, J., Scott, C., & Weathers, F. W. (2005). Peritraumatic and persistent dissociation in the presumed etiology of PTSD. *American Journal of Psychiatry, 162,* 2295–2301.

Bruce, N., Shapiro, S. L., Constantino, M. J., & Manber, R. (2010). Psychotherapist mindfulness and the psychotherapy process. *Psychotherapy: Theory, Research, Practice, Training, 47,* 83–97.

Cahill, S. P., Rothbaum, B. O., Resick, P. A., & Follette, V. M. (2009). Cognitive-behavioral therapy for adults. In E. B. Foa, T. M. Keane, M. J. Friedman, & J. A. Cohen (Eds.), *Effective treatments for PTSD: Practice guidelines from the International Society for Traumatic Stress Studies* (pp. 139–222). New York: Guilford Press.

Chödrön, P. (2002). *The places that scare you: A guide to fearlessness in difficult times.* Boston: Shambhala.

Cioffi, D., & Holloway, J. (1993). Delayed costs of suppressed pain. *Journal of Personality and Social Psychology, 64,* 274–282.

Cloitre, M., Stovall-McClough, K. C., Miranda, R., & Chemtob, C. M. (2004). Therapeutic alliance, negative mood regulation, and treatment outcome in child-abuse-related posttraumatic stress disorder. *Journal of Consulting and Clinical Psychology, 72,* 411– 416.

Coelho, H. F., Canter, P. H., & Ernst, E. (2007). Mindfulness-based cognitive therapy: Evaluating current evidence and informing future research. *Journal of Consulting and Clinical Psychology, 75,* 1000–1005.

Courtois, C. A., & Ford, J. D. (2012). *Treatment of complex trauma: A sequenced, relationship-based approach.* New York: Guilford Press.

Dalai Lama & Goleman, D. (2003). *Destructive emotions: How can we overcome them? A scientific dialogue with the Dalai Lama.* New York: Bantam Books.

Dutton, M. A., Bermudez, D., Matas, A., Majid, H., & Myers, N. L. (2013). Mindfulness-based stress reduction for low-income, predominantly African American women with PTSD and a history of intimate partner violence. *Cognitive and Behavioral Practice, 20,* 23–32

Epstein, M. (2008). *Psychotherapy without the self: A Buddhist perspective.* New Haven, CT: Yale University Press.

Foa, E. B., Huppert, J. D., & Cahill, S. P. (2006). Emotional processing theory: An update. In B. O. Rothbaum (Eds.), *Pathological anxiety: Emotional processing in etiology and treatment* (pp. 3–24). New York: Guilford Press.

Follette, V. M., & Vijay, A. (2009). Mindfulness for trauma and posttraumatic stress disorder. In F. Didonna (Ed.), *Clinical handbook of mindfulness* (pp. 299–317). New York: Springer.

Fulton, P. R. (2005). Mindfulness as clinical training. In C. K. Germer, R. D. Siegel, & P. R. Fulton (Eds.), *Mindfulness and psychotherapy* (2nd ed., pp. 55–72). New York: Guilford Press.

Germer, C. K., & Siegel, R. D. (Eds.). (2012). *Wisdom and compassion in psychotherapy.* New York: Guilford Press.

Gier, N. F., & Kjellberg, P. (2004). Buddhism and the freedom of the will: Pali and Mahayanist responses. In J. K. Campbell, J. Keim, M. O'Rourke, & D. Shier (Eds.), *Freedom and determinism* (pp. 277–304). Boston: MIT Press.

Gilbert, P. (2009). Introducing compassion-focused therapy. *Advances in Psychiatric Treatment, 15,* 199–208.

Gold, D. B., & Wegner, D. M. (1995). Origins of ruminative thought: Trauma, incompleteness, nondisclosure, and suppression. *Journal of Applied Social Psychology, 25,* 1245–1261.

Grossman, P., Niemann, L., Schmidt, S., & Walach, H. (2004). Mindfulness-based stress reduction and health benefits: A meta-analysis. *Journal of Psychosomatic Research, 57,* 35–43.

Hanh, T. N. (1987). *Interbeing: Fourteen guidelines for engaged Buddhism* (3rd ed.). Berkeley, CA: Parallax Press.

Harvard Health Publications. (2009). Yoga for anxiety and depression. Retrieved December 13, 2012, from *www.health.harvard.edu/newsletters/Harvard_Mental_Health_Letter/2009/April/Yoga-for-anxiety-and-depression.*

Hayes, S. C., Follette, V. M., & Linehan, M. M. (Eds.). (2004). *Mindfulness and acceptance: Expanding the cognitive-behavioral tradition.* New York: Guilford Press.

Hayes, S. C., Strosahl, K. D., & Wilson, K. G. (2011). *Acceptance and commitment therapy: The process and practice of mindful change* (2nd ed.). New York: Guilford Press.

Hembree, E. A., & Foa, E. B. (2003). Interventions for trauma-related emotional disturbances in adult victims of crime. *Journal of Traumatic Stress, 16,* 187–199.

Hofmann, S. G., Sawyer, A. T., Witt, A. A., & Oh, D. (2010). The effect of mindfulness-based therapy on anxiety and depression: A meta-analytic review. *Journal of Consulting and Clinical Psychology, 78,* 169–183.

Horowitz, M. J. (1986). *Stress-response syndromes* (2nd ed.). New York: Jason Aronson.

Kabat-Zinn, J. (1982). An outpatient program in behavioral medicine for chronic pain patients based on the practice of mindfulness meditation: Theoretical considerations and preliminary results. *General Hospital Psychiatry, 4,* 33–47.

Kabat-Zinn, J. (2003). Mindfulness-based interventions in context: Past, present, and future. *Clinical Psychology: Science and Practice, 10,* 144–156.

Kar, N. (2011). Cognitive-behavioral therapy for the treatment of post-traumatic stress disorder: A review. *Neuropsychiatric Disease and Treatment, 7,* 167–181.

Kearney, D. J., McDermott, K., Malte, C. A., Martinez, M., & Simpson, T. L. (2012). Association of participation in a mindfulness program with measures of PTSD, depression and quality of life in a veteran sample. *Journal of Clinical Psychology, 68,* 101–116.

Kimbrough, E., Magyari, T., Langenberg, P., Chesney, M. A., & Berman, B. (2010). Mindfulness intervention for child abuse survivors. *Journal of Clinical Psychology, 66,* 17–33.

Lambert, M. J., & Barley, D. E. (2001). Research summary on the therapeutic relationship and psychotherapy outcome. *Psychotherapy, 38,* 357–361.

Lambert, M. J., & Okishi, J. C. (1997). The effects of the individual psychotherapist and implications for future research. *Clinical Psychology: Science and Practice, 4,* 66–75.

Linehan, M. M. (1993). *Cognitive-behavioral treatment of borderline personality disorder.* New York: Guilford Press.

Lynch, T. R., Trost, W. T., Salsman, N., & Linehan, M. M. (2007). Dialectical behavior therapy for borderline personality disorder. *Annual Review of Clinical Psychology, 3,* 181–205.

Marlatt, G. A., & Gordon, J. R. (1985). *Relapse prevention: Maintenance strategy in the treatment of addictive behaviors.* New York: Guilford Press.

Martin, D. J., Garske, J. P., & Davis, M. K. (2000). Relation of the therapeutic alliance with outcome and other variables: A meta-analytic review. *Journal of Consulting and Clinical Psychology, 68,* 438–450.

Morgan, W. D., Morgan, S. T., & Germer, C. K. (2005). Cultivating attention and empathy. In C. K. Germer, R. D. Siegel, & P. R. Fulton (Eds.), *Mindfulness and psychotherapy* (2nd ed., pp. 73–90). New York: Guilford Press.

Morina, N. (2007). The role of experiential avoidance in psychological functioning after war-related stress in Kosovar civilians. *Journal of Nervous and Mental Disease, 195,* 697–700.

Nader, K. (2006). Childhood trauma: The deeper wound. In J. P. Wilson (Ed.), *The posttraumatic self: Restoring meaning and wholeness to personality* (pp. 117–156). London: Routledge.

Ogden, P., Minton, K., & Pain, C. (2006). *Trauma and the body: A sensorimotor approach to psychotherapy.* New York: Norton.

Pietrzak, R. H., Harpaz-Rotem, I., & Southwick, S. M. (2011). Cognitive-behavioral coping strategies associated with combat-related PTSD in treatment-seeking OEF-OIF Veterans. *Psychiatry Research, 189,* 251–258.

Queen, Q. S. (1995). *Engaged Buddhism in the West.* Somerville, MA: Wisdom.

Rosenthal, J. Z., Grosswald, S., Ross, R., & Rosenthal, N. (2011). Effects of transcendental meditation in veterans of Operation Enduring Freedom and Operation Iraqi Freedom with posttraumatic stress disorder: A pilot study. *Military Medicine, 176,* 626–630.

Rothbaum, B. O., & Davis, M. (2003). Applying learning principles to the treatment of post-trauma reactions. *Annals of the New York Academy of Sciences, 1008,* 112–121.

Salzberg, S. (1995). *Lovingkindness: The revolutionary art of happiness.* Boston: Shambhala.

Schneider, K. S., Bugental, J. F. T., & Pierson, J. F. (2002). *The handbook of humanistic psychology: Leading edges in theory, research, and practice.* Thousand Oaks, CA: Sage.

Schore, A. N. (1994). *Affect regulation and the origin of the self: The neurobiology of emotional development.* Hillsdale, NJ: Erlbaum.

Schottenbauer, M. A., Glass, C. R., Arnkoff, D. B., Tendick, V., & Gray, S. H. (2008). Nonresponse and dropout rates in outcome studies on PTSD: Review and methodological considerations. *Psychiatry, 71,* 134–168.

Scott, C., Jones, J., & Briere, J. (2014). Psychobiology and psychopharmacology of trauma. In J. Briere & C. Scott (Eds.), *Principles of trauma therapy: A guide to symptoms, evaluation, and treatment* (2nd ed., DSM-5 update). Thousand Oaks, CA: Sage.

Segal, Z. V., Williams, J. M. G., & Teasdale, J. D. (2002). *Mindfulness-based cognitive therapy for depression: A new approach to preventing relapse.* New York: Guilford Press.

Semple, R. J., & Lee, J. (2011). *Mindfulness-based cognitive therapy for anxious children: A manual for treating childhood anxiety.* Oakland, CA: New Harbinger.

Shapiro, D. H. (1992). Adverse effects of meditation: A preliminary investigation of long-term meditators. *International Journal of Psychosomatics, 39*, 62–66.

Shapiro, S. L., & Carlson, L. E. (2009). *The art and science of mindfulness: Integrating mindfulness into psychology and the helping professions.* Washington, DC: American Psychological Association.

Shay, J. (2005). *Achilles in Vietnam: Combat trauma and the undoing of character.* New York: Simon & Schuster.

Siegel, D. J. (2007). *The mindful brain: Reflection and attunement in the cultivation of well-being.* New York: Norton.

Steil, R., Dyer, A., Priebe, K., Kleindienst, N., & Bohus, M. (2011). Dialectical behavior therapy for posttraumatic stress disorder related to childhood sexual abuse: A pilot study of an intensive residential treatment program. *Journal of Traumatic Stress, 24*, 102–106.

Thanissaro, B. (Trans.). (1997). *Sallatha Sutta: The arrow.* Retrieved December 27, 2011, from *www.accesstoinsight.org/tipitaka/sn/sn36/sn36.006.than.html*.

Thompson, N., & Walsh, M, (2010). The existential basis of trauma. *Journal of Social Work Practice: Psychotherapeutic Approaches in Health, Welfare and the Community, 24*, 377–389.

Thompson, B. L., & Waltz, J. (2007). Everyday mindfulness and mindfulness meditation: Overlapping constructs or not? *Personality and Individual Differences, 43*, 1875–1885.

Treanor, M. (2011). The potential impact of mindfulness on exposure and extinction learning in anxiety disorders. *Clinical Psychology Review, 31*, 617–625.

van der Kolk, B. A., Pelcovitz, D., Roth, S., Mandel, F. S., McFarlane, A., & Herman, J. L. (1996). Dissociation, somatization, and affect dysregulation: The complexity of adaptation of trauma. *American Journal of Psychiatry, 153*(Suppl.), 83–93.

van der Kolk, B. A., Roth, S. H., Pelcovitz, D., Sunday, S., & Spinazzola, J. (2005). Disorders of extreme stress. *Journal of Traumatic Stress, 18*, 389–399.

Wagner, A. W., & Linehan, M. M. (1998). Dissociative behavior. In V. M. Follette, J. I. Ruzek, & F. R. Abueg (Eds.), *Cognitive-behavioral therapies for trauma* (pp. 191–225). New York: Guilford Press.

Williams, J. M. G., & Swales, M. (2004). The use of mindfulness-based approaches for suicidal patients. *Archives of Suicide Research, 8*, 315–329.

Yehuda, R. (Ed.). (1998). *Psychological trauma.* Washington, DC: American Psychiatric Press.

2

Healing Traumatic Fear

The Wings of Mindfulness and Love

Tara Brach

In my practice as a psychotherapist and Buddhist meditation teacher working with people who have endured trauma, I have found that for healing to occur, the painful emotions buried in the body must be directly recontacted, but from a fresh and enlarged perspective. This is a delicate process that only can be accomplished after establishing an environment of sufficient safety, care, and connection and helping to fortify the client's own inner resources. When combined with a trusting therapeutic relationship, meditations that awaken mindfulness and a sense of loving presence offer much potential to facilitate healing from trauma.

Trauma is the experience of extreme stress—physical or psychological—that overwhelms an individual's normal capacities to process and cope. When people are in a traumatized state, gripped by primitive survival strategies, they are cut off from their own inner wisdom and the resources of the world around them. Their entire reality is confined to the sense of the self in isolation, helpless and afraid. This profound state of disconnection is the core characteristic of trauma.

Neuroscience tells us that traumatic abuse causes lasting changes by affecting physiology, the nervous system, and brain chemistry. In the normal process of forming memories we evaluate each new situation in terms of the cohesive worldview that we have formulated. With trauma, this cognitive process is short-circuited by a surge of painful and intense stimulation. Instead of "processing the experience" by fitting it into our understanding of how the world works and thereby learning from it, people who have been traumatized revert to a more primitive form of encoding—through physical sensations and visual images. The trauma, undigested and locked in the brain and body, is experienced as randomly breaking into consciousness. For years after the actual danger is past, the traumatic event may be relived as if it were continually occurring in the present.

Unprocessed pain keeps the traumatized person's system of self-preservation on permanent alert. In addition to sudden intrusive memories, a wide range of situations—many nonthreatening—may activate the alarmingly high levels of pain and fear stored in the body. Someone's partner might raise her voice in irritation, and the full force of traumatic past wounds—all the terror or rage or hurt that lives in the body—can be unleashed, even when there is no present danger.

In order to endure the reawakened pain, some victims of trauma dissociate from their bodies, numbing their sensitivity to physical sensations. Some people feel "unreal," as if they are disembodied and experiencing life from a great distance. They do whatever they can to keep from feeling the raw, physical sensations of fear and pain. They might lash out in aggression or freeze in depression or confusion. Some may have suicidal thoughts or drink themselves senseless, while others may overeat, use drugs, or lose themselves in mental obsessions. Yet the pain and fear do not go away. Rather, they lurk in the background and from time to time suddenly take over.

Dissociation, while protective, creates suffering. When people who have suffered trauma leave their bodies, they leave home. By rejecting pain and pulling away from the ground of their being, they experience the disease of separation—loneliness, anxiety, and shame. They are cut off from a wholeness of being.

A Caring Presence

When I work with individuals who have been traumatized, there is a natural progression. The first step is for my clients to be able to take comfort in my presence—physically, emotionally, energetically. This can take several months or even longer. The traumatized self is fragile and needs an external resource. Yet because the original traumatic wounding often occurred in relationship, relationships may have become associated with danger. For this reason, it is essential to develop trust in the therapeutic relationship.

Dana had been coming to my weekly meditation group for 4 months when she approached me one evening after class. She told me that she needed more help in dealing with her fear. "Trust doesn't come easy for me," she said, "but listening to you calms me down. I get the sense that I'd feel safe working with you."

Dana did not appear insecure or easily intimidated. A tall, robust African American woman in her late 20s, she had a tough job as a parole officer in a state prison. She also had an easy smile and lively eyes, but her words told a different story. "I can be just fine, Tara," she said, "and then if I get tripped off, I'm a totally dysfunctional person." This was especially true when a strong male got angry with her. "It's like I'm a scared little girl, a basket case. I get tongue-tied."

In our first session I asked Dana to tell me about some recent times when she had been tongue-tied with fear. She began nervously tapping the floor with one foot. When she spoke, it was in a rush of words. "One place it happens is with my boyfriend. He drinks—too much—and sometimes he'll start yelling, accusing me of things that aren't true, like I'm flirting with other men or talking about him behind his back." She stopped for a moment, then added, "When he gets on my case, threatening me, my insides just huddle up into a tight little ball, and it's like the real me disappears." At such times she was unable to think or talk. All she was aware of was the pounding of her heart and a choking feeling in her throat.

Her boyfriend was not the first man to violate her. It soon emerged that Dana had disappeared into that tight ball repeatedly, ever since she was 11 years old and her uncle began to molest her. For 4 years, until he moved out of state, Dana had lived in fear that he would drop by when her mother was at work. After each assault, he would swear her to secrecy and threaten to punish her if she told on him. He accused her of "asking for it." Even then, a part of Dana knew this was not true, but something else in her believed him. "It still does," she said. "It's like there's some badness in me that's always waiting to come out."

Dana was clear about the source of her fear, but that clarity did not protect her from feelings of anxiety, guilt, and powerlessness. The next time I saw her, she reported that after our first session, the old terrors had resurfaced. Now, just being in my office plunged her into an old and familiar spiral of fear. She stopped talking, her face froze, and her eyes became fixed on the floor. She was trembling and her breathing had become shallow. "Are you disappearing inside?" I asked. She nodded without looking up. It was clear that Dana was having a posttraumatic stress reaction. She seemed to have tumbled back into the past, as defenseless and endangered as when her uncle abused her.

I've found that what a person needs when fear is this intense is to have a sense of what I call "being accompanied"—an experience of another person's caring, accepting presence. The core of vulnerability is feeling alone in one's pain; connection with another person eases fear and increases the sense of safety. However, when someone experiences posttraumatic stress disorder (PTSD), it is also important that he or she control the degree of contact. Otherwise, contact itself could be associated with the traumatizing situation.

"Dana," I said gently, "would you like me to sit next to you?" She nodded. When I moved to her side, I asked her if it was okay for me to sit so close, and she whispered, "Sure. Thanks." I suggested that she make herself as comfortable as possible in order to feel her body being supported by the sofa and her feet resting against the floor. I encouraged her to notice the felt sense of what it was like for us to be sitting together.

Over the next few minutes, I checked in several times and let her know that I was there with her. She remained silent but gradually stopped trembling, and her breathing became more regular. When I asked again how she was doing, she turned her head enough to catch my eye and smiled slightly. "I'm settling down, Tara. It's better now." I could tell by the way she was engaging—with her eyes and her smile—that she no longer felt so trapped inside her fear.

I returned to my chair facing her so that we could discuss what had happened. "I don't know what's wrong with me," she began. "I should be able to get it together on my own, but when I get stuck like that, it's embarrassing. I just feel so broken." Dana knew that she had been traumatized, yet she still considered her "episodes," as she called them, to be a sign of weakness and cowardice. Worse, they were evidence that she was spiritually bereft. As she put it, "I have no spiritual center, it's just darkness there . . . no soul."

De-Shaming Trauma

One of the most painful and lasting legacies of trauma is self-blame. Students and clients often tell me that they feel broken, flawed, like "damaged goods." They may understand the impact of trauma rationally, but still they experience self-revulsion and shame when they feel or act out of control. Their underlying belief seems to be that no matter how awful their inner firestorm, they should be able to subdue its terror, quiet their catastrophic thinking, and avoid false refuges like addictive behavior. In other words, the self, no matter how distressed, should always be in control.

But if the client feels a therapist's acceptance and trusts that there is no hidden judgment, in time that acceptance can become internalized. For Dana, that trust grew as she felt my care and acceptance during moments when the raw feelings of trauma were arising. Our close contact during those disturbing moments in my office was an important first step.

For Rosalie, a client who had been severely abused by her father during childhood and at 35 still suffered from extreme anxiety, her strongest ally was an imagined "good fairy" that she came in contact with during a guided journey in my office. The fairy promised to protect Rosalie by touching and closing off various parts of her body with a magic wand so that Rosalie—and the little girl still living inside her—could bear all the terrible feelings bound up in her body until she was ready to deal with them. The fairy explained that in the meantime Rosalie would have to find ways to keep the buried feelings at bay. What's more, the fairy said that although Rosalie's strategies for managing her pain—anorexia, avoiding intimacy, dependence on marijuana and sleeping pills—filled her with shame, she was doing the best she could. The fairy predicted that the day would come when Rosalie had the resilience to contact her painful feelings and heal them. Before leaving, the fairy assured her of her intrinsic goodness, of being lovable.

The fairy's message was a source of profound relief for Rosalie. Until that point Rosalie had felt nothing but self-hatred for the strategies that had made it possible for her young, wounded self to survive. This understanding is key for anyone troubled by the deep shame that generally accompanies trauma. For Rosalie, the message helped her move toward self-acceptance and compassion, and opened the way to healing.

Cultivating Inner Refuge

While initially the sense of acceptance—or safety, worth, or love—may be offered through an external (or imagined) other, for healing to occur and be sustained, these states must be experienced from within.

Through meditative strategies, the outer refuge—the caring presence of the therapist—can become a bridge to unfolding a trustworthy inner refuge of love and well-being that dwells—though often unrealized—in each client's own heart.

Once a positive mindstate has been generated in therapy, it can continue to be strengthened outside the clinical setting. This is where attentional training—meditation—comes in. If a client practices focusing and sustaining attention on the felt sense of the positive experience, it can become internalized as a self-sustaining pattern in the brain and nervous system. Researchers are discovering what happens in the brains of meditators when their attention is focused on love. Sophisticated brain scans show that the left frontal cortex, a part of the brain that is deactivated during trauma, lights up during loving-kindness and compassion meditations. According to both research and subjective reports, when this region of the brain "turns on," there is a correlation with feelings of happiness, openness, and peace. Neuroscientists report that "neurons that fire together, wire together." The more individuals practice such meditations, the more this cluster of positive emotions takes hold.

Intentionally internalizing and strengthening positive inner resources allows clients to develop an inner refuge where they feel loved and safe. When they're able to contact an inner refuge through internally generated words, images, or self-touch, their neurobiology shifts. Characteristic fight–flight–freeze reactivity no longer overwhelms potentially adaptive responses, and the mind becomes more spacious and receptive. As the intensity of traumatic fear is reduced, new associations, new inner resources, new ways of coping and understanding begin to emerge spontaneously. The most basic outcome is a growing sense of self-efficacy, confidence, or trust; clients begin to discover that they have within themselves whatever is needed to meet their life circumstances with increased equanimity.

When I teach meditations for the heart, I often include visualizing being held by a loved one, or gentle self-touch, as part of the practice. Research shows that a 20-second hug stimulates production of oxytocin, the hormone associated with feelings of love, connectedness, and safety (Grewen, Girdler, Amico, & Light, 2005). Yet we do not need a physical hug from another: As many of my clients and meditation students have discovered, either imagining a hug or feeling our own touch—on our cheek, on our heart—can awaken similar feelings of well-being. Whether through visualization, words, or touch, meditations on love can shift brain activity in a way that arouses positive emotions and reduces traumatic reactivity. This, in turn, brings a healing, mindful presence to the energetic layers of trauma in the body.

After we had established a sense of safety and care, my next goal in working with Dana was to help her access feelings of love and safety on her own. She was already practicing a traditional version of loving-kindness meditation, but now we would personalize it, identifying the particular images and words that would allow her to feel held in love.

When I asked her who in her life made her feel safe inside, Dana's eyes lit up. "That's easy. Marin, my friend, or my little sister Serena. I trust both of them, they've totally got my back. And I feel safe with you." She said this a little shyly and I smiled, letting her know that I felt honored to be counted in.

Next, I suggested that she picture her "allies" right here in the room and imagine that she was surrounded by the three of us. Closing her eyes, Dana concentrated for a few moments, then said softly, "Okay, I see each of you. You and Marin are on either side. Each of you is holding one of my arms, and my sister's right behind me."

When I asked her what that felt like, she responded without hesitation. "It's like being in a warm bath!"

"Good," I said. "Now let yourself just soak that warmth in, feel how deep it can go, how it can relax the places inside that most need it." Then: "As you let in the warmth of your allies' presence, what words might be most comforting to hear and remember?"

"It's that I'm safe, that I'm loved. That's my prayer: May I feel safe, may I feel loved."

I waited a few moments, then suggested, "Dana, if you contract inside and get huddled up in fear, just imagine each of us here. Feel the warmth surrounding you and let your prayer comfort you. Let the feeling of being safe and loved sink into you. Let your body have the felt sense of being loved. You can practice that now if you'd like."

Dana settled back in her chair and was quite still. When she looked up at me again, she smiled. "This reminds me that it's possible to relax. It's like there's a net around me and I can't fall too far. I feel better than I've felt in a long time."

Before she left, I encouraged Dana to practice calling on her allies at some point each day, during a time of low stress. "Experiment with what helps you feel our presence, our company," I suggested. "You might whisper our names, visualize our faces, feel our touch supporting you, whatever connects you with this sense of ease. Then remember your prayer for safety and love, and let it fill you."

Like Dana, some people immediately identify an individual—a family member or friend, healer or teacher—whose presence creates the feeling of being "at home." For others, home is a spiritual community, a 12-step group, or a circle of intimate friends. Sometimes the feeling of belonging is strongest with someone who has died, or with someone the person reveres but has never met, such as the Dalai Lama, Gandhi, or Mother Teresa. Many people feel drawn to an archetypal figure like the Buddha, Jesus, or the Virgin Mary. I have also known a good number of people who feel comfort and belonging when they call to mind their dog or cat. I assure my clients and students that no one figure is more spiritual or elevated than another. All that matters is choosing a source of safe and loving feelings and through a meditative attention—sustaining focus and staying in the present moment—strengthening those feelings. Key to these instructions is feeling the positive experience in the body.

In addition to asking students and clients to identify an ally, there are some other questions I pose to help them develop an inner refuge of safety and love—always with the caveat that these questions are best considered when the student or client is not in the grip of fear. Practiced regularly, they can become important pathways to a sense of refuge during difficult times.

• *"When and where do you feel most at home—safe, secure, relaxed, or strong?"* Some people find a sense of sanctuary in the natural world and are able to relax when they are in the woods or by the ocean. Others have a sense of safe space when they are at their church or temple. Still others feel more secure when surrounded by the noise and vibrancy of a big city. The feeling of "at home" may occur anywhere. Even if clients almost never feel truly relaxed or secure, by carefully reviewing their day-to-day lives, they can probably identify several settings and situations where they are closest to feeling at home.

• *"What events or experiences or relationships have best revealed to you your strength, your courage, your potential?"* Sometimes what arises is a memory of a particularly meaningful experience—an artistic or work endeavor, a service offered, an athletic feat—that was a source of personal gratification or accomplishment. For one client it was the part she played in a school play, while another remembered that at age 12 he had confronted his father for yelling and physically threatening his mother. Whatever the experience, clients can use it to explore how it deepens their trust in themselves and can help awaken a sense of ease, safety or care.

- *"What about yourself helps you to trust your goodness?"* When we are in the grip of trauma or very strong emotion, it may not be possible to reflect on goodness, our own or others'. But when the body and mind are less agitated, this inquiry can be a powerful entry to inner refuge. I often ask clients or students to consider the qualities they like about themselves—humor, kindness, patience, creativity, curiosity, loyalty, honesty, wonder. I suggest that they recall their deepest life aspirations—loving well, realizing truth, happiness, peace, serving others—and sense the goodness of their hearts' longing. And I invite them to sense the goodness of their very essence, their experience of aliveness, awareness, and heart.

- *"When you are caught in fear, what is it that you most want to feel?"* When I ask this question, people often say that they just want the fear to go away. But when they pause to reflect, they often name more positive states of mind. Like Dana, they want to feel safe or loved. They want to feel valued or worthwhile. They long to feel peaceful, at home, or trusting. Or they want to feel physically held, embraced. The words that name their longings and the images that arise with them can become a valuable entry to inner refuge. Often the starting place is to offer wishes or prayers such as, "May I feel safe and at home." Like the phrases in the classic loving-kindness meditation, they serve as reminders to care for one's inner life and help to soften and open the heart.

Sometimes, however, people feel so isolated, so disconnected from love and security, that they cannot initially find any inner resources to build on. Especially when they are frightened, offering themselves phrases of well-wishing does not seem to make a dent. Still, I have found that even when there is only a fragile tendril of connection to a larger sense of belonging—to what is experienced as life's goodness—the refuge of the heart can be cultivated. The key is sincere willingness to look for whatever warms and opens the heart and then to practice bringing attention there over and over again.

Deepening Loving Refuge

For 3 months, Dana practiced faithfully, calling on her allies daily during moments of relative calm. She reported feeling embraced by their warmth and her own prayers for safety and love. When this capacity to draw on inner resources got tested, Dana came out the other end with a confidence she had not thought possible.

"I'm learning what it means to trust myself," she began, after a life-changing episode. Then she told me what had happened. After downing a six-pack, Dana's boyfriend had taunted her, then egged her on to react. "You don't like my talk? Go ahead, bitch, try shutting me up and see what happens." Dana felt her gut instantly seize up with fear, and she knew that if she stayed, she would only become more frightened and frozen. Before she walked out the door, she told her boyfriend that this time it was over between them.

And then the fear slammed into her. Afraid to be at home alone, she went to her friend Marin's apartment and asked to stay the night. Marin welcomed her, and they spent an hour talking. But after Marin went to sleep, Dana lay awake on the couch. "I couldn't stop thinking about how he might try to punish me." Feeling a rising tide of terror, Dana found herself curled up in a ball and shaking. "That was when I remembered that time in your office when I freaked out and we sat on the sofa together. I knew I had to call on my allies."

Dana sat up and wrapped her blanket around her. She focused on the support of the sofa under her, as I had suggested she do when she felt her fear arise, and she planted her feet squarely on the ground, feeling its solidity. "Then I called out for help," Dana said. "I whispered Marin's name, my sister's name, and yours. I was gathering my women allies, having them surround me. But even then my heart still felt like it was exploding with fear."

Dana likened the fear to "hot, broken glass" tearing up her chest, but she kept whispering her allies' names and bringing her attention to her feet on the ground. She hugged herself and imagined that we were there hugging her, even as her body trembled uncontrollably and fear continued to rip through her. Yet, as she put it, "I kept feeling you all there caring—like I was surrounded by a presence that was caring about me—while my insides were being broken apart. Even though I was freaked out, I didn't feel alone. I could hear the words 'May I feel safe, may I feel loved' going through my mind."

Gradually Dana noticed that something was shifting. "The fear was still there, but it was no longer taking over. There was some space. It was that space of loving that was larger than this scared self. And as I settled down a little, and the minutes went by, that space became more and more filled with light. It was like I was part of that light. And then I realized my soul was back. That lit-up space was inside me. I started crying, feeling how all these years I'd been lost, living without this light, living in a broken self."

Dana fell silent. Her hands pressed together as if in prayer and she bowed her head, allowing the tears to flow. When she looked up and spoke, her voice was soft, yet full. "Tara," she said, "I'm sad, and that's okay. There's something new growing in me. When I told you I am learning to trust myself, what I meant is that I'm trusting that caring place that lets in love, that is loving—my soul. That's where the safety is. Even though I'll probably have that broken feeling again, even though I'll feel lost, I'll find my way back. This light, this love, is part of what I am."

Although the pain of trauma may lead us to believe that our spirit has been tainted or destroyed, that is not so. No amount of violence can corrupt the timeless and pure presence that is the very ground of our being. Waves of shame or fear may possess us temporarily, but as we continue to entrust ourselves to loving presence, as we let ourselves feel loved, our lives become more and more an expression of who or what we are. This is the essence of grace—homecoming to who we are.

Dana's journey back to herself is a good example of the phrase "Where attention goes, energy flows." When through meditative training we repeatedly direct our minds toward thoughts and memories that evoke feelings of love or safety or strength, the very structure of our brains is altered. On a physical and energetic level, new neural connections are formed that serve as vital channels for healing. As Dana discovered by meditating on love and staying present with her moment-to-moment experience, she was carried home to the light and love of her own soul—the part of herself that had felt lost to her for so long.

Awakening the Wing of Mindfulness

In both psychotherapy and meditation, once sufficient outer and inner resources are in place, the next phase of the critical transformational work begins. That is to bring a clear and compassionate attention to the experience that has been dissociated, unfelt and left "frozen" in the body. Although any therapeutic process involving somatic presence requires mindfulness on the part of both client and therapist, in many instances there is a lack of explicit training to cultivate a mindful awareness. Such training would entail teaching the client how to bring a nonjudging attention to her or his moment-to-moment experience. When included in therapy, training in mindfulness deepens self-compassion and empowers the client to continue the process of healing independently.

I recently counseled a young man who had served in Iraq and was suffering from PTSD. When he first came to me, paying attention to any part of his body other than his feet triggered terror. We worked together to build two inner resource anchors: the sensations in his feet—which helped to ground him—and a mantra, or set of sacred words, that reminded him of the protection of a loving universal spirit. For many months, his primary practice was to reflect on his mantra, repeating it inwardly over and over again, and to feel his feet on the ground. After about 6 months, when he was feeling more grounded and protected, he gradually began to mindfully name and include the sensations in the rest of his body in his awareness. This occurred during our sessions as well as on his own. In time he was able to bring an alert, curious, and kind attention to the areas that felt most vulnerable and raw. He called this his "journey back to being alive and whole" and developed confidence in his capacity to be present with the strong feelings that continued to arise.

When I started working with Rosalie—my client who had been sexually abused by her father—it was clear that her body was presenting its bill.

The guided journey in which she discovered her "good fairy" was part of the process, and the combination of our relationship and the sense of an inner benevolent presence allowed her more access to a felt experience of safety. Rosalie was now ready to begin systematically cultivating mindful awareness of the places in her body that were holding deep wounds.

I introduced her to a "sweeping meditation," guiding her attention slowly up and down her body, focusing on each region—feet and legs, torso, shoulders, arms and hands, neck, head. I encouraged her to imagine breathing energy and light into the part of the body she was attending to, then letting go and relaxing as she breathed out. As Rosalie deepened her attention in each area, I suggested that she bring mindfulness to whatever sensations she felt there, accepting them exactly as they were. Most important, if the experience felt like "too much," Rosalie could remind herself of us being in the room together, or turn toward her inner resources.

During one session, when she said that she was having a hard time feeling sensations in her stomach and pelvic area, I asked her what color felt healing to her. She remembered a shimmering blue that had surrounded the fairy. I suggested that she imagine feeling those areas of her body bathed in that blue, letting the color wash through her with each breath. After some moments Rosalie nervously reported, "I do feel some movement, some tingling," and then, "That's enough for now." Although she was not able to sustain her attention in that newly awakening area for long, Rosalie was proud of her first efforts. It had taken courage to reenter the places that had felt so dangerous.

Rosalie arrived at one of our final sessions excited about a new man she had met. But by the following week the excitement had turned to anxiety, and her body appeared rigid with terror. She really liked this man and did not want to retreat in fear, as she had done repeatedly in the past. "If I can't make peace with this fear, Tara, I won't hang in there," she said. Rosalie knew that she needed to meet and accept her body's fearful reaction.

I suggested that she pause and, feeling into her body, sense what was most asking for her attention and acceptance. This was new for Rosalie. Up to this point she had only explored a mindful presence in her body when she was relatively relaxed. That had felt safe, but to experience raw fear had many painful associations. Closing her eyes, she fell silent and still. After about a minute she placed her hand on her stomach. "In here," she said. "I'm really scared. I feel like I could throw up." I encouraged her to let the warmth of her hand, her own gentle touch, help her bring her full awareness to the unpleasant feelings. I asked her if she could feel that area from the inside and just notice what was happening.

Rosalie took several full breaths and sank back into the sofa. For the next few minutes she named what she was experiencing and just let it be there: the soreness and squeezing tightness in the center of her belly; the feelings of her chest rising and falling with several deep breaths; the loosening and dissolving of the hard knot in her gut; a quaking and jumpiness spreading throughout her stomach; the thought "Maybe he's the right one"; stabbing fear, shaking; the image of a young child alone in a closet, hiding from her father; the thought, *I can't stand this*; heat spreading up into her chest and throat; a strangling feeling in her throat; breathing in blue; opening and softening in her throat; an upwelling of sadness. When she finally looked up, her eyes were glistening. "Tara, all this is happening inside me, and I'm just holding the little girl I was in my arms." She paused, then added, "I feel like I can accept this pain. I can handle whatever I'm feeling."

At the core of Buddhist psychology is the understanding that we suffer when we forget our wholeness and identify with a limited, deficient sense of self. When a client has been traumatized, very often he or she feels cut off from the flow of life and trapped in a narrow, endangered, and powerless sense of self. The process of healing, as discussed throughout this chapter, is one of supporting clients to reconnect with the intrinsic resources of love and presence. Therapists provide that support as we offer our care and acceptance, while also helping clients to strengthen their inner sense of being safe and lovable, and pay mindful attention to their unfolding experience.

In moments when the two wings of mindfulness and loving presence come together, there is a shift in identity. As Rosalie put it, "all this is happening inside me, and I'm just holding the little girl I was in my arms." She was no longer identified with her small, fearful self. She had enlarged her perception of herself to occupy the mindful and loving presence that could hold the fear. This shift in identity is the true release from suffering discovered through all healing therapies and pointed to in all spiritual texts.

Acknowledgment

This chapter is adapted from *Radical Acceptance* (New York: Bantam Books, 2003), copyright 2003 by Tara Brach, and *True Refuge* (New York: Bantam Books, 2013), copyright 2013 by Tara Brach, by permission of Bantam Books, an imprint of Random House, a division of Random House LLC.

Reference

Grewen, K. M., Girdler, S. S., Amico, J., & Light, K. C. (2005). Effects of partner support on resting oxytocin, cortisol, norepinephrine, and blood pressure before and after warm partner contact. *Psychosomatic Medicine, 67*(4), 531–538.

3

Cultivating Self-Compassion in Trauma Survivors

Christopher K. Germer and Kristin D. Neff

> Whatever your difficulties—a devastated heart, financial loss, feeling assaulted by the conflicts around you, or a seemingly hopeless illness—you can always remember that you are free in every moment to set the compass of your heart to your highest intentions.
>
> —JACK KORNFIELD (2011)

Most of us treat ourselves rather unkindly when bad things happen to us. Rather than offering ourselves the same sympathy and support we would give to a loved one, we tend to criticize ourselves ("What's the matter with you!"), we hide from others or ourselves in shame ("I'm worthless"), and we get stuck in our heads trying to make sense of what happened to us ("Why me?"). And when *very* bad things happen, we attack ourselves from two directions saying, for example, "I'm bad because I was abused" and "I was abused because I'm bad." If we do not numb ourselves through dissociation, we may try drugs, alcohol, or self-injury. And no matter how much we wish to get out of our heads and get on with our lives, we find ourselves locked in a struggle with intrusive memories, nightmares, and flashbacks.

Such reactions make our suffering persist and even amplify it, but they're not our fault. They're how we're wired (Gilbert, 2009a). When we feel threatened by *external* danger, our survival often depends on our capacity to fight, flee, or freeze. But when we're threatened *internally* by intense emotions such as dread or shame, the fight–flight–freeze response turns into an unholy trinity of self-criticism, self-isolation, and self-absorption.

Fortunately, we also have a hardwired capacity to respond to our own

43

suffering in a soothing, healing way—*self-compassion*. The Dalai Lama (1995) defines compassion as "an openness to suffering with the wish to relieve it," and *self*-compassion is that same attitude directed toward oneself. This may seem like a tall order to a person suffering from childhood abuse, neglect, or later trauma, but self-compassion has been linked to so many measures of psychological well-being and mental health, including emotional resilience in the face of negative events, that it warrants careful consideration. Additionally, therapists working in any treatment model— cognitive-behavioral, psychodynamic, humanistic, family systems—can help their clients *cultivate* self-compassion. This chapter reviews our current understanding of self-compassion and offers suggestions for helping traumatized clients treat themselves with greater care, understanding, and respect.

What Is Self-Compassion?

Self-compassion is a relatively new psychological construct derived from ancient Buddhist contemplative psychology. Neff (2003), a developmental psychologist and student of Buddhist meditation, first defined the concept and developed the Self-Compassion Scale (SCS) that is used in most research. Self-compassion has three main components: (1) self-kindness, (2) a sense of common humanity, and (3) mindfulness. *Self-kindness* entails being warm and caring toward ourselves when things go wrong in our lives. *Common humanity* recognizes the shared nature of suffering when difficult situations arise, rather than feeling desperately alone. And *mindfulness* refers here to the ability to open to painful experience ("this hurts!") with nonreactive, balanced awareness. Taken together, self-compassion is precisely the opposite of our typical reaction to internal threat—self-criticism, self-isolation, and self-absorption.

Even in ancient times, the Buddha prescribed kindness, a sense of common humanity, and mindfulness as an antidote to unrealistic fear and dread. Our current method of practicing loving-kindness meditation derives from a talk given by the Buddha to a group of monks who were too terrified to live in the forest and practice meditation during the rainy season. An excerpt from that discourse (*metta sutta*) reads as follows:

> Let no one work to undo another.
> Let no one think badly of anyone.
> Either with anger or with violent thoughts,
> One would not wish suffering on others.
> Just as a mother would watch over her
> Son—her one and only son—with her life,
> In just the same way develop a mind

> Unbounded toward all living creatures.
> Develop a mind of loving kindness
> Unbounded toward the entire world:
> Above and below and all the way 'round,
> With no holding back, no loathing, no foe.
>   (Olendzki, 2008)[1]

By shifting their mind-set from fear to loving-kindness, the monks were able to return to the forest and meditate until they could resume their wanderings when the monsoon season ended.

In those days, a "mind of loving-kindness, unbounded toward the entire world" included oneself as well. Because everyone is born with the wish to be happy and free from suffering, the practice of cultivating compassion toward others traditionally begins by anchoring our awareness in how we naturally feel toward ourselves. Ironically, in modern times, it is easier to evoke loving states of mind by remembering how we feel toward *others*—special people or other living beings—and then sneak ourselves into that circle of compassion to evoke love for ourselves. Self-compassion feels especially foreign to people suffering from shame and self-criticism as a consequence of trauma, but it is no less essential.

Self-Compassion and Trauma

Three symptom clusters commonly found in posttraumatic stress disorder (PTSD) are (1) arousal, (2) avoidance, and (3) intrusions. Interestingly, these three categories closely correspond to the stress response (fight–flight–freeze) and to our reactions to internal stress (self-criticism, self-isolation, and self-absorption) mentioned earlier (see Figure 3.1). Together they point toward self-compassion as a healthy, alternative response to trauma. Self-kindness can have a calming effect on autonomic hyperarousal, common humanity is an antidote to hiding in shame, and balanced, mindful awareness allows us to disentangle ourselves from intrusive memories and feelings.

Research shows that people who lack self-compassion are likely to have critical mothers, to come from dysfunctional families, and to display insecure attachment patterns (Neff & McGeehee, 2010; Wei, Liao, Ku, & Shaffer, 2011). Childhood emotional abuse is associated with lower self-compassion, and individuals with low self-compassion experience more emotional distress and are more likely to abuse alcohol or make a serious suicide attempt (Tanaka, Wekerle, Schmuck, Paglia-Boak, & the MAP Research Team, 2011; Vettese, Dyer, Li, & Wekerle, 2011). Research also indicates that self-compassion mediates the relationship between childhood maltreatment and later emotional dysregulation, meaning that abused

---

[1]Reprinted with permission from Andrew Olendzki.

Stress Response	Stress Response Turned Inward	PTSD Symptoms	Self-Compassion
Fight	Self-Criticism	Arousal	Self-Kindness
Flight	Self-Isolation	Avoidance	Common Humanity
Freeze	Self-Absorption	Intrusions	Mindfulness

FIGURE 3.1. Components of the stress response, PTSD, and self-compassion.

individuals with higher levels of self-compassion are better able to cope with upsetting events (Vettese et al., 2011). This relationship holds even after accounting for history of maltreatment, current distress level, or substance abuse, suggesting that self-compassion is an important resiliency factor for those traumatized as children.

In a study of undergraduate students who met criteria for PTSD (mostly with adult traumas such as accidents or deaths), Thompson and Waltz (2008) found that only the "avoidance" cluster of symptoms was negatively correlated with self-compassion. Self-compassion may protect against the development of PTSD by decreasing avoidance of emotional discomfort and facilitating desensitization.

Early trauma, such as childhood neglect or abuse, is more likely to lead to self-criticism and shame because those people did not receive sufficient warmth, soothing, and affection in childhood (Gilbert & Proctor, 2006). Paul Gilbert, the leading force behind compassion-focused therapy (CFT; Gilbert, 2009b, 2010), notes that survivors of childhood maltreatment can readily identify their maladaptive thought patterns ("I'm unlovable") and provide alternative self-statements ("*Some* people love me") but that they do not necessarily find cognitive restructuring emotionally reassuring. Therefore, the goal of CFT is to "warm up the conversation" (Gilbert, personal communication, 2011). In a pilot study of compassionate mind training (CMT; a structured program based on compassion-focused therapy; Gilbert & Irons, 2005), hospital day treatment clients struggling with shame and self-criticism showed significant decreases in depression, self-attacking, shame, and feelings of inferiority (Gilbert & Procter, 2006).

Self-compassion seems to be a mechanism of action in different forms of therapy (Baer, 2010). For example, following short-term psychodynamic treatment, decreases in anxiety, shame, and guilt and increases in the willingness to experience sadness, anger, and closeness were associated with higher self-compassion (Schanche, Stiles, McCollough, Swartberg, & Nielsen, 2011). In the same study, increases in self-compassion predicted fewer psychiatric symptoms and interpersonal problems. Because self-compassion is predicated upon connecting with difficult emotions without self-judgment, it appears to lead to healthier psychological functioning.

Mindfulness and Self-Compassion

In Buddhist psychology, compassion is one of the four *Brahmaviharas*, or wholesome attitudes, that contribute to psychological well-being. The other three are loving-kindness, empathic joy, and equanimity. Whereas loving-kindness is "the wish that all sentient beings be *happy*," "compassion is the wish that all sentient beings be *free from suffering*" (Dalai Lama, 2003, p. 67). Compassion emerges when love meets suffering (and the loving attitude remains!). Suffering is a prerequisite for compassion.

Ironically, when we suffer, we may be the last to know it. Usually we shoot up into our heads and ruminate about the problem ("Why did this happen to me?" "What does this say about me?" "What should I do about it?"), losing touch with the simple experience of emotional pain ("ouch!"). That is where mindfulness comes in—the moment-to-moment opening to emotional pain that can trigger a compassionate response. In this way, mindful awareness is the foundation of compassion.

Mindfulness is "awareness of present experience with acceptance" (Germer, 2005), and self-compassion may be considered the *heart of mindfulness*—the emotional attitude of mindfulness—especially in the context of psychotherapy, in which suffering is the focus of our attention. Self-compassion is a particular kind of acceptance: It is *self*-acceptance in the face of sorrow and pain. Mindfulness typically focuses on acceptance of moment-to-moment *experience,* whereas self-compassion focuses on acceptance of the *experiencer.* Mindfulness says, "Feel your pain with spacious awareness." Self-compassion adds, *"Be kind to yourself* in the midst of the pain." When a traumatized individual is drowning in negative emotions such as dread, confusion, or hopelessness, he or she cannot stay open to emotional pain long enough to investigate and transform it. That is when a trauma therapist needs to help the client to feel safer and more comfortable in the body, perhaps through yoga (Emerson & Hopper, 2011), focused awareness exercises (e.g., sensing one's feet on the floor, feeling the breath; R. D. Siegel, 2010), or self-soothing techniques such as petting the dog, loving-kindness meditation, or compassionate self-talk.

Self-compassion may be considered the heart of mindfulness from a research perspective, as well. For example, the multicomponent definition of self-compassion (which includes mindfulness but also kindness and a sense of common humanity) reflected in the SCS accounts for 10 times more variance than the Mindful Attention Awareness Scale (MAAS; Brown & Ryan, 2003) when predicting depression, anxiety, and overall quality of life (Van Dam, Sheppard, Forsyth, & Earlywine, 2011). Additionally, although mindfulness-based cognitive therapy (MBCT; Segal, Williams, & Teasdale, 2002) reduces depression through enhancement of mindfulness and self-compassion, self-compassion was the only factor associated with the decoupling of depressive thinking and positive outcome (Kuyken et al., 2010).

A common healing element found in both mindfulness and self-compassion is the gradual shift from resistance to friendship with emotional pain. Mindfulness primarily invites the question "What are you *experiencing?*" and self-compassion asks, "What do you *need?*" It is often difficult for survivors of severe trauma to know what they need or to be kind to themselves, so the therapist can keep those questions in mind until the client can do it for him- or herself.

Mindfulness is a way of inclining toward the sharp points in our lives, slowly and safely, and gradually desensitizing them. Self-compassion adds an explicit element of comfort and warmth to the process of desensitizing. Together, mindfulness and self-compassion allow us to engage difficult thoughts, feelings, and sensations with open eyes and an open heart. When mindfulness is in full bloom, it is naturally full of self-compassion whenever we're suffering.

What Self-Compassion Isn't

There are some common misconceptions about self-compassion that are worth addressing, as they can interfere in the treatment of traumatized individuals. As a platform for healing, traumatized individuals need to reestablish a sense of safety and control over their lives. A common misconception about self-compassion is that it's something weak, similar to submissiveness, complacency, resignation, or passivity. But compassion can actually be an incredibly powerful agent of change (just think of Martin Luther King, Jr., or Mahatma Gandhi). Self-compassion is a force of will, too—goodwill. It's about providing care and support and demanding fair treatment, not feeling inferior or subordinating ourselves to others (McEwan, Gilbert, & Duarte, 2012). When we're self-compassionate, we validate our own suffering and are more likely to respond in a decisive manner. If a victim of domestic violence can assert "This hurts, this *really* hurts! And it's not okay!" and is committed to caring for her- or himself, that person is less likely to make excuses for the perpetrator ("He had a difficult childhood"), engage in denial ("It's not so bad. It will get better"), and place her- or himself in jeopardy again and again.

Many people believe that self-compassion is selfish. Paradoxically, self-compassion is needed to sustain compassion for others:

> For someone to develop genuine compassion towards others, first he or she must have a basis upon which to cultivate compassion, and that basis is the ability to connect to one's own feelings and to care for one's own welfare. . . . Caring for others requires caring for oneself.

To use an airplane analogy, when cabin air pressure drops, we need to put the oxygen mask on ourselves first. This isn't easy for some victims of trauma.

Childhood trauma survivors may also equate self-compassion with self-pity or self-centeredness. They may have been told as children to "get over yourself" when they suffered and complained. It is important to understand that by entering into our emotional pain with kindness, we are *less* likely to wallow in self-pity. The reason is that self-compassion recognizes the shared nature of human suffering and avoids egocentrism. Sometimes only a few minutes is all that is needed to validate our pain and disentangle ourselves from it.

Even individuals with a minimum of trauma in their lives assume that self-criticism has certain benefits (Gilbert, McEwan, Matos, & Rivis, 2011). Without self-criticism, the argument goes, we will never correct our mistakes and improve. But there is an alternative to self-criticism—*self-encouragement*. Like a good coach, we can say to ourselves, "That didn't work, but it was a good try. At least you learned something. Would you like to try a different approach?" rather than "You fool! What's the matter with you!" Self-criticism is closely associated with feelings of shame, anxiety, and depression (Gilbert & Proctor, 2006), as well as underachievement and self-handicapping strategies such as procrastination (Powers, Koestner, & Zuroff, 2007).

Self-compassion is often confused with narcissistic self-love, although research indicates that there is no link between narcissism and self-compassion (Neff, 2003; Neff & Vonk, 2009). Narcissism is a reactive attempt to bolster our self-image when we fail ("I'm smart—it was just a stupid test!"), whereas self-compassion implies openness to failure, the ability to comfort ourselves, to assess the situation, and to work to improve it (Neff, Hseih, & Dejitthirat, 2005; Neff & McGeehee, 2010). Self-compassion is a healthy inner response to misfortune that makes us feel better, yet it is relatively independent of social evaluation—praise and blame, success and failure (Neff & Vonk, 2009). This is particularly important for trauma survivors who suffer from shame and wish to rebuild their shattered sense of self on a solid foundation.

Victims of childhood trauma often do not have *enough* narcissism, feeling that meeting their own basic survival needs is a forbidden indulgence. Anxiety may arise from the looming possibility of breaking an invisible bond with a primary caregiver who thought the child should suffer for his or her misdeeds or bad nature. Self-deprivation becomes "safety behavior" (Gilbert & Proctor, 2006). It is a necessary compromise made by an abused child in order to survive, so the client becomes frightened, viscerally and unconsciously, when he or she breaks the contract. For this reason, sincere efforts by therapists to help abused or neglected clients may be met with resistance. These clients first need to contact their emotional pain, see how it originated through no fault of their own ("you're not to blame!"), and then gradually bring the same tenderness to themselves that they are likely to give to other, vulnerable beings.

For example, Beth's mother was physically abusive during her childhood and often punished her by withholding food. As an adult, Beth took excellent care of her daughter, despite living on a limited budget, but she deprived herself of food until her hair fell out. She felt that nourishing herself was unnecessary. Beth had internalized the messages of powerful, threatening caregivers ("You get what you deserve, and you don't deserve anything!") to remain connected and survive. In therapy, Beth was determined to reverse her pattern of self-deprivation. Toward that end, Beth started saying loving-kindness phrases for her daughter ("May *you* be safe," "May *you* be healthy"), which flowed easily for her. Then she tucked herself into the circle of compassion, understanding that her daughter could not be well if she weren't ("May *you and I* be safe," "May *you and I* be healthy"), and finally Beth could put her hand over her heart and say to herself ("May *I* be safe," "May *I* be healthy").

Self-Compassion in Trauma Treatment

Self-compassion is a challenge and an opportunity for trauma survivors. It gets to the heart of how we instinctively treat ourselves after catastrophic events, yet it also has the potential to tip the fragile emotional balance between turning toward and turning away from traumatic memories. Self-compassion is a double-edged sword—it cuts through the pain of the present as it opens the pain of the past. Therefore, self-compassion in the broadest clinical sense refers to taking very good care of oneself in both the short run and the long run. In the short run, we want to build the client's capacity to tolerate and transform traumatic memories, and in the long run we want to encourage safe exposure and nonavoidance of the same memories.

"What Do I Need Now?"

The main question of self-compassion training is "What do I need now?" For some clients, simply asking this question can trigger traumatic memories.

I (C. K. G.) had a client, Sarah, who was so severely traumatized as a child that auditory hallucinations ("You are garbage!") arose whenever she asked herself "What do I need?" Earlier on, Sarah reported that stroking her cat made her feel calmer, but when she *noticed* that she felt calmer, she stopped what she was doing. Care and comfort gave way to visceral fear. Intellectually, Sarah knew that she *should* be able to pet her cat, but as a child she had been beaten for so many years by her angry, depressed mother whenever she smiled or felt happy that Sarah became afraid to feel good. During a year of therapy, Sarah courageously increased the length of time that she stroked her cat, starting with a few seconds, allowing herself to experience the comforting sensation of her cat's soft fur while a storm of threats and recriminations raged on in her mind. Gradually Sarah discovered that she could feel good without consequence. She let the voices in her mind storm on without reacting to them, and she could ask herself what else she needed.

Self-compassion can come in an infinite variety of ways, such as drinking a cup of tea, taking a hot bath, talking with friends, exercising, or listening to music. Such behavioral self-care is often safer than mind-training practices such as meditation. Taking antianxiety medication can also be what a person really needs, although in the long run it can be a form of experiential avoidance. If a trauma client is able to meditate, that will probably increase the likelihood that he or she will meet the challenges of daily life in a self-compassionate way. Self-compassion meditation (see Germer, 2009, and Neff, 2011) cultivates the intention or attitude of goodwill. The ultimate goal is to be in the presence of personal suffering with a sense of safety, so that the pain is felt and the process of healing can begin.

Progress in self-compassion training can be measured by the refinement of intention. We all start out by striving to feel better through self-compassion, then we become disillusioned when we still feel bad at times, and finally we learn to embrace ourselves "not to feel better, but *because* we feel bad." It's a riddle, a koan. When self-compassion training is used to manipulate our moment-to-moment experience, it will inevitably fail, because this is a subtle form of resistance that tends to amplify our symptoms. Try to fight sleeplessness, and we develop insomnia. Struggle with grief, and we become depressed. But when we're kind to ourselves simply *because* we feel bad, as we might be toward a child with the flu, then profound relief can occur as an inevitable side effect. As meditation teacher Rob Nairn put it, our goal is not to become perfect; it is to "become a compassionate mess" (Nairn, 2009)—fully human, struggling and uncertain, with great compassion.

Self-Compassion in the Therapy Relationship

Most emotional suffering is created in relationship and is alleviated in relationship. The healing power of empathic attunement with another person who has a soothing presence cannot be overstated (D. Siegel, 2007, 2010). In therapy, a client's hardwired capacity to subjectively experience the feelings and intentions of a therapist in the client's own body can downregulate a hyperaroused, traumatized brain (Cozolino, 2010; Iacoboni et al., 2005).

Compassion is a resource that allows clients to tolerate and transform suffering, but it's also a personal resource for therapists to help them bear vicarious suffering. Some trauma therapists worry that they might have too much compassion, leading to compassion fatigue. In that case, we're talking about "empathy fatigue" rather than "compassion fatigue" (Klimecki & Singer, 2011; Ricard, 2010). Empathy is an "accurate understanding of the [client's] world as seen from the inside" (Rogers, 1961, p. 284), whereas compassion has the added element of warmth and goodwill. Compassion is a positive emotion, and it is usually energizing. The ability to feel inner warmth for our clients and for ourselves, even as we listen to horrific reports of abuse and trauma can be a powerful buffer against compassion fatigue.

Of course, every human being has limits, and a compassionate stance means knowing our own limits and the limits of our clients. When do we orient together *toward* suffering and when do we *turn away*, sharing a light reflection, respectfully noting the feelings in the room, reminding the client that he or she is not to blame, anchoring a disturbing feeling in body sensation, musing about the universality of suffering, or simply changing the subject? Psychotherapy is a bait and switch—the client usually comes to therapy with the desire to be free of suffering, yet the healing process occurs by moving together into difficult thoughts, feelings, and sensations in a supportive, responsive, compassionate, transformative relationship.

Over time, compassion seems to rub off on the client in the form of a new relationship to traumatic experience and to him or herself. How does this happen? One explanation is that our clients bring us their emotional suffering and sense of personal brokenness, we "receive" it all with open eyes (mindful awareness) and open hearts (compassion), we "hold" the client and his or her struggle in compassionate awareness throughout the course of therapy, and gradually "lend" back a more benign attitude which can be carried into daily life.

Backdraft

Most clinicians have witnessed how difficult memories resurface when a client feels truly seen, heard, and loved in therapy. A metaphor for this process is "backdraft." Backdraft occurs when a firefighter opens a door with a hot fire behind it. Oxygen rushes in, causing a burst of flame. Similarly, when the door of the heart is opened with compassion, intense pain can sometimes be released. Unconditional love reveals the conditions under which we were unloved in the past (see earlier example of Sarah). Therefore, some clients, especially those with a history of childhood abuse or neglect, are fearful of compassion (Gilbert et al., 2011).

Backdraft is an intrinsic part of healing, but what if a client leaves the therapy office and does not have the capacity to contain the feelings that arose? Without the skill of self-compassion, a client may find it necessary to fight off disturbing emotions by self-medicating or other forms of self-harm. A compassion-based therapist needs to have the ability to stop a client from opening too much in session, especially during trauma treatment (Herman, 1997; Rothschild, 2010). Our clients only need to "contact" underlying emotional pain, not necessarily dive into it, and then apply the emotional resource of comforting and soothing themselves. Soothing and comfort are prerequisites for safe exposure and desensitization.

Self-Compassion Interventions

It's often helpful to teach traumatized clients specific skills for soothing and comforting themselves when they need it the most. Consider the following example of mild to moderate trauma:

Rachel was an introspective, middle-aged woman who discovered to her horror that her husband had been conducting a 2-year affair with a mutual friend at the summer home owned by her family for generations. Overnight her lifelong place of refuge became a trigger for traumatic images of her husband having sex in their bed, enjoying leisurely walks with his lover, and sharing dinner at sunset on their porch. Two years later, Rachel presented in therapy with nightmares and with intrusive thoughts occurring 10–100 times each day; she had not visited the summer home since receiving this shocking news. Visibly shaking in my office after telling her story, Rachel wondered aloud if she would ever recover the safe world she had lost. Rachel was otherwise okay: She had been in individual and couples therapy, she was taking antianxiety medication, her husband was deeply regretful about the affair, they were making love again, and her family relationships were otherwise solid.

After listening to Rachel's story, and not wanting to send her home without support, I (C. K. G.) asked Rachel if she'd like to learn a way to comfort and soothe herself when disturbing images arose in her mind. She agreed, so we practiced the following exercise, the *self-compassion break* (Neff & Germer, 2013; Neff, 2011). I asked Rachel to take a deep breath and slowly say to herself, "*This is a moment of suffering*" followed by "*Suffering is a part of life.*" Rachel was also invited to reflect for a moment on the fact that many people around the globe were also suffering from the trauma of marital betrayal, just like she was.

Then I asked Rachel to put both hands over her heart and (1) feel the warmth of her hands, (2) notice the gentle touch of her hands over her heart, and (3) feel the rhythmic rising and falling of her chest as she breathed. After a minute, I invited Rachel to repeat the following two phrases to herself, or similar ones that might fit better with her: "*May I be kind to myself*"; "*May I live with ease.*" She was told to simply place the words *on* her heart, not expecting them to go right in. Practicing in this way over the following months, Rachel discovered that her intrusive thoughts, nightmares, and anxiety gradually diminished.

The three components of the self-compassion break correspond to the three elements of self-compassion mentioned earlier: (1) mindfulness ("*This is a moment of suffering*"), (2) common humanity ("*Suffering is a part of life"*), and (3) self-kindness (*"May I be kind to myself"*). Each element allowed Rachel to let go of her ruminations and soften into her distress, gradually desensitizing it.

Of course, no single practice works for everyone. For example, a client with severe childhood trauma, Elissa, discovered that she felt more and more hatred toward her abusive father as she slowly moved her hands toward her heart. The "backdraft" was too intense for her. Elissa modified the exercise to simply noticing her breathing in the chest region, then placing her hand on her chest to feel her breathing, and finally offering goodwill to herself because of the pain she carried in her heart. Some people find they are better able to soothe themselves by cupping their faces in their hands, or by placing a hand on the abdomen. In self-compassion training, we try to stay on the side of comfort and soothing—building resources— until the client feels safe and strong enough to open to his or her trauma.

Some therapists feel uneasy about teaching self-compassion exercises to clients during therapy. For example, some trauma clients just want a witness to hear their story and may not be ready to practice self-compassion at home. Other clients feel ashamed that they have difficulty evoking self-compassion and may withdraw from therapy. It is important that therapists working within the mindfulness- and compassion-based paradigm have personal experience of the transformational process before teaching it, especially to navigate the paradox of suffering in order to alleviate it (see Briere, Chapter 1, this volume) and knowing how to modify the practices for clients, as needed. Personal practice is especially critical when working with trauma clients for whom the stakes of opening to emotional pain are higher than usual.

Self-Compassion Training Programs

Some trauma clients may be candidates for structured programs that directly or indirectly teach self-compassion, such as mindfulness training (Briere, 2012). Research has demonstrated that the mindfulness-based stress reduction program (MBSR; Kabat-Zinn, 1991) significantly increases self-compassion (Shapiro, Astin, Bishop, & Cordova, 2005; Shapiro, Brown, & Biegel, 2007; see also Kearney, Chapter 17, this volume), as does the mindfulness-based cognitive therapy program for treating recurrent depression (MBCT; Kuyken et al., 2010; see also Semple & Madni, Chapter 18, this volume). People who practice mindfulness meditation are more self-compassionate than those who are less experienced (Lykins & Baer, 2009; Neff, 2003; Orzech, Shapiro, Brown, & McKay, 2009), and self-compassion appears to be a "crucial attitudinal factor" in the relationship between mindfulness training and positive mental health (Hollis-Walker & Colosimo, 2011).

There are a number of training programs that are specifically designed to cultivate compassion: the compassion-cultivation training program (Rosenberg, 2011), cognitive-based compassion training (see Williams & Barnhofer, Chapter 6, this volume), and nonviolent communication (NVC; Rosenberg, 2003). Programs that focus on cultivating *self*-compassion are mindful self-compassion training (MSC; Germer & Neff, 2013; Neff & Germer, 2013; see also *www.CenterForMSC.org*) and compassionate mind training (CMT; Gilbert & Proctor, 2006; see also *www.Compassionate-Mind.co.uk*). The latter two programs have different origins—MSC developed out of mindfulness, and CMT arose primarily out of evolutionary psychology—but there is some overlap among the exercises and meditation practices of the two programs.

The MSC program has structural elements similar to Kabat-Zinn's MBSR course (eight sessions plus a retreat day; formal and informal meditation). In a randomized controlled study of the MSC program, results indicated that participation in the course significantly increased self-compassion, mindfulness, compassion for others, and life satisfaction while significantly decreasing depression, anxiety, stress, and emotional avoidance. The degree to which participants' self-compassion level increased was significantly linked to how much informal and formal self-compassion practice they did over the course of the program (Neff & Germer, 2013).

Finally, while reading through the subsequent chapters in this book, you may discover elements of self-compassion, explicit or implicit, in each approach. For example, the dialectical behavior therapy (DBT) program was specifically designed to "radically accept" clients who have difficulty with emotion regulation and trauma histories (see Fiorillo & Fruzzetti, Chapter 5, this volume). Acceptance and commitment therapy (ACT), which encourages an accepting, compassionate response to our own pain, has been successfully applied to trauma treatment (see Engle & Follette, Chapter 4, this volume), and internal family systems (IFS) is an emerging treatment model based on compassion for the many different parts of ourselves which have suffered, sometimes intensely, in our lifetimes (see Schwartz & Sparks, Chapter 8, this volume). Each program offers an array of interventions that enhance self-compassion.

In conclusion, self-compassion provides a promising vision for trauma treatment derived from the ancient wisdom of Buddhist psychology. Self-compassion is strongly linked to emotional well-being, is an important mechanism of change in psychotherapy, and touches the core of trauma-related symptomatology. Our modern, scientific understanding of self-compassion opens the possibility of developing uniquely effective self-compassion-based treatments designed specifically for survivors of childhood and adult trauma.

References

Baer, R. (2010). Self-compassion as a mechanism of change in mindfulness and acceptance-based treatments In R. Baer (Ed.), *Assessing mindfulness and acceptance processes in clients: Illuminating the theory and practice of change* (pp. 135–153). Oakland, CA: Context Press/New Harbinger.

Briere, J. (2012). Working with trauma: Mindfulness and compassion. In C. K. Germer & R. D. Siegel (Eds.), *Wisdom and compassion in psychotherapy: Deepening mindfulness in clinical practice* (pp. 265–279). New York: Guilford Press.

Brown, K. W., & Ryan, R. M. (2003). The benefits of being present: Mindfulness and its role in psychological well-being. *Journal of Personality and Social Psychology, 84,* 822–848.

Cozolino, L. (2010). *The neuroscience of psychotherapy: Healing the social brain.* New York: Norton.

Dalai Lama. (1995). *The power of compassion.* New Delhi, India: HarperCollins.

Dalai Lama. (2003). *Lighting the path: The Dalai Lama teaches on wisdom and compassion.* South Melbourne, Australia: Thomas C. Lothian.

Dalai Lama. (2012). *Training the mind: Verse 7.* Retrieved March 3, 2012, from *www.dalailama.com/teachings/training-the-mind/verse-7.*

Emerson, D., & Hopper, E. (2011). *Overcoming trauma through yoga: Reclaiming your body.* Berkeley, CA: North Atlantic Books.

Germer, C. K. (2005). Mindfulness: What is it? What does it matter? In C. K. Germer, R. D. Siegel, & P. F. Fulton (Eds.), *Mindfulness and psychotherapy* (pp. 3–27). New York: Guilford Press.

Germer, C. K. (2009). *The mindful path to self-compassion.* New York: Guilford Press.

Germer, C. K., & Neff, K. D. (2013). Self-compassion in clinical practice. *Journal of Clinical Psychology, 69*(8), 856–867.

Gilbert, P. (2009a). Introducing compassion-focused therapy. *Advances in Psychiatric Treatment, 15,* 199–208.

Gilbert, P. (2009b). *The compassionate mind: A new approach to life's challenges.* Oakland, CA: New Harbinger Press.

Gilbert, P. (2010). *Compassion focused therapy.* London: Routledge.

Gilbert, P., & Irons, C. (2005). Focused therapies and compassionate mind training for shame and self-attacking. In P. Gilbert (Ed.), *Compassion: Conceptualisations, research and use in psychotherapy* (pp. 263–325). London: Routledge.

Gilbert, P., McEwan, K., Matos, M., & Rivis, A. (2011) Fears of compassion: Development of three self-report measures. *Psychology and Psychotherapy: Theory, Research, and Practice, 84,* 239–255.

Gilbert, P., & Proctor, S. (2006). Compassionate mind training for people with high shame and self-criticism: Overview and pilot study of a group therapy approach. *Clinical Psychology and Psychotherapy, 13,* 353–379.

Herman, J. (1997). *Trauma and recovery: The aftermath of violence—from domestic abuse to political terror.* New York: Basic Books.

Hollis-Walker, L., & Colosimo, K. (2011). Mindfulness, self-compassion, and happiness in non-meditators: A theoretical and empirical examination. *Personality and Individual Differences, 50*(2), 222–227.

Iacoboni, M., Molnar-Szakacs, I., Gallese, V., Buccino, G., Mazziotta, J., & Rizzolatti, G. (2005). Grasping the intentions of others with one's own mirror neuron system. *PloS Biology, 3*(3), e79.

Kabat-Zinn, J. (1991). *Full catastrophe living: Using the wisdom of your body and mind to face stress, pain, and illness.* New York: Dell.

Klimecki, O., & Singer, T. (2011). Empathic distress fatigue rather than compassion fatigue?: Integrating findings from empathy research in psychology and social neuroscience. In B. Oakley, A. Knafo, G. Madhavan, & D. S. Wilson (Eds.), *Pathological altruism* (pp. 368–384). New York: Oxford University Press.

Kornfield, J. (2011). Set the compass of your heart. *Tricycle.* Retrieved March 14, 2012, from *www.tricycle.com/brief-teachings/set-compass-your-heart.*

Kuyken, W., Watkins, E., Holden, E., White, K., Taylor, R., et al. (2010). How does mindfulness-based cognitive therapy work? *Behaviour Research and Therapy, 48,* 1105–1112.

Lykins, E., & Baer, R. (2009). Psychological functioning in a sample of long-term practitioners of mindfulness meditation. *Journal of Cognitive Psychotherapy: An International Quarterly, 23,* 226–241.

McEwan, K., Gilbert, P., & Duarte, J. (2012.). An exploration of competitiveness and caring in relation to psychopathology. *British Journal of Clinical Psychology, 51*(1), 19–36.

Nairn, R. (2009, September). *Foundation training in compassion, Kagyu.* Lecture presented as part of Foundation Training in Compassion, Kagyu Samye Ling Monastery, Dumfriesshire, Scotland.

Neff, K. (2003). Development and validation of a scale to measure self-compassion. *Self and Identity, 2,* 223–250.

Neff, K. (2011). *Self-compassion: Stop beating yourself up and leave insecurity behind.* New York: Morrow.

Neff, K. D., & Germer, C. K. (2013). A pilot study and randomized controlled trial of the mindful self-compassion program. *Journal of Clinical Psychology, 69*(1), 28–44.

Neff, K. D., Hseih, Y., & Dejitthirat, K. (2005). Self-compassion, achievement goals, and coping with academic failure. *Self and Identity, 4,* 263–287.

Neff, K. D., & McGeehee, P. (2010). Self-compassion and psychological resilience among adolescents and young adults. *Self and Identity, 9,* 225–240.

Neff, K. D., & Vonk, R. (2009). Self-compassion versus global self-esteem: Two different ways of relating to oneself. *Journal of Personality, 77,* 23–50.

Olendzki, A. (Trans.). (2008). *Metta Sutta, Sutta Nipata 145–151.* Barre, MA: Barre Center for Buddhist Studies.

Orzech, K., Shapiro, S., Brown, K., & McKay, M. (2009). Intensive mindfulness training-related changes in cognitive and emotional experience. *Journal of Positive Psychology, 4,* 212–222.

Powers, T. A., Koestner, R., & Zuroff, D. C. (2007). Self-criticism, goal motivation, and goal progress. *Journal of Social and Clinical Psychology, 26,* 826–840.

Ricard, M. (2010). *The difference between empathy and compassion.* Retrieved October 15, 2010, from *www.huffingtonpost.com/matthieu-ricard/could-compassion-meditati_b_751566.html.*

Rogers, C. (1961). *On becoming a person.* New York: Houghton Mifflin.

Rosenberg, E. (2011, July 21). *Compassion Cultivation Training Program (CCT)*. Paper presented at the conference on "How to Train Compassion," Max-Planck Institute for Human and Cognitive Brain Sciences, Berlin, Germany.

Rosenberg, M. (2003). *Nonviolent communication: A language of life*. Encinitas, CA: Puddle Dancer Press.

Rothschild, B. (2010). *8 keys to safe trauma recovery: Take-charge strategies to empower your life*. New York: Norton.

Schanche, E., Stiles, T., McCollough, L., Swartberg, M., & Nielsen, G. (2011). The relationship between activating affects, inhibitory affects, and self-compassion in patients with cluster C personality disorders. *Psychotherapy: Theory, Research, Practice, Training, 48*(3), 293–303.

Segal, Z., Williams, J., & Teasdale, J. (2002). *Mindfulness-based cognitive therapy for depression: A new approach to preventing relapse*. New York: Guilford Press.

Shapiro, S. L., Astin, J. A., Bishop, S. R., & Cordova, M. (2005). Mindfulness-based stress reduction for health care professionals: Results from a randomized trial. *International Journal of Stress Management, 12*, 164–176.

Shapiro, S. L., Brown, K. W., & Biegel, G. M (2007). Teaching self-care to caregivers: Effects of mindfulness-based stress reduction on the mental health of therapists in training. *Training and Education in Professional Psychology, 1*(2), 105–115.

Siegel, D. (2010). *The mindful therapist: A clinician's guide to mindsight and neural integration*. New York: Norton.

Siegel, D. J. (2007). *The mindful brain: Reflection and attunement in the cultivation of well-being*. New York: Norton.

Siegel, R. D. (2010). *The mindfulness solution: Everyday practices for everyday problems*. New York: Guilford Press.

Tanaka, M., Wekerle, C., Schmuck, M., Paglia-Boak, A., & the MAP Research Team. (2011). The linkages among childhood maltreatment, adolescent mental health, and self-compassion in child welfare adolescents. *Child Abuse and Neglect, 35*, 887–898.

Thompson, B. L., & Waltz, J. (2008). Self-compassion and PTSD symptom severity. *Journal of Traumatic Stress, 21*, 556–558.

Van Dam, T., Sheppard, S., Forsyth, J., & Earleywine, M. (2011). Self-compassion is a better predictor than mindfulness of symptom severity and quality of life in mixed anxiety and depression. *Journal of Anxiety Disorders, 25*, 123–130.

Vettese, L., Dyer, C., Li, W., & Wekerle, C. (2011). Does self-compassion mitigate the association between childhood maltreatment and later regulation difficulties? A preliminary investigation. *International Journal of Mental Health and Addiction, 9*(5), 480–491.

Wei, M., Liao, K., Ku, T., & Shaffer, P. A. (2011). Attachment, self-compassion, empathy, and subjective well-being among college students and community adults. *Journal of Personality, 79*, 191–221.

Part II

ADAPTING CONTEMPLATIVE APPROACHES

4

Mindfulness and Valued Action

An Acceptance and Commitment Therapy Approach to Working with Trauma Survivors

Jessica L. Engle and Victoria M. Follette

Trauma survivors face a variety of challenges in the wake of a traumatic event, and in some cases these challenges are not recognized as trauma-related suffering. Much of the empirical work on treatments for trauma-related suffering has focused on the alleviation of the three main symptom clusters of posttraumatic stress disorder (PTSD): reexperiencing the event, avoidance of event-related cues, and hyperarousal. In addition to these symptoms, trauma sequelae constitute a range of problems, including depression, substance use, anxiety, suicide, and more general inter- and intrapersonal problems (Polusny & Follette, 1995).

Among available treatments for PTSD, exposure therapy has the largest base of empirical evidence supporting its effectiveness (Cahill, Rothbaum, Resick, & Follette, 2008; Cahill, Foa, Hembree, Marshall, & Nacash, 2006). However, there is evidence that relatively few practitioners use it to treat PTSD (Cahill et al., 2006). Some are concerned about exposure therapy's nearly exclusive focus on PTSD symptoms despite the importance of treating co-occurring problems (Orsillo & Batten, 2005). Others (e.g., Twohig, 2009) have noted that one-third of participants in randomized trials do not respond to exposure treatments (Bradley, Greene, Russ, Dutra, & Westen, 2005). Significant rates of treatment refusal and attrition from exposure therapies also present challenges in research and clinical work

(Schottenbauer, Glass, Arnkoff, Tendick, & Gray, 2008). Although there are other factors that may contribute to problems of low utilization, non-response to treatment, and attrition, many of them are subjects of debate (Mulick, Landes, & Kanter, 2011 2005), and a full discussion of these topics is beyond the scope of this chapter. However, these complications suggest that there is a need for research on treatments that target PTSD and other trauma sequelae that go beyond manualized exposure (Mulick, Landes, & Kanter, 2011; Orsillo & Batten, 2005). To this end, mindfulness-based therapies have been considered as potential alternatives and adjuncts to traditional exposure treatments (Thompson, Arnkoff, & Glass, 2011; Follette, Palm, & Pearson, 2006).

Within the past two decades, mindfulness has been increasingly incorporated into treatments for PTSD and other psychological problems (Follette et al., 2006; Baer, 2003; Mace, 2007). In the treatment of PTSD, mindfulness facilitates healing by promoting acceptance of experiences (Follette et al., 2006), a process that is antithetical to avoidance; avoidance is believed to maintain posttraumatic suffering (Orsillo & Batten, 2005). According to a behavioral model, avoidance-related suffering in the wake of trauma develops in a 2-step process. First, experiences and events that are associated with traumatic incidents acquire distressing properties through the process of classical conditioning (Mowrer, 1960). These associated experiences and events—referred to as conditioned stimuli—are not typically harmful, and yet their presence may elicit an intense emotional response. As the trauma survivor avoids these aversive conditioned stimuli, trauma-related symptoms are then maintained and/or exacerbated.

One behavioral therapy that directly targets avoidance and includes a strong emphasis on awareness/mindfulness is acceptance and commitment therapy (ACT; Hayes, Strosahl, & Wilson, 2012). ACT provides structured guidance to develop mindful awareness and acceptance of both past and present experiences. The central goal in ACT is increasing *psychological flexibility*: the ability to be aware, in the present moment, as a conscious being who has a history, of what is present both internally (e.g., thoughts, feelings, values) and externally (e.g., the objective situation) and to effectively change or persist in behavior in service of one's chosen values (Hayes et al., 2012). ACT targets *experiential avoidance,* which is conceptualized as any attempt to avoid or change the form or frequency of internal experiences (e.g., thoughts, memories, emotions, sensations; Hayes et al., 2012). From the perspective of ACT and other contemporary behavioral theories, experiential avoidance is at the root of suffering in PTSD and many other psychological disorders (Hayes, Wilson, Gifford, Follette, & Strosahl, 1996; Orsillo & Batten, 2005).

Currently, outcome data on ACT for PTSD are limited to the findings of single case studies (e.g., Twohig, 2009; Batten & Hayes, 2005). However, ACT has been shown to be effective in alleviating many psychological problems, including depression, obsessive– compulsive disorder, psychosis, panic disorder, social phobia, generalized anxiety disorder, chronic pain, polysubstance abuse, and much more (as reviewed in Smout, Hayes, Atkins, Clausen, & Duguid, 2012; Hayes, Luoma, Bond, Masuda, & Lillis, 2006). Furthermore, studies have indicated that experiential avoidance is negatively associated with posttraumatic growth (Kashdan & Kane, 2008) and quality of life in trauma survivors (Kashdan, Morina, & Priebe, 2008). Given these data, more research on the effectiveness of ACT for PTSD is warranted, particularly to examine its effectiveness in individuals with coexisting problems and individuals who did not respond to exposure therapy.

Targeting Experiential Avoidance with ACT for Trauma Survivors

The continual struggle to change or banish unwanted internal experiences is evident in statements we often hear from our clients: They have been trying to "put the past behind" them or "just forget about what happened," and it has not worked. Trauma survivors have intense, emotionally evocative memories and may spend a considerable amount of time avoiding them. Avoidance of unwanted trauma-related memories and emotions may involve several strategies, one of which is the avoidance of any environmental stimulus that has become a conditioned stimulus for trauma-related memories and emotions. For example, survivors of rape often report being reminded of a perpetrator when exposed to certain stimuli such as smells (e.g., cologne), physical appearances, visual characteristics of locations (e.g., a dark room), or hearing the footsteps of a person walking behind them. Avoidance of the various locations, activities, or situations that trigger aversive memories may help alleviate the unwanted distress that may arise in the presence of these stimuli.

Although attempts to avoid emotions and memories may work in the short term, avoidance strategies often backfire in several different ways. For instance, one successful, albeit temporary, way to avoid emotions is to use mind-altering substances, many of which, over time, may cause health problems and interfere with relationships, careers, and general well-being. Studies have shown that one avoidance strategy in particular, suppression, may not be successful in the long term and often has the effect of increasing the saliency of the avoided content (Wegner, Schneider, Carter, & White, 1987; Salkovskis & Campbell, 1994). Furthermore, when trauma survivors avoid physical reminders of trauma by restricting their activities, they may lose opportunities to engage in meaningful and beneficial life experiences. Attempts to avoid trauma-related experiences often perpetuate suffering and lead individuals to spend the majority of their time fighting an internal battle against their emotions to no avail. In ACT, we work with clients to help them let go of the struggle with internal experience and choose instead to live a valued life *with* their histories, emotions, and memories as they are.

Mindfulness engenders awareness of the ways in which one's history, internal experiences, and the external environment are relevant in the current moment, creating the opportunity to respond more flexibly and effectively in the present situation. Right now is the *only* moment in which actions can be taken. However, humans spend a great deal of time thinking about the past and the future, and trauma survivors may be particularly susceptible to being stuck in thoughts about the past. Being mindful allows one to notice that one is situated *here and now* as opposed to *there and then*. This is especially important in work with trauma survivors, who often feel as though their existence is defined by past experiences and who frequently feel "retraumatized" by memories of the trauma. They might even feel as though their history has taken over their lives and that controlling thoughts and feelings is the only way to survive. ACT addresses this problem by refocusing the way in which control is understood; we can't always control what we *feel*, but we do have power over what we *do in the present moment*. The solution to regaining a life worth living paradoxically calls for relinquishing the effort to control our inner experiences. Mindfulness in ACT is about being present to all that *is* and choosing to move forward with one's history and experiences in a valued direction.

ACT Processes

Mindfulness is one of the six core processes of ACT and overlaps significantly with each of the other core processes: acceptance, defusion, self as context, values, and commitment (see Figure 4.1 for an illustration of these processes). Within ACT, mindfulness practices are employed in service of each of the processes, which together work to help clients identify ways to live a more valued life.

Many have commented on the similarities between ACT processes and Buddhist principles (Hayes, 2002). Although ACT did not originate from Buddhist philosophies or practice, it shares commonalities with ancient Buddhist traditions (Hayes, 2002). The originator of ACT, Steven Hayes, has noted its relationship to the Four Noble Truths of Buddhism that involve orienting humans toward engagement in their life's values by cultivating awareness of suffering, relinquishing attachment, and doing good deeds (Hayes, 2002). It is important to note that cultivating awareness of suffering or letting go of attachment are not necessarily goals in and of themselves, but they can be understood as processes that bring individuals into contact with important values in life and allow them to act effectively in service of these values.

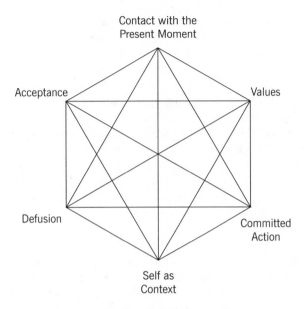

FIGURE 4.1. The ACT model. Copyright by Steven C. Hayes. Used by permission. *The figure may be copied and reused freely.*

Acceptance

Acceptance involves a willingness to be *with* uncomfortable memories, thoughts, sensations, and emotions without attempts to suppress or minimize them (Hayes et al., 2012). This process encourages openness to internal experiences, including experiences that are uncomfortable, without judging them or trying to change them. As discussed earlier, acceptance is an alternative strategy to experiential avoidance and involves receptiveness toward experiences. Many mindfulness practices facilitate attention to and awareness of experiences as they are, and thus experiential avoidance is incompatible with being truly mindful.

For trauma survivors with trauma-related distress, acceptance exposes them to a host of uncomfortable emotions that have been avoided for some time. It is believed that acceptance may facilitate habituation to emotions such as fear and anxiety and eventually extinguish avoidance responses over time (Hayes et al., 1996). By reducing avoidance, acceptance facilitates engagement in behaviors that may increase quality of life.

Defusion

Fusion is defined as the process by which thoughts are perceived as objective truths (Hayes et al., 2012). In other words, one can *fuse,* or overidentify, with a thought such that its mere existence is regarded as sufficient evidence for its veracity. Fusion may lead to strong emotional and behavioral reactions to cognitive processes. For instance, fusion with a thought, such as "I'm stupid," may be the sole basis upon which important decisions are made, as in "I can't go back to school or apply for a higher position in the company; I'm too stupid." In this way, fusion can restrict opportunities to explore new experiences by limiting one's behaviors.

An antithetical process to fusion, *defusion*, involves the development of a new relationship to one's thoughts, namely being able to acknowledge the content of thoughts without overidentifying with them. Thoughts such as "I'm worthless," if taken to be true, can have a profound effect on one's emotional state, as well as on how one chooses to engage in life. Defusion works to create psychological distance between the content of thoughts and behavioral reactions to them.

Defusion can be developed through practicing awareness of thoughts by observing them with less investment in their content. As encouraged in many traditional meditations, ACT promotes the practice of "just noticing" thoughts without attachment to them. Many ACT therapists also encourage their clients to acknowledge thoughts as "just thoughts" that one is having (Hayes et al., 2012), helping to further decrease reactivity to one's own thoughts. Clients may be reminded that thoughts are not necessarily true, no matter how convincing they are, and that being fused with them can get in the way of living the life the client wants.

Self as Context

In ACT, self as context is a perspective from which life's events can be observed without overly identifying with experiences (Hayes et al., 2006). Self as context is experienced as the quiet, conscious "observer" that has watched life's events, thoughts, and emotions flow through awareness over time, and this experience has been labeled as feeling transcendent to many individuals (Hayes et al., 2012). The opposite of self as context is called the *self as concept*, which is the self as understood through one's roles, behaviors, thoughts, emotions, and other experiences. Culturally, we are accustomed to defining ourselves according to our self-concepts, even though they are in constant flux over time, and this can result in an inherently unstable or rigid sense of the self.

Many individuals are attached to self-concepts that are not effective for them (Hayes et al., 2012). For example, someone who has been proudly defined as "independent" and "strong" may have difficulty reconciling his or her identity after a tragic accident leaves him or her handicapped and in need of others' help. Self as context broadens one's understanding of who he or she is by bringing awareness to the experience of consciousness; we sometimes refer to this part of one's experience as the "observer self." Mindfulness exercises that bring awareness to this "observer self" ask the meditator to remember events and related thoughts and feelings throughout life while simultaneously noticing the ongoing flow of quiet, observing awareness that was there all along. The meditator may then be asked to notice how experiences have flowed through awareness, constantly moving forward in time, and yet the "observer self" remained unchanged.

Values

In Buddhism, the eightfold path prescribes specific ways to conduct one's life that are thought to alleviate human suffering (Nhat Hanh, 1998). Similarly, ACT seeks to alleviate human suffering by encouraging individuals to conduct their lives in accordance with their chosen values (Hayes et al., 2012). In contrast to Buddhism, which identifies specific pathways, ACT is more person-centered in helping the client to identify *his or her own* values and values-consistent behaviors.

In ACT, values are freely chosen, dynamic, and ongoing (Wilson, Sandoz, Flynn, & Slater, 2010). In other words, values are constructed by the individual and are not motivated by "shoulds," or the avoidance of negative consequences. They may involve goals, but are distinguished from goals in that they are ongoing ways of living. Valuing lifelong learning, for example, may involve the goals of going to school and earning a degree, but learning remains to be valued after the degree is earned.

Clients often need support in identifying and clarifying values, and therapists can assist in this process in many ways. Various measures have been developed to facilitate clinical conversations about values (see Wilson, Sandoz, Flynn, Slater, & DuFrene, 2010). The Valued Living Questionnaire (VLQ; Wilson, Sandoz, Kitchens, & Roberts, 2010) is a paper-and-pencil questionnaire that can be useful in guiding clinical work on values. Other values assessments include the Personal Values Questionnaire (PVQ; Blackledge & Ciarrochi, 2006) and the Values Compass (Dahl, Wilson, Luciano, & Hayes, 2005).

It is often true that committing to values, let alone identifying them, can be a source of some psychological distress. It can be difficult to come into contact with the pain of not having lived in accordance with values. Furthermore, pain can arise as a result of choosing to live a valued life and coming into contact with the difficulties in making choices associated with those values. For example, a value of maintaining a loving relationship with a family member might necessitate tolerating some harmless but annoying behaviors of that family member without expressing ones frustration—easier said than done. For this reason, acceptance of thoughts and emotions is an integral part of living a valued life. Being present with what the mind, body, and world bring to bear and consciously choosing to act according to values calls for the ability to be mindfully aware and accepting of what one is feeling in the moment.

Committed Action

Committed action is a core process in ACT involving engagement in actions that are consistent with one's chosen values (Hayes et al., 2012). In ACT, commitment involves more than just motivation to engage in valued action; it *is* behavioral engagement in valued action. Commitment in ACT involves behavioral activation and is essential to the goal of ACT: living a valued life (Hayes et al., 2012).

Commitment to living a valued life may be facilitated through present-moment awareness. Present-moment awareness of values and goals, in addition to what arises internally and exists externally in the environment, enhances the ability to choose effective values-directed actions. In other words, being aware of goals and values *while* sustaining attention to the present moment may help one to best ascertain and engage in behaviors that are committed to values. Being able to approach the present environment with focus and flexibility may provide the best opportunity for change (Hayes et al., 2012), and this is precisely what ACT processes are intended to facilitate.

Assessment

Although a thorough discussion of clinical assessments for each process is beyond the scope of this chapter, it is important to notice that core concepts in ACT are intertwined and considered to be essential to successful outcomes. ACT utilizes a functional approach to analyzing behavior instead of a topographical approach (Hayes et al., 1996); in other words, it focuses on how a behavior functions, or works for the client, as opposed to focusing on the form of the behavior (i.e., what the behavior looks like). In determining the behaviors that are functionally related to the problem (e.g., determining that the behaviors of substance abuse, isolation, and self-harm all function as avoidance), ACT therapists can ascertain the extent to which each of the six processes should be targeted in treatment. Each process promotes experiential acceptance, which facilitates committed engagement in behaviors that are consistent with chosen values.

ACT in Practice

For therapists, practicing ACT with trauma survivors most effectively begins with basic didactic and experiential training in the ACT model.

Understanding ACT's core theory and processes is thought to engender a greater degree of therapy competence and can avoid various therapy pitfalls, such as failing to see the interconnectedness of the six processes, among others (Luoma, Hayes, & Walser, 2007).

The Therapist's Role

Among the many therapies that have been empirically examined, it has long been known that the therapeutic relationship is a strong predictor of therapy success (Hayes et al., 2012). Clients have noted that working with an effective ACT therapist often results in a deep sense of connection and validation. It is believed that this closeness develops, in part, because ACT therapists believe that psychological problems are the result of normal psychological processes, and the therapist does *not* consider the client to be abnormal or broken. Instead, both the client *and* the therapist are thought to be susceptible to the same pitfalls of learning and language processes. This theoretical stance engenders an understanding and compassionate stance toward the client. Also, many ACT therapists develop a desire to be aware of their own values, thoughts, and emotions as they are relevant in the present moment, both when working with the client and in other areas of their lives. A parallel aspiration to live a valued life by engaging in the ACT processes is typically evident in the therapist's interactions with the client, and this helps to build a shared sense of the struggle to live a life worth living.

The efficacy of ACT is believed to be enhanced when the therapist practices ACT in his or her own life (Hayes et al., 2012; Luoma et al., 2007). There are many reasons for this, the first of which is that it is difficult to cultivate a space for acceptance when the therapist is unwilling to accept what arises in the room (Hayes et al., 2012). Therapists we know who work with trauma survivors have admitted at times that they felt significant discomfort after encouraging clients to come into contact with immensely painful thoughts and emotions. Working with survivors of trauma is often painful work, and how therapists manage their own pain can be as important as how they manage the painful reactions of the client. The therapist's failure to be mindfully aware of reactions to suffering, to defuse from self-judgments, and to accept the emotion that arises in order to engage in values-oriented behavior (in this case, the values-oriented behavior is helping the client improve) could potentially hinder therapeutic progress for the client. For instance, a therapist who is fused with "I am hurting this client" may easily become stuck in emotions—likely sadness and guilt—and may choose to avoid approaching further emotional work with the client. In this way, a therapist's attempts to avoid his or her own emotions in therapy may reinforce the client's avoidance of emotions as well.

Another reason therapists are encouraged to maintain personal practices that are consistent with ACT is that, through modeling ACT-consistent behaviors, the therapist can facilitate learning for the client (Hayes et al., 2012). This is not to suggest that the therapist is expected to be perfect in living an ACT-consistent life, but rather that the therapist is able to share in the struggle of self-development with the client, growing in his or her own skills. Lastly, the authors suggest that incorporating ACT into our own lives honors the immense strength of our clients by helping us to bear witness to the authenticity and emotional courage our clients bring to the difficult work of therapy.

Targeting ACT Processes with Mindfulness

There are many mindfulness practices in ACT that can be useful for acceptance, present-moment awareness, and defusion work with trauma survivors. For example, one way for the therapist to facilitate mindfulness and acceptance for the client is to periodically prompt the client to describe his or her present-moment emotional experiences (Engle & Follette, 2012). In some cases, the client may be unable to label his or her current feelings. If this happens, the therapist may then ask the client to describe any bodily sensations or thoughts that are occurring. Next, the client is asked to "sit with" these experiences for a period of time. By asking the client to bring the experience of an emotion, thought, or sensation into his or her awareness and to focus on it, this exercise works against avoidance processes that, often with trauma survivors, can appear to happen almost automatically after an aversive emotion occurs (e.g., dissociating during discussion of the traumatic event). As the client becomes better able to experience aversive emotions without avoiding them, he or she may become increasingly aware of the situations, cognitions, and physical experiences that indicate the emotion may be present. This general awareness of one's pattern of experiences fosters flexible responding in the presence of the emotion. It also has the additional effect of creating a slight experiential distance between the emotion and the observer self. Although relief from the emotional state is not the primary goal of mindfulness, it is often a potential relief to be experienced.

Another mindfulness exercise that targets acceptance, present-moment awareness, and defusion involves sitting quietly and noticing the thoughts, emotions, and sensations that are being experienced in the present moment. This exercise can be instructed in a number of ways, although it is often helpful to incorporate some imaginary setting in which to envision the flow of experiences, especially for clients who are new to mindfulness meditation. For example, an exercise that is commonly used by ACT therapists and clients is called "leaves on a stream." This exercise begins by asking clients to envision a stream and a tree next to it. In this initial part of the exercise, any amount of time can be spent filling in the imaginary setting, for example, imagining what the leaves look like, how fast the stream is flowing, and so forth. Once the setting is established, the client is asked to notice any thoughts, emotions, or sensations that arise. Then, the client is instructed to place these experiences on leaves and watch them float away down the stream without trying to push them away or hold on to them. An additional instruction can be added, asking clients to label each experience as a thought, emotion, or sensation. These types of exercises develop present-moment awareness, acceptance of internal experience, and defusion. By labeling internal experiences, clients are able to see the experiences for their true nature—just thoughts, emotions, or sensations—without getting stuck in them or overly fused with them. In our experience, trauma survivors often find this exercise to have a soothing quality to it, and they find it to be a helpful way to not get caught up in their internal experiences as they happen.

The self-as-context process can also be targeted through specific metaphors and exercises (e.g., the chessboard metaphor, the *Whole, Perfect, Complete* exercise; see Walser & Hayes, 2006; Hayes et al., 2012). However, a simple way to integrate this process with existing mindfulness exercises is to ask clients during the exercises to notice "who" is noticing their internal experience. Developing an awareness of the observer self can be especially helpful for survivors of trauma because confusion or dissatisfaction with one's sense of identity often occurs in the aftermath of traumatic experiences. Many individuals feel that they are empty and have lost their sense of self in the wake of the trauma, or that they dislike the "person they have become." Some people, especially individuals who suffered trauma of an interpersonal nature, may find that their sense of self seems to exist only in the perceptions of others. Becoming aware of the transcendent part of the self that is not defined by labels and that simply "is" can help to transform one's understanding of the self and facilitate defusion from self-judgments. Defusing from self-content can help empower individuals to move forward and build a life worth living as opposed to remaining limited by what the mind tells them about who they are and what they can do.

Building a life worth living in ACT involves the identification of chosen values and incorporating behavioral commitment to those values in one's everyday practice. Commitment is not just a statement of what one will do—it is doing it. It is choosing to take actions that matter in the present moment. Therefore, mindfulness of what is happening *now* and what one values *now* is critical to engaging in committed, values-oriented actions.

Conclusion

Although more research is needed to determine the efficacy of ACT in the treatment of PTSD and trauma-related problems, there is reason to believe that ACT may be effective; experiential avoidance has been demonstrated to have a relationship to trauma-related outcomes (Palm & Follette, 2011). ACT's process of acceptance promotes engagement in valued activities for trauma survivors, even when those activities provoke unwanted internal experiences. In this way, ACT works to minimize the avoidance that maintains trauma symptoms and related problems while also increasing engagement in valued activities that can increase quality of life.

Being present in the world is a key process in ACT; it allows one to fully participate in one's own life, and yet it is more than that. When we commit to living life according to our values, we accept the difficult experiences that are encountered along the way. The practice of acceptance yields a sense of compassion for ourselves as we are able to accept our histories, thoughts, and emotions without judgment. This compassion for the self often leads to an extension of our compassion toward others. Many trauma survivors we have worked with have expressed their compassion through a desire to reach out and help minimize others' suffering. Their strength and dedication to living their valued lives continue to inspire our work.

References

Baer, R. A. (2003). Mindfulness training as a clinical intervention: A conceptual and empirical review. *Clinical Psychology: Science and Practice, 10*, 125–143.

Batten, S. V., & Hayes, S. C. (2005). Acceptance and commitment therapy in the treatment of substance abuse and post-traumatic stress disorder: A case study. *Clinical Case Studies, 4*, 246–262.

Blackledge, J. T., & Ciarrochi, J. (2006, May). *Personal Values Questionnaire.* Paper presented at the annual conference of the Association for Behavior Analysis, Atlanta, Georgia.

Bradley, R., Green, J., Russ, E., Dutra, L., & Westen, D. (2005). A multidimensional meta-analysis of psychotherapy for PTSD. *American Journal of Psychiatry, 162*, 214–227.

Cahill, S. P., Foa, E. B., Hembree, E. A., Marshall, R. D., & Nacash, N. (2006). Dissemination of exposure therapy in the treatment of posttraumatic stress disorder. *Journal of Traumatic Stress, 19*, 597–610.

Cahill, S. P., Rothbaum, B. O., Resick, P. A. & Follette, V. M. (2008). Cognitive-behavioral therapy for adults. In E. B. Foa, T. M. Keane, & M. J. Friedman (Eds.), *Effective treatments for PTSD* (2nd ed., pp. 139–222). New York: Guilford Press.

Dahl, J., Wilson, K. G., Luciano, C., & Hayes, S. C. (2005). *ACT for chronic pain.* Reno, NV: Context Press.

Engle, J. L., & Follette, V. (2012). Acceptance and commitment therapy for trauma. In R. A. McMackin, T. M. Keane, E. Newman, & J. Fogler (Eds.), *Trauma therapy in context: The science and craft of evidence-based practice* (pp. 353–372). Washington, DC: American Psychological Association.

Follette, V., Palm, K., & Pearson, A. (2006). Mindfulness and trauma: Implications for treatment. *Journal of Rational-Emotive and Cognitive-Behavior Therapy, 24,* 45–61.

Hayes, S. C. (2002). Buddhism and acceptance and commitment therapy. *Cognitive and Behavioral Practice, 9,* 58–66.

Hayes, S. C., Luoma, J. B., Bond, F. W., Masuda, A., & Lillis, J. (2006). Acceptance and commitment therapy: Model, processes, and outcome. *Behaviour Research and Therapy, 44,* 1–25.

Hayes, S. C., Strosahl, K. D., & Wilson, K. G. (2012). *Acceptance and commitment therapy: The process and practice of mindful change.* New York: Guilford Press.

Hayes, S. C., Wilson, K. W., Gifford, E. V., Follette, V. M., & Strosahl, K. (1996). Experiential avoidance and behavioral disorders: A functional dimensional approach to diagnosis and treatment. *Journal of Consulting and Clinical Psychology, 64*(6), 1152–1168.

Kashdan, T. B., & Kane, J. Q. (2008). Post-traumatic distress and presence of post-traumatic growth and meaning in life: Experiential avoidance as a moderator. *Personality and Individual Differences, 50,* 84–89.

Kashdan, T. B., Morina, N., & Priebe, S. (2008). Post-traumatic stress disorder, social anxiety disorder and depression in survivors of the Kosovo war: Experiential avoidance as a contributor to distress and quality of life. *Journal of Anxiety Disorders, 23,* 185–196.

Luoma, J. B., Hayes, S. C., & Walser, R. D. (2007). *Learning ACT: An acceptance and commitment therapy skills training manual for therapists.* Oakland, CA: New Harbinger.

Mace, C. (2007). Mindfulness in psychotherapy: An introduction. *Advances in Psychiatric Treatment, 13,* 147–154.

Mowrer, O. H. (1960). *Learning theory and behavior.* New York: Wiley.

Mulick, P. S., Landes, S. J., & Kanter, J. W. (2011). Contextual behavioral therapies in the treatment of PTSD: A review. *International Journal of Behavioral Consultation and Therapy, 7,* 23–32.

Nhat Hanh, T. (1998). *The heart of the Buddha's teaching: Transforming suffering into peace, joy, and liberation.* Berkeley, CA: Parallax Press.

Orsillo, S. M., & Batten, S. V. (2005). Acceptance and commitment therapy in the treatment of posttraumatic stress disorder. *Journal of Behavior Modification, 29,* 95–129.

Palm, K. M., & Follette, V. F. (2011). The roles of cognitive flexibility and experiential avoidance in explaining psychological distress in survivors of interpersonal victimization. *Journal of Psychopathology and Behavioral Assessment, 33*(1), 79–86.

Polusny, M. A., & Follette, V. M. (1995). Long-term correlates of child sexual abuse: Theory and review of the empirical literature. *Applied and Preventive Psychology, 4,* 143–166.

Salkovskis, P. M., & Campbell, P. (1994). Thought suppression induces intrusions in naturally occurring negative intrusive thoughts. *Behaviour Research and Therapy, 32,* 1–8.

Schottenbauer, M. A., Glass, C. R., Arnkoff, D. B., Tendick, V., & Gray, S. H. (2008). Nonresponse and dropout rates in outcome studies on PTSD: Review and methodological considerations. *Psychiatry, 71,* 134–168.

Smout, M. F., Hayes, L., Atkins, P. W. B., Clausen, J., & Duguid, J. D. (2012). The empirically supported status of acceptance and commitment therapy: An update. *Clinical Psychologist, 16,* 97–109.

Thompson, R. W., Arnkoff, D. B., & Glass, C. R. (2011). Conceptualizing mindfulness and acceptance as components of psychological resilience to trauma. *Trauma, Violence, and Abuse, 12,* 220–235.

Twohig, M. P. (2009). Acceptance and commitment therapy for treatment-resistant posttraumatic stress disorder: A case study. *Cognitive and Behavioral Practice, 16,* 243–252.

Walser, R. D., & Hayes, S. C. (2006). Acceptance and commitment therapy in the treatment of posttraumatic stress disorder: Theoretical and applied issues. In V. M. Follette & J. I. Ruzek (Eds.), *Cognitive-behavioral therapies for trauma* (2nd ed., pp. 146–172). New York: Guilford Press.

Wegner, D. M., Schneider, D. J., Carter, S. R., & White, T. L. (1987). Paradoxical effects of thought suppression. *Journal of Personality and Social Psychology, 53,* 5–13.

Wilson, K. G., Sandoz, E. K., Flynn, M. K., Slater, R., & DuFrene, T. (2010). Understanding, assessing, and treating values processes in mindfulness and acceptance-based therapies. In R. Baer (Ed.), *Assessing mindfulness and acceptance: Illuminating the processes of change* (pp. 77–106). Oakland, CA: New Harbinger.

Wilson, K. G., Sandoz, E. K., Kitchens, J., & Roberts, M. (2010). The Valued Living Questionnaire: Defining and measuring valued action within a behavioral framework. *Psychological Record, 60,* 249–272.

5

Dialectical Behavior Therapy for Trauma Survivors

Devika R. Fiorillo and Alan E. Fruzzetti

Dialectical behavior therapy (DBT; e.g., Linehan, 1993) is considered the standard of care treatment for a range of difficulties associated with severe emotion dysregulation, including the prototypic borderline personality disorder (BPD), along with self-harm, suicide attempts, depression, substance use, and other difficulties (Feigenbaum, 2007; Robbins & Chapman, 2004). The prevalence of PTSD among individuals with BPD varies from 33% in community samples to as high as 58% in an inpatient sample (Swartz, Blazer, George, & Winfield, 1990; Zanarini, Frankenburg, Hennen, & Silk, 2004). Thus, as the standard of care for BPD, DBT is also a key point of intervention for survivors of trauma (Wagner & Linehan, 1994; Harned & Linehan, 2008). Mindfulness is the "core" skill in DBT and is utilized across intervention strategies. When treating people with trauma-related problems in DBT, mindfulness is employed specifically to facilitate exposure-oriented interventions, to help block or redirect away from avoidance, to increase acceptance (of the events and of oneself), and to help clients learn other skills for regulating emotions and building the quality of life they desire. In this chapter we present a brief overview of DBT interventions for trauma-related problems and then detail the specific uses of mindfulness in DBT interventions related to treating trauma-related problems.

Overview of DBT

Although DBT was originally designed to treat chronically suicidal women diagnosed with BPD with multiple, complex, and severe co-occurring psychological problems (Linehan, 1993), in recent years DBT has been shown to be effective in treating people with a broad array of problems related to emotion dysregulation. DBT is based on a biosocial or transactional theory in which problems characteristic of BPD develop from the transactions between temperamental vulnerability to emotional dysregulation and an invalidating social and family environment in which individuals' communications about their private experiences are frequently punished, ignored, or misunderstood (Fruzzetti, Shenk, & Hoffman, et al., 2005; Fruzzetti & Worrall, 2010). Both vulnerabilities (e.g., emotion sensitivity, reactivity, and slow return to baseline) and invalidating responses in the social environment are seen as transacting in a reciprocal and iterative manner to produce and maintain difficulties with emotion regulation.

In addressing the core problem of emotion dysregulation, DBT is heavily influenced both by the principles of behavioral science, such as classical and operant conditioning, positive and negative reinforcement, the development of stimulus and response classes of behaviors, and exposure-based interventions, and by the importance of mindfulness, acceptance, and validation. Accordingly, the treatment emphasizes the development of skills to change or replace problematic behaviors and improve social relationships and environments. DBT also draws from the principles of dialectics and balances change by balancing and synthesizing acceptance, in particular in the development of mindfulness skills, with problem solving and behavior therapy.

When applied as a treatment for individuals with a significant trauma history, DBT can be useful for individuals with PTSD and other trauma-related problems, both to facilitate stabilization in preparation for exposure-based interventions and to augment those procedures. It is also well suited to address the range of additional, complex problems that extend beyond those that are directly related to traumatic experiences, including substance use problems, relationship problems, depression, anxiety, low self-esteem, eating disorders, and so on.

Mindfulness in DBT

DBT explicitly integrates cognitive-behavioral therapy (CBT) change strategies with mindfulness, based in part on Zen Buddhist principles (e.g., Hanh, 1976) but also compatible with most other Eastern spiritual practices and Western contemplative and experiential traditions (e.g., Binswanger, 1963). Mindfulness practice in DBT emphasizes observation or self-monitoring of public (action) and private (thoughts, sensations, emotions) behaviors, which is similar to most of CBT's mindfulness interventions adopted in recent years. The most common definitions of mindfulness in CBT (e.g., Bishop et al., 2004; Kabat-Zinn, 1994) are compatible with DBT mindfulness skills and practices: Mindfulness has key components of (1) paying attention on purpose, or intentionally; (2) paying attention without judgments; and (3) bringing attention to the present moment. However, DBT is somewhat different from other CBT approaches to mindfulness in two ways: (1) DBT includes greater emphasis on awareness of internal experiences and acting from a mindful perspective, or "wise mind"; and (2) mindfulness practice of any behavior (public or private) is encouraged and the use of meditation is not emphasized or required, so mindfulness is ideally fully integrated into daily living. Mindfulness skills also are woven into all the other skill modules (distress tolerance, emotion regulation, and interpersonal effectiveness).

Mindfulness is also a core skill in treating trauma within DBT, facilitating other interventions geared toward trauma. First, as an acceptance strategy, mindfulness leads to awareness and acceptance of the current moment and counterbalances the emphasis on change (e.g., exposure), which is part of the dialectical processes essential to DBT. Second, "straight" exposure interventions, although effective, are difficult, and dropout rates are high. Mindfulness may help reduce dropout. Third, mindfulness can increase awareness and the client's capacity to stay focused, which improves the ability to notice, describe, and communicate experiences. This enhanced attention can help interventions that rely on monitoring, in which individuals are expected to have some capacity to observe, remember, and relay their experiences in therapy. This capacity to attend is particularly relevant for DBT with trauma victims, in part because increased awareness functions as informal exposure to sensations and emotions, reducing secondary reactions to painful emotions. This, in turn, can make formal exposure more efficient and easier to manage for patients and thus more effective. Finally, mindfulness can also enhance learning and the use of other skills. Thus mindfulness can promote significant life improvements and engagement in previously avoided, yet meaningful, activities.

Mindfulness skills as taught in DBT are well suited to survivors of trauma, including those who have experienced childhood sexual and physical abuse. Benefits of mindfulness include attention control, which is relevant for individuals with a history of trauma who are distracted by experiencing thoughts or memories of trauma and a variety of intense emotions, helping to reduce ruminative or hypervigilant preoccupation with past events. Mindful practice focusing on present awareness further helps reduce reexperiencing of traumatic events. Some individuals who engage in problematic behaviors (self-harm, substance use, etc.), which almost always serve escape and avoidance functions, may benefit significantly from increased attention to present emotion (especially primary emotions) or even alternative stimuli, as well as emotion-regulation skills (Harned, Korslund, Foa, & Linehan, 2012). Others may benefit from increased attention to present situations and the positive emotions that may be elicited. Finally, mindfulness skills may also help increase awareness of interpersonal cues, including danger-related cues, which can be essential in preventing revictimization (Fruzzetti & Lee, 2011).

Mindfulness as a "Core" Skill

Mindfulness is the "core" skill that is taught in DBT, meaning that mindfulness is an essential component of other skills (e.g., emotion regulation, distress tolerance, interpersonal skills). Three states of mind are identified: (1) *reason* mind, or the mind state one is in when approaching awareness or "knowing" from an intellectual, rational, logical, empirical, and/or planning perspective; (2) *emotion* mind refers to moments when awareness (and thinking and behavior) are controlled mainly by states of high emotional arousal; and (3) *wise* mind refers to more pure awareness, or even intuitive knowing, based on the integration or synthesis of both reason and emotion. Wise mind awareness and behavior is present in everyone's repertoires, although in many situations it may be difficult to find or use this perspective. One way to think about mindfulness skills in DBT is as steps or means for achieving wise mind, leading to effective action, in part by helping to stabilize or moderate (or prevent) dysregulated emotions and cognition. This process has been developed into teachable skill steps by Linehan (1993), which describe both *what* a person does when being mindful and *how* the person engages in those tasks mindfully.

Mindfulness "What" Skills

This set of mindfulness skills identifies what one does with his or her attention when actually being mindful. These skills include observing, describing, and participating and are geared toward developing a capacity to participate in one's own life and experiences with awareness and skill (including both acceptance- and change-oriented skills).

   Observing refers to the process of simply noticing or paying attention (in the present moment) both to events outside the person and to thoughts, sensations, and emotions inside the person. When observing, the person does not engage in any attempts (at least at that moment) to alter his or her experience or the events—including neither prolonging them when pleasant nor escaping or terminating them when unpleasant. Observing includes bringing attention to something, just noticing. As clients become better able to sustain attention and tolerate their internal experiences, mindfulness can also include awareness of thoughts, sensations, and emotions. Mindfulness practice is essential because it strengthens one's ability to experience the moment, no matter how distressing, rather than engaging in dysfunctional escape behaviors. This focus on "experiencing the moment" facilitates non-reinforced exposure (e.g., Foa & Rothbaum, 1998) by helping to extinguish automatic escape and fear responses and increasing habituation. Additionally, the experience of observing an event is discriminated from the event itself (e.g., feeling fearful is differentiated from being in danger). For survivors of abuse, this ability to attend to certain events (e.g., memories, images or flashbacks of traumatic events) with a simultaneous ability to step back from them into the reality of the present moment (safety) is essential for successful outcomes.

Describing requires using words in a descriptive, rather than judgmental or evaluative, manner and is particularly important in dealing with thoughts and feelings. Simply labeling a thought as a thought and emotion as emotion reduces their literality and importance in the client's interpretation of present experience. For example, the thought "I must have done something to cause the abuse" and the feelings of guilt and shame can be observed and described as thoughts and emotions, respectively, and discriminated from actually deserving to have been abused. Furthermore, these thoughts and feelings can be validated (and self-validated) as normative, albeit painful and undeserved, consequences of abuse rather than "attaching" to the individuals as true in content. Using verbal labels to refer to external and internal events is also critical for establishing a more internal locus of self-control. Being able to observe sensations, feelings, and urges and to describe them can help the client understand the contexts in which they occur while also understanding that they do not have to dictate behavior. The accurate use of descriptive words to understand experiences is also helpful both for regulating emotion and for effective communication. Accurate, descriptive expression makes it easier for others to understand and validate, in part because it reduces the likelihood that personal interpretations, inaccurate "descriptions," and other misleading communication will cloud the message being conveyed (Fruzzetti & Worrall, 2010).

Participating is being engaged in the activity in the current moment, without separating from the activities that are ongoing, and without self-consciousness (i.e., not focusing on observing and describing or other higher cognitive activities while participating). This encourages authentic connection with events, processes, and activities in the present moment and the reduction of excessively automated or habitual responses. The idea is simple, though the practice can be difficult: bring full attention to walking while walking, taking a shower while taking a shower, eating while eating, driving while driving, and so on (rather than judging, evaluating, being distracted, etc., while engaging in those activities).

Mindfulness "How" Skills

The second set of mindfulness skills describes "how" to do things mindfully and explains the manner in which one observes, describes, and participates mindfully.

A *nonjudgmental* stance is emphasized in which all experiences and events are acknowledged as they are (descriptively), without being labeled as "good" or "bad" or "right" or "wrong." In mindfulness, there are no "should" or "shouldn'ts" in the past. In this way, mindfulness in DBT is directed toward accepting experiences, events, and people as they are (and thus not putting energy into "fighting the reality" of the past). It should be noted that being nonjudgmental or accepting of reality does not mean that negative judgments need to be replaced with positive ones or that painful or unpleasant experiences need to be approved of or negative experiences invalidated. For survivors of trauma, a nonjudgmental and accepting stance should not be mistaken for forgiveness or justification of the abuse. In fact, a nonjudgmental perspective could help the person to acknowledge harmful (or even possibly useful) consequences or positive or negative feelings, but emphasis is certainly placed on acceptance of the entire experience as it is. For a significant proportion of trauma survivors who tend to engage in extreme judgments, particularly about themselves, learning to let go of judgments (and instead to notice, describe, and/or participate in their experience and thus themselves) is an essential alternative to patterns of self-recrimination and paves the way for other behavior changes.

The nonjudgmental characteristic of mindfulness can help in the reduction of self-stigma, self-invalidation, and self-blame associated with trauma and can help people still living in unsafe and/or invalidating social situations to change them. Individuals with a history of trauma frequently also have difficulties accepting certain behaviors in themselves and in their histories. Nonjudgmental practice can thus be utilized as a method for promoting greater acceptance of oneself, leading to reduced suffering internally and greater connection with safe and loving other people.

Learning to be nonjudgmental of perpetrators can be difficult for trauma survivors and also for therapists. In a mindfulness sense, saying the perpetrator was not a bad or evil person (i.e., taking away the judgment) *does not mean* that he or she is a good person. There is no good or bad. Rather, it may help lead to a description that facilitates healing: The person was abusive (even describing in some detail what he or she did), and it had multiple and long-lasting negative consequences (describing physical and emotional pain that resulted). This helps the individual to accept the reality of the abuse and leads to a focus on repairing the consequences, rather than getting stuck in the "abuse dichotomy" that flips back and forth between the judgmental positions that either the perpetrator was evil or the victim deserved it (Linehan, 1993). Nevertheless, bringing a nonjudgmental stance to work with trauma survivors can be challenging.

Being *one-mindful* refers to focusing attention on one thing at a time in the present moment, rather than splitting attention either behaviorally or cognitively between tasks or being distracted (nonpurposeful attention). Survivors of trauma in particular are likely to be affected by thoughts and images related to trauma or sequelae of trauma, along with rumination about current troubles, self-invalidation and shame, preoccupation with negative mood, or concerns about the future, and they are likely to need skills to focus attention on one activity at a time in an alert and awake manner. This skill can be practiced in a number of day-to-day activities, such as eating, driving or bus riding, engaging in a hobby, and spending time with a friend or partner.

Acting in an *effective* manner means behaving in a way that is effective, that is needed in a particular situation to be consistent with a person's long-term goals and closely held (wise mind) values. It includes identifying one's goals and acting in a balanced, principle-oriented, rather than in an exclusively outcome-oriented, manner. Thus it is not possible, within this definition, to engage in self-destructive behaviors mindfully, even if done so with great attention. Clients with a history of trauma may also struggle with trusting their own perceptions, judgments, and decisions and may be overly focused on what is supposed to be "right" (rather than effective). Effectiveness mindfulness can help the client make more "wise mind" decisions.

Use of Mindfulness in Treatment

Therapist Relationship Mindfulness

It is essential that therapists utilizing DBT have experience with mindfulness to effectively teach skills and create a strong therapeutic relationship. Much of mindfulness involves experiential exercises, along with some more didactic training. The experiential practice of mindfulness on the part of the therapist, particularly during times of his or her own difficulties, builds his or her deep knowledge about its fundamental principles and practice, which helps the therapist to understand the clients' problems better and consequently affords greater opportunities to address their concerns. Practice of mindfulness by the therapist can help the therapist maintain focus and direction, which can be important when working with clients with a history of abuse who may have chronic and severe difficulties. Increased ability to stay focused is helpful when the client presents in an overwhelmed state, is tangential, or reports a wide range of problems. The practice of mindfulness can also help therapists manage their own physical, cognitive, and emotional experiences in response to working with clients. Providers working with survivors of abuse may have to deal with challenging behaviors such as passivity and hopelessness, in addition to their own judgments (about clients, perpetrators, themselves, or others). Additionally, trauma therapists are also at unique risk for experiencing secondary traumatic reactions from being exposed regularly to sensitive abuse material as related by the client, especially while conducting formal exposure treatment. Many of the basic mindfulness skills taught to clients in DBT can be used in session by therapists for the purposes of titrating attention and maintaining emotion regulation and balance. The therapist can simply notice slight changes in his or her bodily sensations, thoughts, and emotions and bring awareness to the breath in order to act in an effective rather than reactive manner.

Mindfulness can also help the therapist cope with his or her negative self-evaluation. Because many clients with a history of abuse have long-standing behavioral patterns that are sometimes difficult to change, the therapist may begin to doubt his or her abilities and may experience increased hopelessness and urges to give up that can in turn affect the therapist's capacity to motivate the client and stay focused on goal-directed activity. The practice of mindfulness also helps the therapist achieve balance between continuing to work toward goals and developing an attachment to outcomes. Retaining a sense of nonattachment is critical. When goals are not met, or at least not to the extent that the therapist desires, the suffering and burnout of the therapist may be prevented or ameliorated by maintaining this sense of nonattachment.

Mindfulness in the Session

With regard to survivors of trauma, the principles of mindfulness may be employed by the therapist in session to facilitate exposure. Although traditional exposure-based interventions for specific traumatic experiences are also used in DBT, exposure (to a variety of situations) is also carried out more informally under the intervention labeled "opposite action." The purposes of opposite action are to reduce dysfunctional avoidance and associated negative mood and also to increase new adaptive behaviors and build positive emotions associated with them (Rizvi & Linehan, 2005). Upon cue exposure, the therapist blocks problematic responses such as escape and avoidance behaviors and feelings of guilt, shame, and anger and helps the client to engage in emotion-regulation strategies. Much of the work with trauma survivors is focused on opposite action, and the principles of mindfulness are used throughout the intervention to facilitate change.

Opposite action is based on observation that all emotions have an associated action urge and that when that emotion is secondary or unjustified by what is happening in the present moment, engaging in an alternative action that is opposite of the action urge will lessen the negative emotion. To facilitate this process, the therapist stays alert and welcomes *in vivo* cues when working with clients who often become overwhelmed with negative emotions, have difficulties identifying emotions, tend to experience dysregulated secondary emotional responses, become stuck in their experience of a single emotion, or become aware of their emotions only after the fact.

The therapist also observes passive and subtle behavior indications on the part of the client that may suggest that he or she is avoiding or inhibiting emotional responses, often inquiring about emotional reactions and blocking "escape" patterns. Because the client has to be able to make a connection between the emotion and the action urge and has learned opposite actions, the therapist can help the client observe and label emotional states by using mindfulness. This often includes raising awareness of internal and external prompting events, thoughts and interpretations related to the event, physical and sensory responses associated with the experience of emotions, desires or urges associated with the emotions, associated action tendencies, and aftereffects of the emotions. The client is also asked to pay attention to overt reactions that may reflect certain emotions, such as facial expressions and body posture or movements and other actions that may betray the experience of a particular emotion. Because survivors of abuse often present with difficulties in labeling and identifying emotions accurately, mindfulness also plays an integral role in improving knowledge and awareness of emotion.

To counterbalance change-based strategies, such as opposite action, the DBT therapist also focuses on mindfulness, distress tolerance, and validation (and self-validation) as acceptance-oriented skills. Mindfulness is essential when the client is practicing "radical acceptance" or the use of a nonjudgmental stance toward him- or herself and the situation, including the abuse itself. The therapist also validates the client's experience, which reflects understanding of the world from the client's perspective and communicates the legitimacy of his or her emotions, thoughts, and behaviors. Validation should not be mistaken for actions that function to soothe or comfort the patient per se, although validation does help reduce negative emotional arousal (Shenk & Fruzzetti, 2011). Rather, one of the key goals of validation is to help the client learn how to self-validate, which is important for increasing his or her sense of self and for diminishing self-judgments and secondary emotions such as shame and guilt.

The therapist utilizes mindfulness principles and frequent practice with clients to help them observe and label their emotions and other experiences accurately. By learning to describe private experiences (thoughts, feelings, wants, etc.) and overt behaviors without added judgment and evaluation, the client is able to block or prevent self-invalidating responses, so common in survivors of abuse. The client can also be guided to notice and describe self-imposed behavioral demands, unrealistic expectations for acceptable behavior, and the related experiences of guilt and shame as ineffective strategies that lead to increased and unnecessary suffering.

An active role is assumed by the therapist in helping clients observe and describe their thought processes, underlying assumptions about themselves and the world, and "crazy-making" experiences in their social worlds. These efforts ultimately help clients accept themselves as they are.

Case Example

The following is a fictionalized case example (aggregated from common client features and presentations). Angie is a 32-year-old female. She was sexually abused by her stepfather for several years, beginning in early childhood, and also reports severe physical abuse at the hands of her brother, who is 7 years older. Angie meets criteria for major depression, generalized anxiety disorder, and alcohol abuse and has significant interpersonal difficulties. She divorced several years ago and shares legal custody of her 10-year-old daughter with her ex-husband. He has primary physical custody, and Angie spends time with her daughter several times per week. Her relationship with her ex-husband is mostly collaborative around their daughter. Angie has been dating another man for the past 2 years and has regular contact with him, although she indicates that they are not in any formal or committed relationship. According to Angie, her ex-husband tends to "baby" her and treat her like a child at times, whereas the man she is currently dating is often overbearing and controlling.

The following is an example of an early session highlighting the use of mindfulness, both as an intervention itself and to augment other intervention strategies.

THERAPIST: All right, now let's figure out our agenda for today. Your diary card seems to show that today might have been your most difficult day this week. Let's look at the chain of things that happened to get you overwhelmed. What else do you want to put on the agenda?

CLIENT: I think this is the most important thing I need help with right now. It really all began this morning. I think I was doing just fine until I picked Chelsea [daughter] up from Tim [ex-husband] to take her to school because Tim had an early meeting at work. You know, he asked me to be careful about what I tell her teachers during my quick scheduled meeting with them about Chelsea's performance at school. It was like there was something he was trying to warn me about, and I was pretty sure it was because I've been stupid with them before. I felt so dumb that he had to give me these subtle reminders to be careful about what I might say to people. I'm just not a very intelligent person, you know, and I began to worry that I'd ruin it for Chelsea, mess it up, and do something terrible with her teachers, so I dropped by the house to get Stewart [current boyfriend] to go to the school with me for some support.

THERAPIST: Whoooa. Slow down a little.

CLIENT: OK . . .

THERAPIST: All right, let's stop here for a second and let me get this. It sounds like you were rather judgmental of yourself this morning, and maybe again just now.

CLIENT: What do you mean? Tim was right . . . I do screw these things up. Tim didn't mean any harm. I do think I'm kind of crazy sometimes in how I interact with others, you know.

THERAPIST: All right, I'm not trying to minimize your problems here, but let's compare your experiences this morning, the event, your thoughts, judgments, feelings to an orange. Now let's say you've never had an orange or seen someone eat an orange before. You might just assume that you are supposed to eat the whole thing. You may not know it is made up of different parts, some you can eat and others not. What I'd like you to do is to peel apart the judgments and other experiences from the event itself, much like you'd peel the cover off the orange to separate it from the part that you can eat. It doesn't mean the peel isn't part of the orange or that your judgments aren't part of your experience, it just means that they can still be separated. And then you can pay less attention to them, and more to the descriptive part of your experience.

CLIENT: I guess I can try to do that. I know I've said things to Chelsea's teachers that have made them frustrated and angry before. It's because I get nervous when I talk to them because I'm so concerned, you know, about being a good mom and I want Chelsea to be OK, and to know that I'm a good mom. I tend to be very direct in my interactions, because it hides my nervousness; you see, I don't want to seem passive, which was something I had problems with for several years and something I don't want Chelsea to develop. Sometimes, I'm just so direct now that I don't think of how people may take my words. That's gotten me in trouble many times with Chelsea's teachers and with Tim, other places too. The judgments, well, I had many. I always think I'm a bad mom, I'm too stupid to interact with Chelsea's teachers, I'm not capable of asserting my needs so I shouldn't even try doing that for my daughter, I'm not as good enough as her father and she'd probably be better off with him. I guess I also just assumed Tim was referring to me being stupid, although I didn't even ask what he was thinking about exactly.

THERAPIST: Awesome work here, Angie, with separating your judgments from the event itself. You're right. "Stupid" is a judgment. "Bad mom" is a judgment. Sure, maybe you get upset and sometimes assert yourself a little beyond what might be effective. That's both descriptive and a solvable problem, something we can work on.

CLIENT: But it seems so real, though, that I *am* a bad mom. I don't know how to, like, separate what's real from my judgments sometimes. They feel so real and then I'm just overpowered by these thoughts I'm having. And then it's like a tornado inside.

THERAPIST: Yes, exactly. It seems that way. Everyone has judgments sometimes, and it can be really hard to tell the difference between description and judgments. Remember when we talked about Teflon pans and Teflon mind? Can you try being like a Teflon pan, noticing the judgments that pop up but not letting them stick? They can then fall off without doing so much damage. Can you try right now? You really did this well before.

CLIENT: OK . . . I'm doing that right now. And I can remember to try next time.

THERAPIST: Great!

[Further discussion for a couple of minutes about using these two strategies, sorting judgments from description, "Teflon" mind in daily life, and orienting and committing to more practice. This might include more direct practice in the session, with coaching.]

THERAPIST: So moving on, what happened? You were saying you went to get Stewart to help out.

CLIENT: Right. But reaching out to Stewart only made things worse because he went with me but ended up cutting me off every time I tried to say something. Not only that, he even rambled on about how I have difficulties with speaking up, and how he thinks I'm bad at parenting. Chelsea was right there, too! I kind of got overwhelmed and don't even remember what happened the last few minutes in the car with him. (*Silence; hunches her back, decreases eye contact.*)

THERAPIST: What just happened? Can you notice you're behaving differently right now?

CLIENT: I just feel terrible about myself (*in a soft voice*).

THERAPIST: Yes, I can see that. Try to let the judgments go again, and maybe this time just notice your sensations and observe that this would have been a really unpleasant situation for anyone, facing all that second guessing and criticism or invalidation. What emotion are you feeling now?

CLIENT: I'm not sure, I just feel I'm not worthy of much and I just don't think I'm a good mother, you know (*softer voice*). I guess I feel really ashamed.

THERAPIST: Yes, you look like you do. We all feel embarrassed or ashamed when others are judgmental of us, or when we judge ourselves. But there often are other emotions, too.

CLIENT: I think I feel shameful a lot. I just wanted some support and I ended up making a fool of myself in front of everyone. Not only that, Chelsea is probably thinking I'm the worst mom someone could have now (*barely audible, no eye contact*).

THERAPIST: OK, try to stop and notice again (*pause*). Let's try to see what else you might be feeling by observing the judgments, not attaching to them. What else can you notice? Not just the orange peel . . . what else?

CLIENT: I don't know. I just feel so terrible about myself. Maybe some fear. I'm really sad, too. Maybe you're thinking I'm a bad mom, too. I kind of feel like leaving right now. It's hard.

THERAPIST: So when you're shameful, it's hard to see anything else, and you maybe want to run away or hide from the world, including me. Let's try some opposite action here. I want you to look at me, OK? And sit up even though you're feeling shameful.

CLIENT: If you say so. (*Slowly looks up, sits up in the chair.*)

THERAPIST: What do you notice when you look at me? Am I judging you?

CLIENT: I don't think so.

THERAPIST: Right, of course I'm not. And it's easier to see that when you act opposite to your urges to run away, and notice, right now, right here, what's going on. When you really bring your attention to me, it's hard to think or feel that I'm judging you. Your wise mind knows. You've got to point your attention and notice. You look like something is different inside, something emotionally?

CLIENT: Yes, I feel less ashamed and overwhelmed.

THERAPIST: Great. I know shame can feel overwhelming, but now you're really starting to ride this bucking bronco of shame, rather than being knocked off and crashed into the stone wall. Can you take a moment and be mindful of any other emotions you may be having now, or may have had this morning during the time at Chelsea's school, or when you were with Tim or Stewart?

CLIENT: I'm frustrated that Stewart talked for me instead of just being by my side, and I'm just so hurt that he aired my dirty laundry, telling everyone I have trouble with parenting.

THERAPIST: Of course, regardless of his intentions, that's a tough spot to be in, and frustration and hurt make a lot of sense. You wanted support, but it went really differently. It was in public and with your daughter's teachers. Nobody would want to be discussed in this way. It seems like you had some ideas about what you wanted to communicate to them, and yes, I'd be frustrated—anyone would—if I were cut off or not given a chance to talk.

CLIENT: Yes. I'm not really sure how to talk with Stewart about this, either, but I think I have to.

THERAPIST: Well, what emotions or other things would you want to communicate to him, would you want him to understand?

CLIENT: I really want him to understand how undercut I felt, how sad and disappointed and hurt I am in him about all of this.

THERAPIST: That makes a lot of sense. Maybe we should turn our attention to how you can communicate these things really effectively? Seems like if you can do that, you'll feel a lot less disempowered. How's your emotion right now? Your own judgments about yourself?

CLIENT: I'm feeling kind of motivated to talk with Stewart, and my judgments are kind of quiet. But I notice now that I'm a little afraid of just blasting him.

THERAPIST: Right. So, let's find a way for you to communicate really clearly and assertively, without blasting him . . . a way to be true to yourself and really skillful in asserting yourself, so he understands. And also so he doesn't feel completely attacked. Great. Remember the skills we have for this kind of situation?

[Therapist and client go on to organize and practice what and how Angie will talk with Stewart. At the end of the session, Angie reports feeling motivated and committed to talk effectively with Stewart, less ashamed, and that she's looking forward to her evening with Chelsea.]

Conclusion

DBT is a skill-based program of intervention appropriate for individuals whose psychological difficulties are assumed to be maintained by emotion dysregulation, primarily in the context of an invalidating environment either historically, presently, or both. Mindfulness is an integral part of DBT and is used to facilitate skills training and generalization and to augment other procedures and strategies (e.g., exposure) to help clients feel empowered, present, and authentic (in their "wise minds"). The problems targeted by DBT overlap considerably with those commonly reported by survivors of child abuse. In fact, a unique subset among those who have experienced trauma, who also seem resistant to exposure-based interventions, may be particularly suited to the use of DBT. Mindfulness is taught as the core skill to the client and is also used by the therapist to engage the client in the process of developing a repertoire to tolerate distress and regulate emotions and to engage life in a meaningful, skillful, and empowered way.

References

Binswanger, L. (1963). *Being-in-the-world: Selected papers of Ludwig Binswanger* (J. Needleman, Trans.). New York: Basic Books.

Bishop, S. R., Lau, M., Shapiro, S., Carlson, L., Anderson, N. D., Nicole, D. et al. (2004). Mindfulness: A proposed operational definition. *Clinical Psychology: Science and Practice, 11*(3), 230–241.

Feigenbaum, J. (2007). Dialectical behaviour therapy: An increasing evidence base. *Journal of Mental Health, 16*(1), 51–68.

Foa, E. B., & Rothbaum, B. O. (1998). *Treating the trauma of rape: Cognitive behavioral therapy for PTSD.* New York: Guilford Press.

Fruzzetti, A. E., & Lee, J. E. (2011). Multiple experiences of domestic violence. In M. P. Duckworth & V. M. Follette (Eds.), *Retraumatization: Assessment, treatment, and prevention* (pp. 345–376). New York: Routledge Press.

Fruzzetti, A. E., Shenk, C., & Hoffman, P. D. (2005). Family interaction and the development of borderline personality disorder: A transactional model. *Development and Psychopathology, 17,* 1007–1030.

Fruzzetti, A. E., & Worrall, J. M. (2010). Accurate expression and validation: A transactional model for understanding individual and relationship distress. In K. Sullivan & J. Davila (Eds.), *Support processes in intimate relationships* (pp. 121–150). New York: Oxford University Press.

Hanh, T. N. (1976). *The miracle of mindfulness: A manual on meditation.* Boston: Beacon.

Harned, M. S., Korslund, K. E., Foa, E. B., & Linehan, M. M. (2012). Treating PTSD in suicidal and self-injuring women with borderline personality disorder: Development and preliminary evaluation of a dialectical behavior therapy prolonged exposure protocol. *Behavior Research and Therapy, 50,* 381–386.

Harned, M. S., & Linehan, M. M. (2008). Integrating dialectical behavior therapy and prolonged exposure to treat co-occurring borderline personality disorder and PTSD: Two case studies. *Cognitive and Behavioral Practice, 15*(3), 263–276.

Kabat-Zinn, J. (1994). *Wherever you go, there you are: Mindfulness meditation in everyday life.* New York: Hyperion.

Linehan, M. M. (1993). *Cognitive-behavioral treatment of borderline personality disorder.* New York: Guilford Press.

Rizvi, S. L., & Linehan, M. M. (2005). The treatment of maladaptive shame in borderline personality disorder: A pilot study of "Opposite Action." *Cognitive and Behavioral Practice, 12,* 437–447.

Robbins, C. J., & Chapman, A. L. (2004). Dialectical behavior therapy: Current status, recent developments, and future directions. *Journal of Personality Disorders, 18,* 73–89.

Shenk, C., & Fruzzetti, A. E. (2011). The impact of validating and invalidating responses on emotional reactivity. *Journal of Social and Clinical Psychology, 30,* 163–183.

Swartz, M. S., Blazer, D., George, L., & Winfield, I. (1990). Estimating the prevalence of borderline personality disorder in the community. *Journal of Personality Disorders, 4,* 257–272.

Wagner, A. W., & Linehan, M. M. (1994). Relationship between childhood sexual abuse and topography of parasuicide among women with borderline personality disorder. *Journal of Personality Disorders, 8,* 1–9.

Zanarini, M. C., Frankenburg, F. R., Hennen, J., & Silk, K. R. (2004). Mental health service utilization by borderline personality disorder patients and Axis II comparison subjects followed prospectively for 6 years. *Journal of Clinical Psychiatry, 65*(1), 28–36.

6

Mindfulness-Based Cognitive Therapy for Chronic Depression and Trauma

J. Mark G. Williams
and Thorsten Barnhofer

Depression is a global problem, afflicting about 5% of the world's population at any one time. It is not limited to rich countries: Depression is the leading cause of years lost to disability in both high- *and* low- to middle-income countries, yet fewer than 25% of those affected have access to effective treatments (Mathers, Boerma, & Ma Fat, 2008). A major reason for the large global burden of depression is that the first onset of depression most commonly occurs in adolescence and early adulthood, and thereafter there is a high risk of recurrence (50% after the first episode and rising to 70–80% risk after subsequent episodes; Boland & Keller, 2009). The most commonly used treatment for depression is antidepressant medication, but once the treatment is finished, the risk of another episode returns to the level prior to the start of treatment (Geddes et al., 2003). In this chapter, we examine the reasons that depression sometimes takes a chronic course, focusing on the role of adversity and trauma on psychological processes (particularly autobiographical memory) that make chronicity more likely. Finally, we draw on our experience of teaching mindfulness to chronically depressed, suicidal people to consider what changes to a mindfulness program might be made to address the specific issues raised.

Depression and the Problem of Chronicity

Major depression is diagnosed when a person experiences a number of symptoms that co-occur for most of the time over a 2-week period in such severity that it impairs normal functioning. This means that, over this period, people experience either or both of the core symptoms of major depression—low mood and lack of interest—as well as at least four of the noncore symptoms (changes in eating patterns, changes in sleep, agitation or retardation, guilt, concentration difficulties, fatigue, and suicidal ideas or actual suicidal behavior). In fact, it is rare for depression to last only 2 weeks, and the normal expectation is for it to last between 6 and 9 months. In addition, not only is the course of depression often recurrent, but also the risk of relapse increases with number of episodes and needs fewer and fewer life events to trigger it (for an overview, see Tennant, 2002).

The magnitude of the burden suffered by those who have recurrent depression has become clear only in the past few years as very-long-term studies are completed. Judd et al. (2008), in their long-term follow-up of clients recruited in the National Institute of Mental Health (NIMH) Collaborative Depression Study (CDS), found that over 15 years, clients with depression experienced some degree of disability in more than 50% of months, including about 20% of months with moderate and almost 10% of months with severe impairment. Particularly after severe episodes, residual symptoms remain (Kennedy, Abbott, & Paykel, 2004). About 20% of all clients with depression (and 47% of clients with depression treated in mental health systems) suffer from chronic depression as defined by current classification systems; that is, an episode of major depression that lasts more than 2 years. Rate of prevalence of chronic depression alone in adult populations of Western countries is reported to be at about 3% and would likely be considerably higher if the definition were broadened to take into account lifetime symptom courses in which symptoms are present most of the time. Chronic courses often begin at an early age, tend to self-perpetuate as the psychological mechanisms underlying maintenance of symptoms become increasingly habitual over time, and have a severe impact on quality of life. The reason is that once clients have entered such a chronic course of the disorder, they are significantly less responsive to established treatments. A recent meta-analysis of psychotherapeutic treatments for chronic depression that included 16 studies found a significant but small pre- to posttreatment effect size of only $d = 0.23$ (Cuijpers et al., 2010), with only one recently developed treatment for chronic depression producing better effects (Keller et al., 2000).

Although they differ with regard to their particular course configuration, recent research has found chronic forms of depression to be highly homogeneous with regard to a broad range of demographic, clinical, psychosocial, family history, and treatment response variables while at the same time differing in important ways from episodic forms of the disorder. What are the factors involved in whether depression persists in this way, or remits?

Chronic courses tend to be characterized by *increased familiality,* with findings being most pronounced when rates of familial clustering are estimated based on assessments of lifetime symptom course (taking into account residual and subthreshold symptom states) rather than current DSM-5 categories. Furthermore, research has consistently demonstrated chronic depression to be associated with *increased temperamental vulnerabilities,* such as increased neuroticism and increased dispositional negative affect (for an overview, see Klein, 2010). Third, and of interest for this chapter, chronicity is associated with *increased levels of early adversity* (Lizardi et al., 1995).

However, the relevance of these factors for treatment development is restricted, as they are impossible to modify. The question, therefore, is: Can we identify what long-term changes in a person might be produced by a history of trauma and adversity that, once they occur, later act to *increase the risk* of depression and then to *maintain* mood disturbance if depression has occurred? We turn now to one such variable: overgeneralized memory.

Autobiographical Memory Overgenerality, Trauma, and Chronicity of Depression

Our methodology for studying memories is to elicit events from the past using the Galton cue-word paradigm. This involves giving a positive, negative, or neutral word to a participant and asking him or her to retrieve a specific memory that the word reminded him or her of. The instructions ask people to come up with an event, which could be important or trivial, from a long time ago or from recently. The only constraint is that it should be a *specific* memory of an event that occurred within one day. In other words, to the cue word *enjoy,* it would not be acceptable to say "I always enjoy a good party." But it would be fine to say "I remember enjoying Jane's party five months ago" or "I remember my first birthday party when I was eight."

The original discovery by Williams and Broadbent (1986) was that, whereas people in general, when given cues such as *happy, safe, sorry,* or *interested,* would have very little difficulty coming up with specific memories, people who feel hopeless and suicidal would make a nonspecific response; for instance, to the word *safe,* "being in my home."

One of the first questions we asked after the original work with suicidal clients was whether this was true of other clinical groups as well. We set about to see whether this finding was also true in those with a diagnosis of major depression, finding that overgeneralized memory was present among them, too (Williams & Scott, 1988). Similarly, a Harvard study of Vietnam veterans by Richard McNally found that they, too, suffered from overgeneralized memory (McNally et al., 1995). Since McNally's study, the association between overgenerality and a history of trauma has been repeatedly reported. Although some studies are ambiguous (see Moore &

Zoellner, 2007), they continue to show associations between trauma, experiential avoidance, and overgeneralized memory.

Can Overgeneralized Memory Explain the Role of Trauma in Producing Later Emotional Disturbance?

Harvey, Bryant, and Dang (1998) found that people who recalled a road traffic accident in more general terms were more likely to have traumatic reactions a few months later. Similarly, Bryant, Sutherland, and Guthrie (2007) tested firefighters when they first got their jobs, assessing overgenerality in memory. Two years later—after the firefighters had undergone several traumas as part of their jobs—they examined the cohort to see who was more likely to have posttraumatic stress disorder (PTSD). They found that those who showed overgeneralized memories at the outset were more likely to suffer PTSD as a result of their traumas. Similarly, Kleim and Ehlers (2008) found that following an assault, people were more likely to suffer PTSD and depression if they had overgeneralized memories.

Perhaps of greatest interest is the research by Brennen and colleagues (2010) on war trauma. In a first study, they assessed Bosnian adolescents (*n* = 40, current mean age = 18), all of whom had witnessed the 1991–1995 war when they were between 3 and 7 years of age. Of the 40 in the sample, 39 had close family members who fought in the war, 38 had experienced bombing in their vicinities, 29 had their homes bombed or shelled, 33 were forced to leave their homes, 20 lived near a place where a massacre occurred, and 6 lost a parent in the war.

When the researchers compared the adolescents with a matched Norwegian sample, they found that the Bosnian adolescents were much less likely to be specific in their memories and more likely to be overgeneral. However, of course, Brennen and colleagues realized that samples from Bosnia and from Norway might have all sorts of other cultural differences that might explain the difference in their memories. So they returned to the former Yugoslavia to work with colleagues testing Serbian adolescents who were now between 18 and 22 years old who lived in towns bombed by the North Atlantic Treaty Organization (NATO) in 1999 (when they were between 9 and 13 years old). He compared 50 such young adults with 90 people who had lived in other towns that had not suffered bombing by NATO.

The results were striking. First, there were no discernible differences at all between the bombed and the unbombed young adults in terms of their current depression or even of the current impact of events (using the Impact of Event Scale [IES]; Horowitz, Wilner, & Alvarez, 1979). And yet the memory specificity showed exactly the scarring effect that he predicted: The group who had been in towns that were bombed were more likely to have overgeneralized memories.

Because these young people's depression and IES scores showed that they were *not* distressed by this trauma in their past at the time of assessment, one might ask why such nonspecificity matters. It matters because, if overgenerality is a latent vulnerability factor, it will have its impact later, downstream, if a person suffers other stressful events. There are several studies that show that this can occur.

Downstream Consequences of Overgeneralized Memory

Gibbs and Rude (2004) studied 81 young adults (mean age = 21). They assessed their levels of overgeneralized memory and then, 4–6 weeks later, recorded life events that had occurred and examined the probability of depression. They found that there was a prediction of Time 2 depression symptoms (controlling for Time 1 scores) from the frequency of life events for each individual, depending on whether the individual had been above or below the median on overgeneralized memory at the start of the research period.

Similarly, Anderson, Goddard, and Powell (2010) examined 135 young adults (mean age = 22) as to whether life events predicted depression over a 14-week period. They found that if daily hassles were high, it made very little difference in depression symptoms at Time 2 for those who were *specific* in their preexisting memories. However, the depression symptoms at Time 2 rose by 50% in those who had shown overgeneralized memories at Time 1.

Finally, Sumner et al. (2011) studied 55 young people (mean age = 17). They looked at interpersonal stresses and whether they predicted depression over a 16-month period given different levels of overgeneralized memory at the outset. They found that the onset of a major depressive episode (MDE) was much more probable over this period of time as a function of the specificity of memories for those who suffered interpersonal stress. For those with specific memories, the probability of MDE onset was not affected, even if these people had a number of interpersonal stresses. However, with high interpersonal stress *and* overgeneralized memories, the risk of major depression was high.

Williams et al. (2007) proposed that three key variables can account for overgeneralized memory. First, overgeneralized memory is more likely if a person is easily "captured" by self-referential material and then starts to ruminate about it. Second, overgeneralized memory is more likely if people have reduced executive capacity for any reason, as is often the case in depression (Dalgleish et al., 2007). The third factor, which is of interest here, is that people are more likely to be overgeneral if they have suffered trauma or adversity in the past because they attempt to regulate affect by truncating retrieval of memories (Raes et al., 2003). Overgenerality can remain as a scar, a latent vulnerability factor, that is created by trauma in the past and then acts as a moderator in the future of further negative life events, making an *onset* of major depression more likely. Does it also predict *chronicity*?

Brittlebank, Scott, Williams, and Ferrier (1993), Dalgleish, Spinks, Yiend, and Kuyken (2001), and Peeters, Wessel, Merckelbach, and Boon-Vermeeren (2002) all found that people who had overgeneralized memory early on in their depressive illness were more likely to still be depressed at a second time of testing 3–7 months later. Similarly, Hermans et al. (2008) found that overgeneralized memory at the outset of the episode predicted whether clients still met diagnostic criteria for depression months later. This association of overgenerality with chronicity is clearly important, in that it provides a psychological variable that is associated with difficult-to-modify "trait" factors or previous experience but is itself modifiable.

In summary, overgeneralized memory provides an explanation for why some people are at higher risk of depression than others given interpersonal stresses and life events. It can be a scar of previous trauma that remains as a latent vulnerability factor until further life events come along. It is due to a combination of processes: increased capture and rumination, increased avoidance, and increased executive impairment. Of particular interest here is the association between overgeneralized memory and avoidance following previous trauma. But whatever the processes underlying it, there seems compelling evidence that it can remain as a vulnerability factor, not only increasing the risk of depression given further stress but also prolonging that depression and making it more chronic.

How Might Mindfulness Help?

One of the distinctive things about mindfulness is that it provides a mental training that decreases attentional capture and rumination, reduces avoidance, and increases executive control. We would therefore expect mindfulness training to reduce overgeneralized memory and thereby reduce trait vulnerability. Williams, Teasdale, Segal, and Soulsby (2000) found that, compared with the "treatment as usual" (TAU) group, MBCT reduced overgeneralized memory. An important replication of this finding has been conducted by Heeren, Van Broeck, and Philippot (2009). They looked at specific memories before and after mindfulness training and found no difference in the control group but a large change in specificity in the MBCT group, with mindfulness decreasing overgeneralized memories.

Possible Changes in MBCT to Deal with Chronicity Due to Trauma

MBCT was originally designed for relapse *prevention*, offered to those who are between episodes of depression. In this it seems to be remarkably successful: In six randomized controlled trials (total $N = 593$), MBCT has been found to be highly efficacious in preventing relapse in clients with a recurrent course of the disorder, reducing risk of depression by an average of 44% across the trials and being equivalent to antidepressant medication in two of these trials (Piet & Hougaard, 2011).

However, MBCT is now being increasingly used in those for whom other treatments have failed. These studies have shown that MBCT may be successfully extended to the treatment of clients with acute treatment-resistant (Eisendraht et al., 2008) and chronic (Barnhofer et al., 2009) depression. Understanding the ways in which mindfulness meditation may affect cognitive processes involved in symptom maintenance will help to further develop this approach for the treatment of chronic depression.

Taking into account current symptoms and the fact that chronic symptoms often translate into difficulties in general motivation to initiate any behavior, any new treatment may need to combine intensive training in mindfulness meditation with new elements such as behavioral activation techniques (aimed at reducing symptoms at an early treatment stage). Behavioral activation interventions help clients to reengage in their lives through focused activation strategies, such as activity scheduling and monitoring, that systematically reduce avoidant tendencies (Dimidjian & Davis, 2009).

Second, MBCT may need to take into account the role that trauma has played in producing chronicity. In doing so, it will need to draw on current psychological models of trauma and the treatments that are derived from these models. For example, our current research using MBCT for suicidal depression takes explicit account of how memories of trauma may be qualitatively different from the other distressing thinking and imagery that often arise with depression. Whereas depressive thinking is more verbal and ruminative in nature, traumatic memories often have a "here and now" quality, are more vivid, and may come in the form of images in several sensory modalities. It may seem to clients that techniques that have previously been helpful may not apply here. Meditation teachers need to know the "map of the territory" so that they can respond if and where necessary by explaining the nature of traumatic imagery; in particular, that traumatic memories are more intrusive because (1) they are more fragmented, (2) they are not well integrated in memory, and (3) they occur in response to triggers that may be difficult to identify. Furthermore, traumatic memories are more likely to produce flashforwards as well as flashbacks, especially if there is imagery concerning suicide and suicidal behavior (Holmes, Crane, Fennell, & Williams, 2007; Crane, Shah, Barnhofer, & Holmes, 2012). Finally, traumatic imagery is more likely to produce strongly negative thoughts and feelings (see Figure 6.1) in which the person feels irreversibly damaged and that nothing will change.

Mindfulness teachers may encourage and help clients in a number of ways—for example, to encourage more flexibility, highlighting the possibility of deliberately moving closer *and away again* from distressing images

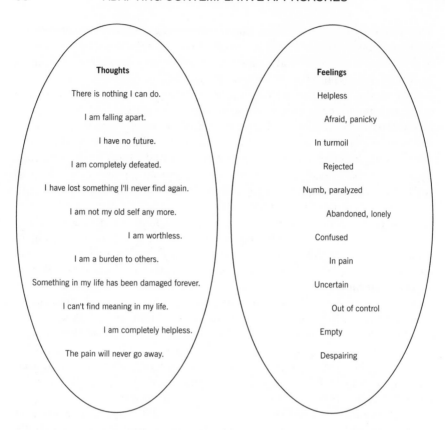

FIGURE 6.1. The territory of despair. Examples of the kinds of thoughts and feelings that arise in people who are highly vulnerable to becoming depressed and suicidal and who may have suffered trauma and adversity in the past. Based on Orbach, Mikulincer, Gilboa-Schechtman, and Sirota (2003).

and their bodily expression; grounding in body sensations or breath; and stressing the role of kindness and compassion in both moving toward and moving away.

Conclusion

Chronic depression is a huge burden to those who suffer from it, to their families, and to society as a whole. It has a genetic component, but it is also closely associated with a history of trauma and adversity. However, knowing about genetic and historical variables cannot help us in treatment. For this, we need to know what effect these biological or historical factors have on psychological variables that are modifiable. We have seen that one candidate variable is overgeneralized memory. It is affected by trauma; it increases the risk of an onset of depression and increases the risk that, once mood is disturbed, it will become chronic. MBCT has been found to reduce overgenerality in memory, but it was designed to prevent relapse in those currently in remission, so modifications to mindfulness programs will need to be made for the specific treatment of chronic and unremitting depression in which trauma has been a factor. These modifications will need to take into account the tendency of memory to be overgeneralized in such clients; the multisensorial nature of trauma memories and flashbacks; the way these may lead to flashforwards (intrusive images of the future); and the extremely aversive negative thoughts and feelings that predict a completely hopeless future.

These are some of the challenges of working with those who suffer such severe and prolonged affective disturbance, but the early indications are that mindfulness and acceptance-based approaches may have more to offer than we have previously seen in the history of psychological treatment research.

References

Anderson, R. J., Goddard, L., & Powell, J. H. (2010). Reduced specificity of autobiographical memory as a moderator of the relationship between daily hassles and depression. *Cognition and Emotion, 24,* 702–709.

Barnhofer, T., Crane, C., Hargus, E., Amarasinghe, M., Winder, R., & Williams, J. M. G. (2009). Mindfulness-based cognitive therapy as a treatment for chronic depression: A preliminary study. *Behaviour Research and Therapy, 47,* 366–373.

Boland, R. J., & Keller, M. B. (2009). Course and outcome of depression. In I. H. Gotlib & C. L. Hammen (Eds.), *Handbook of depression* (2nd ed., pp. 23–43). New York: Guilford Press.

Brennen, T., Hasanovic, M., Zotovic, M., Blix, I., Solheim-Skar, A. M., Prelic, N. K., et al. (2010). Trauma exposure in childhood impairs the ability to recall specific autobiographical memories in late adolescence. *Journal of Traumatic Stress, 23,* 240–247.

Brittlebank, A. D., Scott, J., Williams, J. M. G., & Ferrier, I. N. (1993). Autobiographical memory in depression: State or trait marker? *British Journal of Psychiatry, 162,* 118–121.

Bryant, R. A., Sutherland, K., & Guthrie, R. M. (2007). Impaired specific autobiographical memory as a risk factor for posttraumatic stress after trauma. *Journal of Abnormal Psychology, 116,* 837–841.

Crane, C., Shah, D., Barnhofer, T., & Holmes, E. A. (2012). Suicidal imagery in a previously depressed community sample. *Clinical Psychology and Psychotherapy, 19,* 57–69.

Cuijpers, P., van Straten, A., Schuurmans, J., van Oppen, P., Hollon, S. D., &

Andersson, G. (2010). Psychotherapy for chronic major depression and dysthymia: A meta-analysis. *Clinical Psychology Review, 30,* 51–62.

Dalgleish, T., Spinks, H., Yiend, J., & Kuyken, W. (2001). Autobiographical memory style in seasonal affective disorder and its relationship to future symptoms remission. *Journal of Abnormal Psychology, 110,* 335–340.

Dalgleish, T., Williams, J. M. G., Golden, A. M., Perkins, N., Feldman Barrett, L., Barnard, P., et al. (2007). Reduced specificity of autobiographical memory and depression: The role of executive control. *Journal of Experimental Psychology, 136,* 23–42.

Dimidjian, S., & Davis, K. J. (2009). Newer variations of cognitive-behavioral therapy: Behavioral activation and mindfulness-based cognitive therapy. *Current Psychiatry Reports, 11,* 453–458.

Eisendraht, S. J., Delucchi, K., Bitner, R., Fenimore, P., Smit, M., & McLane, M. (2008). Mindfulness-based cognitive therapy for treatment-resistant depression: A pilot study. *Psychotherapy and Psychosomatics, 77,* 319–320.

Geddes, J. R., Carney, S. M., Davies, C., Furukawa, T. A., Kupfer, D. J., Frank, E., et al. (2003). Relapse prevention with antidepressant drug treatment in depressive disorders: A systematic review. *Lancet, 361,* 653–661.

Gibbs, B. R., & Rude, S. S. (2004). Overgeneral autobiographical memory as depression vulnerability. *Cognitive Therapy and Research, 28,* 511–526.

Harvey, A. G., Bryant, R. A., & Dang, S. T. (1998). Autobiographical memory in acute stress disorder. *Journal of Consulting and Clinical Psychology, 66,* 500–506.

Heeren, A., Van Broeck, N., & Philippot, P. (2009). The effects of mindfulness on executive processes and autobiographical memory specificity. *Behaviour Research and Therapy, 47,* 403–409.

Hermans, D., Vandromme, H., Debeer, E., Raes, F., Demyttenaere, K., Brunfaut, E., et al. (2008). Overgeneral autobiographical memory predicts diagnostic status in depression. *Behaviour Research and Therapy, 46,* 668–677.

Holmes, E. A., Crane, C., Fennell, M. J. V., & Williams, J. M. G. (2007). Imagery about suicide in depression: "Flash-forwards"? *Journal of Behavior Therapy and Experimental Psychiatry, 38,* 423–434.

Horowitz, M., Wilner, N., & Alvarez, W. (1979). Impact of Event Scale: A measure of subjective stress. *Psychosomatic Medicine, 41,* 209–218.

Judd, L. L., Schettler, P. J., Solomon, D. A., Maser, J. D., Coryell, W., Endicott, J., et al. (2008). Psychosocial disability and work role function compared across the long-term course of bipolar I, bipolar II, and unipolar major depressive disorders. *Journal of Affective Disorders, 108,* 49–58.

Keller, M. B., McCullough, J. P., Klein, D. N., Arnow, B., Dunner, D., Gelenber, A. J., et al. (2000). A comparison of nefazodon, the cognitive-behavioral-analysis system of psychotherapy, and their combination for the treatment of chronic depression. *New England Journal of Medicine, 342,* 1462–1470.

Kennedy, N., Abbott, R., & Paykel, E. S. (2004). Longitudinal syndromal and subsyndromal symptoms after severe depression: 10-year follow-up study. *British Journal of Psychiatry, 184,* 330–336.

Kleim, B., & Ehlers, A. (2008). Reduced autobiographical memory specificity predicts depression and posttraumatic stress disorder after recent trauma. *Journal of Consulting and Clinical Psychology, 76,* 231–242.

Klein, D. N. (2010). Chronic depression: Diagnosis and classification. *Current Directions in Psychological Science, 19*, 96–100.

Lizardi, H., Klein, D. N., Ouimette, P. C., Riso, L. P., Anderson, R., & Donaldson, S. K. (1995). Reports of the childhood home-environment in early-onset dysthymia and episodic major depression. *Journal of Abnormal Psychology, 104*, 132–139.

Mathers, C., Boerma, T., & Ma Fat, D. (2008). *The global burden of disease: 2004 update.* Geneva, Switzerland: World Health Organization.

McNally, R. J., Lasko, N. B., Macklin, M. L., & Pitman, R. K. (1995). Autobiographical memory disturbance in combat-related posttraumatic stress disorder. *Behaviour Research and Therapy, 33*, 619–630.

Moore, S. A., & Zoellner, L. A. (2007). Overgeneral autobiographical memory and traumatic events: An evaluative review. *Psychological Bulletin, 133*, 419–437.

Orbach, I., Mikulincer, M., Gilboa-Schechtman, E., & Sirota, P. (2003). Mental pain and its relationship to suicidality and life meaning. *Suicide and Life-Threatening Behavior, 33*, 231–241.

Peeters, F., Wessel, I., Merckelbach, H., & Boon-Vermeeren, M. (2002). Autobiographical memory specificity and the course of major depressive disorder. *Comprehensive Psychiatry, 43*, 344–350.

Piet, J., & Hougaard, E. (2011). The effect of mindfulness-based cognitive therapy for prevention of relapse in recurrent major depressive disorder: A review and meta-analysis. *Clinical Psychology Review, 31*, 1032–1040.

Raes, F., Hermans, D., de Decker, A., Eelen, P., & Williams, J. M. G. (2003). Autobiographical memory specificity and affect regulation: An experimental approach. *Emotion, 3*, 201–206.

Sumner, J. A., Griffith, J. W., Mineka, S., Rekart, K. N., Zinbarg, R. E., & Craske, M. G. (2011). Overgeneral autobiographical memory and chronic interpersonal stress as predictors of the course of depression in adolescents. *Cognition and Emotion, 25*, 183–192.

Tennant, C. (2002). Life events, stress and depression: A review of recent findings. *Australian and New Zealand Journal of Psychiatry, 36*, 173–182.

Williams, J. M. G., Barnhofer, T., Crane, C., Herman, D., Raes, F., Watkins, E., et al. (2007). Autobiographical memory specificity and emotional disorder. *Psychological Bulletin, 133*, 122–148.

Williams, J. M. G., & Broadbent, K. (1986). Autobiographical memory in suicide attempters. *Journal of Abnormal Psychology, 95*, 144–149.

Williams, J. M. G., & Scott, J. (1988). Autobiographical memory in depression. *Psychological Medicine, 18*, 689–695.

Williams, J. M. G., Teasdale, J. D., Segal, Z. V., & Soulsby, J. (2000). Mindfulness-based cognitive therapy reduces overgeneral autobiographical memory in formerly depressed patients. *Journal of Abnormal Psychology, 109*, 150–155.

7

Eye Movement Desensitization and Reprocessing and Buddhist Practice

A New Model of Posttraumatic Stress Disorder Treatment

Deborah Rozelle and David J. Lewis

EMDR Treatment for Posttraumatic Stress Disorder

Eye movement desensitization and reprocessing (EMDR) is a trauma-focused, individual therapy for posttraumatic stress disorder (PTSD) and related maladies. Though its best-known element is bilateral visual, auditory, or tactile stimuli, EMDR is a complete, well-articulated, integrative treatment system with elements from cognitive, behavioral, humanistic, body-based, and psychodynamic therapies (Shapiro & Maxfield, 2003, p. 197; Shapiro, 2002, pp. 5–6), as well as contemplative methods. EMDR posits that PTSD is a memory and information processing disorder (Schubert & Lee, 2009, pp. 119–120; Stickgold, 2008, p. 289; van der Kolk, 1994) and that therapeutic change involves the client exploring and processing personal networks of memories, fears, assumptions, perceptions, and somatic reactions that maintain the chronic dysfunction (Adler-Tapia & Settle, 2008, pp. 3–4; Van der Kolk, McFarlane, & Van der Hart, 1996, pp. 419–420).

Though EMDR stimulated questions from its introduction in 1989 about the quality of research supporting its claims for efficacy (Herbert et al., 2000), numerous studies, meta-analyses, and professional bodies have subsequently established it as a first-line psychological treatment for PTSD, equal in efficacy to prolonged exposure (PE) or trauma-focused cognitive-behavioral therapy (TF-CBT; Spates, Koch, Cusack, Pagoto, & Waller, 2009, p. 288; Bisson et al., 2007). The major remaining substantive issue is the role and even necessity of bilateral stimulation or eye movements, which we consider in this chapter and which is significantly addressed by recent research.

EMDR and Buddhism

EMDR has not to date been considered an explicitly contemplative therapy (Lipke, 2000, p. 83; Smyth & Poole, 2002, p. 159). We propose, however, that there is substantial correspondence between EMDR and a large range of Buddhist practices, including cultivation of both concentrated attention and transformative insight. We can therefore consider EMDR implicitly contemplative, illuminate its mechanisms of action through the lens of Buddhist thought and practice, and cast new light on trauma therapy. This correspondence amounts to a new model of PTSD treatment and might also point the way toward more effective and efficient use of contemplative methods in general for trauma.

We structure this chapter around a case example that presents the basics of EMDR with reflections on its correlations with Buddhist practice.

Case Example: "My World Is Shrinking"

EMDR is used for PTSD at all levels of severity and complexity, but to show the correspondence of EMDR with Buddhism clearly, we present a case of treating debilitating PTSD symptomology due to an isolated traumatic incident, combining and modifying some actual cases. The client, Tina (a pseudonym), was a 40-year-old woman who came to me (D. R.) for treatment of PTSD. Tina was a proud, independent woman with a strong presence and the toughness of a true survivor. Despite earlier significant traumatic events and major life stressors, Tina had been relatively resilient, with a strong, secure attachment history, and did not exhibit clinical PTSD until the tragic death of her best friend 3 years prior. For several reasons Tina requested short-term therapy, so we agreed to target only the recent trauma associated with her current PTSD symptoms.

Tina and her friend were walking on a sidewalk when a drunk driver swerved off the street and struck her friend, who died at the scene in Tina's arms. In the hours and days after the tragedy, Tina developed a wide range of traumatic reactions, many debilitating. But rather than abate on their own, as happens in a majority of trauma survivors, Tina's symptoms worsened, defied her willful attempts to stop them, and had a severe impact on her life. The reactions and their persistence constitute the definition of PTSD, which occurs in a significant minority of trauma survivors.

Characteristically, Tina *reexperienced* the trauma regularly and in various ways: frequent nightmares and unbidden waking images of her friend's death, both spontaneously and in response to *triggers,* such as television car chases, that reminded her of the trauma and evoked maladaptive reactions. The images were replete with vivid details, as if the trauma were happening right then and there, and they produced in the present many of the same reactions—strong horror, despair, and a range of *hyperarousal* and *hypoarousal* reactions—that she experienced during and soon after the traumatic event. Each reexperiencing robbed Tina of whatever calm and perspective she had mustered since the previous episode. She had numerous other *numbing, avoidance,* and *hypervigilance* effects, such as rarely leaving her apartment; inability to feel love for her children and friends and shame at being useless to them, as she had been to her friend; and avoiding the area of the accident or any place like it. Tina's resilience was all but gone, and time was not healing her. As Tina herself said, "My world is shrinking."

PTSD and Buddhism: An Asymmetric Analogy

PTSD touches every aspect of life with a wide range of debilitating symptoms. But reexperiencing in particular threatens to reignite the suffering of trauma at almost any moment and underlies much of the other dysfunction. Like many researchers and clinicians, we therefore regard the phenomenological root of PTSD to be intrusive, persistent, preconceptual reexperiencing of the traumatic event or events and their distress as if they were occurring in the here and now rather than in the past (Brewin, Lanius, Novac, Schnyder, & Galea, 2009, pp. 369–370; Ehlers, 2010; Michael, Ehlers, Halligan, & Clark, 2005; Thompson & Waltz, 2010, p. 409; van der Kolk & MacFarlane, 1996, pp. 9–15).[1] We may thus think of PTSD as a realm of suffering rooted in a kind of delusion, a deep, persistent, preconceptual misapprehension about the nature of the sufferer's experience that significantly distorts his or her experience of place, time, memory, and identity.

On the other hand, Buddhism posits that *everybody's ordinary*

---

[1]Others have proposed that avoidance is the core symptom of PTSD (Thompson & Waltz, 2010, p. 409) from angles such as statistical correlation and justification of therapies that primarily address avoidance. Avoidance and reexperiencing are actually related, because avoidance, deliberate or unconscious, presumably exists largely to prevent the distress of triggers and reexperiencing.

experience is in fact a realm of suffering called *samsara*. The suffering of samsara arises not only overtly from obvious pain and loss but also subtly from clinging to what we ordinarily see as pleasure and gain, because such experiences are transient and will inevitably end. And, as in PTSD, Buddhism conceives the root of samsara and its suffering to be a fundamental delusion, a misapprehension.[2] The samsaric misapprehension, however, is far deeper and more extensive than that of PTSD. According to Buddhism we pervasively misapprehend the true nature of the self, and of all things in the world, as separate, noninterdependent, permanent entities, unconnected with and actually in opposition to one another, when in fact they are intertwined in an ever-changing, interdependent web of cause and effect (Hanh, 2012, pp. 136–137, 518).

Even though the symptoms of PTSD are within samsara, PTSD is a distinct, pervasive, and persistent constellation fueled by the additional misapprehension of traumatic reexperiencing. We therefore draw a phenomenological analogy between samsara and PTSD: Each is a realm of suffering rooted in its respective nonconceptual misapprehension. There is much more to the analogy than we address in this chapter, including the theoretical relationship between the two misapprehensions; here we focus, however, on mechanisms of therapeutic action, comparing Buddhist practice and EMDR, creating, in effect, a new treatment model. The ideal goal of both PTSD therapy and Buddhism is to end a client's respective root misapprehension and thus decisively relieve his or her associated level of suffering. Buddhist practice does that by delivering experiential, nonconceptual insight into the samsaric misapprehension (Bodhi, 2013). EMDR, as we discuss, likewise acts by fostering experiential insight into the traumatic misapprehension, helping the client to realize that the traumatic event is just a memory and no longer threatening.

There is a significant asymmetry to the analogy; it is not an equivalence. Buddhism addresses ultimate questions of reality, existence, roots of all kinds of suffering, overt and subtle, and liberation from those roots, and its goal is enlightenment, a state beyond sorrow. By contrast, the primary goal of trauma therapy is to relieve the relatively overt suffering of PTSD and return the client to common unhappiness (Freud, 1895), that is, samsara. Buddhist practice aims at the realization that the everyday self does not exist in the way we commonly perceive it, as a singular, unitary, independent, unchanging identity, whereas EMDR, indeed any conventional psychotherapy, accepts an everyday self as the ground of ordinary experience.

---

[2]There is no simple English term that captures the complexity of Buddhist words often translated as "delusion" or "ignorance," and of course delusion is also a complex concept in psychology with many overtones. For the remainder of the chapter, we therefore use the more neutral word *misapprehension* with this extended meaning, in both PTSD and Buddhism.

Case Example Continued: The Safe Place Resource

After taking Tina's history and doing an initial assessment, I guide Tina to create an imagined, personal *safe place*, a multimodal image in which she feels calm, grounded, and secure from perceived threats in the present. I explain to her the instructions for working in EMDR: Just let whatever happens happen; there's no right or wrong; she's in charge and can stop any time. This encourages Tina to use primed, mostly silent *free associa-tion* with personal material, a fundamental process in EMDR whereby the client "moves sequentially through related material" that arises spontane-ously, with minimal input from the therapist (Shapiro, 2001, p. 321).

DEBORAH: Think of a place, real or imagined, where you feel calm, con-tent, peaceful, comfortable. Notice if this place is outside or inside, whether you are alone or with someone, what you are doing or not doing, what time of day it is, other details.

TINA: I'm thinking about when I fished with my dad as a kid. We had great conversations, a good time. Sometimes we took a boat ride. I have always liked nature, water.

DEBORAH: Notice what you see, how you feel.

TINA: I see the trees, bank, my dad, our poles.

DEBORAH: What feelings do you notice as you remember this scene?

TINA: Peaceful. Everything is balanced. A great sense of well-being.

DEBORAH: What does your body feel?

TINA: Calming. Soothing. One with the world.

DEBORAH: Good. Think about that as you follow my fingers; let whatever happens just happen.

[I place my left index and middle finger together, upright, about 2 feet from Tina's eyes and move them horizontally back and forth within her visual field, about one cycle per second for 5 or 6 seconds (or up to a minute or two and a bit faster in later sessions). I ask Tina to track my fin-gers with her eyes without moving her head. We do not talk so that Tina can follow her thoughts wherever they take her. This constitutes one *set* of free association with bilateral stimulation (*BLS set*), the fundamental EMDR unit for both resource development and, to come later, trauma processing.]

[I gently stop moving my fingers.]

DEBORAH: Take an easy breath. What is happening now?

TINA: Relaxing. I feel the sun. Enjoying the water.

DEBORAH: Good. Go with that. [We do another BLS set. Afterward Tina appears relaxed and lighthearted.]

DEBORAH: Take another easy breath. What do you notice now?

TINA: I got a tabletop water fountain as a gift. It sits on one of my little tables at home. It's funny. I put it next to my parents' photos. Never realized how they connected before. At home, I listen to my fountain, along with monks chanting. So peaceful.

[Tina makes her first linkage to associated material during free association, a fundamental occurrence that we discuss at length below.]

Safe Place and Other Resources

Safe place is the most prominent example of a *resource* in EMDR (Korn & Leeds, 2002), a positive antidote to negative states, a tool for the client to self-regulate so he or she can approach and stay in contact with his or her traumatic memories and overcome blockages in processing. Developing resources is the *stability phase* of EMDR therapy, which aligns with the initial phase in the consensus model of trauma-informed treatment (Korn & Leeds, 2002). Tina will invoke her safe place to regulate her arousal and reduce her symptoms in reaction to traumatic material, a crucial function for the success of trauma processing.

Trauma Processing

With safe place and other stability phase resources (not covered in this chapter) in hand, Tina begins the *trauma processing phase*. She works directly with traumatic material using EMDR's trauma processing protocol (Leeds, 2009; Shapiro, 2001, pp. 69–75, 222–226). Trauma processing also uses BLS sets, but the protocol is considerably more elaborate. In treatment planning Tina and I chose targets for processing, each a traumatic memory, present-day trigger, or template for future action. Following in condensed form is the processing of the single traumatic memory target for Tina's brief course of treatment.

Case Example Continued: Trauma Processing

DEBORAH: Rally your positive qualities and resources, including your safe place, going fishing with your dad.

TINA: OK, I'm ready. (*Looks at me with gentle determination.*)

DEBORAH: Bring up the image of a worst moment, your friend being killed. What do you see?

TINA: (*Shivers dramatically.*) I couldn't get the blood off of me, and the smell. I threw those clothes away.

[Tina's first intentional engagement with traumatic material is important. I see in her body that she is in contact with the memory, aroused but coping successfully, having already reduced her symptoms somewhat and invoked her safe place at the beginning of the session.]

DEBORAH: As you see that, what's a thought about yourself now that's not so good, a negative belief?

TINA: I can never get clean, I'm unworthy.

[Tina thus identifies the NC (*negative cognition*) for this target, which further articulates and concretizes the traumatic material she has so far failed to process.]

DEBORAH: And when you see that scene, that worst moment, what would you *rather* think about yourself now, instead of "I'm unworthy"?

TINA: I'm worthy. But it's not really true.

DEBORAH: (*reassuringly*) That's OK. On a scale of from 1 to 7, 1 being totally false, 7 completely true, how true are the words "I'm worthy" as you think of this scene?

TINA: 2? 3?

[We thus establish the PC (*positive/preferred cognition*) for this target and begin tracking its strength. Depending on the client's capacity, the PC can reflect the final goal or remain understated for now to avoid unrealistic expectations and despair.]

DEBORAH: As you think of that scene, of the blood and smell, what emotions, feelings do you notice?

TINA: Useless! There was nothing I could do. Helpless.

DEBORAH: So on a scale of 0 to 10, 0 being no distress or neutral, 10 the worst ever, how distressing is this memory to you now?

TINA: An 8.

DEBORAH: Where do you feel that distress in your body, besides the smell?

TINA: Chill up my spine. No sweating.

[We thus locate the body sensations associated with the trauma. Tina is now ready for free association.]

DEBORAH: All right, now let's put the pieces together. Think of the blood and smell, the thought "I'm unworthy," the feelings of being useless, helpless, the chill up your spine.

[We execute a series of BLS sets, with Tina internally following material as it arises. During the third set she shivers again and makes a repulsive face.]

DEBORAH: Take an easy breath. What do you get now?

TINA: Ughhhh, I felt the chill. (*Coughs and sneezes.*)

DEBORAH: (*With a gentle, steady voice*) Yes, just notice. [Another BLS set.]

TINA: I'm trying to stay calm. I kept feeling the chill in my back. Then I thought of my dad, fishing. [Another BLS set.]

[Tina's body is visibly calmer after the distress, presumably through the implicit and explicit use of her safe place and other resources. She is effectively self-regulating, titrating rather than avoiding her reaction to remain in contact with the traumatic material.]

TINA: You know, I can cope, I can handle it. I know what happened. I can deal. (*Reports a drop in distress from 8 out of 10 to 5.*)

DEBORAH: What keeps it at a 5?

TINA: I was useless. I *couldn't* save her!

DEBORAH: So, here is a question. Given what your father knew about you, would he have said you were useless?

TINA: (*Looks a bit perplexed; pauses and says gently*) No.

DEBORAH: Go with that. [A BLS set.]

TINA: That helps. He loved me no matter what.

DEBORAH: Go with that. [A BLS set.]

TINA: I wanted so much to save her. She was a great person. She was my best friend.

[This intervention, called an *interweave*, helps Tina unblock her processing. An interweave is a proactive intervention, used sparingly, that helps the client overcome blocks and cycles in his or her processing (Shapiro, 2001, pp. 244–247). Interweaves can be cognitive, affective, somatic, and presented in many forms; this one is Socratic and uses a corrective self-perception based on Tina's secure attachment.]

Trauma Target, Exposure, and Suffering

Tina primed the session with the memory image, NC, emotions and body sensations associated with the traumatic memory, which constitute the target to be processed. Working directly with traumatic material is called *exposure*. All first-line treatments for PTSD use exposure (Foa, Keane, Friedman & Cohen, 2010, p. 551) in some form, but EMDR entails much less exposure than TF-CBT (Ho & Lee, 2012), and the exposure is less intensive (Lee, Taylor, & Drummond, 2006). In this session Tina consciously or unconsciously contrasted her traumatic memory with present safety, reflecting a classical exposure mechanism (Rauch & Foa, 2006, pp. 63–64) to partly dissolve the traumatic misapprehension. But EMDR adds the subjective safety and calm of safe place and other resources, which arguably enhances the effect. Also, as we discuss, EMDR has other modes of change.

EMDR as Meditation

Buddhist meditation has two aspects: *concentration* (*shamatha, calm abiding*) and *insight* (*vipashyana*; Gunaratana, 2011). Concentration is heightened attention with stability and clarity; the mind neither wanders with excitement nor sinks into dullness (Wallace, 2006, p. 14). Insight meditation uses concentration to cut through misapprehension and experientially realize the true nature of self and phenomena, thereby relieving suffering.

EMDR's mostly silent, interior exploration is not formal meditation, but it has a general meditative quality and, most important, is *functionally* analogous for trauma processing to both aspects of Buddhist practice. Using resources such as safe place, Tina's exclamation, "I can cope, I can handle it" reclaimed capacities lost since her friend's death. She regulated her reactions to traumatic material with resources, staying within her *window of tolerance* between hypoarousal and hyperarousal (Minton, Ogden, & Pain, 2006, pp. 26–29) to remain alert and calm, just as a meditator employs antidotes to dullness and overexcitement to achieve stable and clear concentration. Though the EMDR client's concentration is only modestly heightened by ordinary standards, his or her improved ability to stay in contact with traumatic and related material is as much an accomplishment relative to his or her usual traumatic reactivity as trained concentrative meditation is to ordinary, easily distracted attention. EMDR's resources thus correspond functionally to meditative concentration.

Furthermore, just as the Buddhist meditator's concentration enables nonconceptual insight that undermines samsaric misapprehension, the EMDR client's alert and calm state enables processing and resolution of traumatic material. Tina's flash of experiential insight, "I know what happened," cut through some of her traumatic misapprehension and produced a measurable reduction in reexperiencing and distress. Trauma processing thus corresponds through the analogy to the insight aspect of meditation.

PC and Aspiration

The PC is an aspect of what we call the *positive pole* of EMDR, which also includes resources and affective interweaves. The positive pole is an integral aspect of EMDR therapy (Lipke, 2000, pp. 67, 73–83) with several important functions that correlate with Buddhist practice. At this point

Tina's PC is a concrete expression of her aspiration to heal, corresponding to the equally pivotal function of motivation in Buddhism (Harvey, 2000, pp. 190–191). As with motivation in Buddhist practice, the client invokes the PC near the beginning of each session, and it exerts a vital influence throughout, often below conscious awareness, to keep processing moving in a positive direction and undercut avoidance. My encouragement about Tina's still weak PC helps cultivate self-compassion (Germer & Neff, Chapter 3, this volume), assuring that her suffering can be healed even though it seems entrenched. This corresponds through the asymmetric analogy to the principle of *Buddha Nature* (Makransky, 2007, pp. 3, 35), every being's inherent capacity to end his or her its suffering through enlightenment.

Case Example Continued: Free Association

Tina continues processing the target traumatic memory using EMDR's style of mostly silent free association with no explicit interpretation by either of us. She does not dwell continuously or forcefully on the traumatic image (Greenwald, 2007, p. 41). Instead, she calmly follows sequences of associated thoughts, such as positive and negative memories, feelings and body sensations, from her past, present, and future, sometimes returning to the trauma itself. EMDR imposes no theoretical constraints, and I do not direct the process other than to help choose the initial target and offer interweaves, so Tina mostly goes where her associations take her. EMDR's free association thus appears to mobilize and assist the natural process by which most trauma survivors resolve traumatic distress, failure of which leads to PTSD.

Tina's particular associations revolve around life in her apartment, her friend's family, the neighborhood where the accident happened, childhood events, and other memories. She stops and focuses attention on many of them, gaining realizations small and large that reduce her traumatic distress in various ways. For example, after one set Tina reports thinking about her father's unexpected death years earlier. After several BLS sets processing that and associated memories, she arrives at the realization, "It was hard but I'm OK with it; I miss him, but he's still with me." After more processing she links her father's death explicitly to the recent trauma: "If I can feel that with my father, maybe I can do it with my friend," and with that her distress level for the target image drops significantly.

Free Association and Analytical Meditation

The moving attention of EMDR's free association, engaging and following thoughts as they arise, seems less like meditation, especially in the mindfulness tradition, and more like its antithesis, unrestrained distraction, engaging objects rather than letting them go (Lutz, Slagter, Dunne, & Davidson, 2009, pp. 6–7). An important Tibetan Buddhist insight practice, however, called *analytical meditation,* uses a combination of nondistracted moving and fixed attention (G. K. Gyatso, 1995, pp. 89–94; Gelek, 2005) and is analogous in many ways to EMDR's free association. Meditators use analytical meditation to realize the fundamental misapprehension of noninterdependence, as well as points along the way, such as impermanence, and to develop supporting qualities, such as compassion (G. K. Gyatso, 1995, pp. 394–446; Dodson-Lavelle, Ozawa-De Silva, Negi, & Raison, Chapter 22, this volume). In analytical meditation, they assess a topic from multiple standpoints: part–whole analysis, logical inference, cause and effect, personal experience, introspective observation and questioning, emotions, or any cognitive, affective, or tangible aspects. They move among objects by similar connections. When during this moving attention an intuition or hint of realization arises on a point, the meditator focuses there to strengthen the understanding and gain insights.

The structure for free association is mainly the client's traumatic image and other targets chosen in treatment planning. Analytical meditation, by contrast, uses an extensive, predetermined scaffolding of universal topics such as impermanence, compassion and the misapprehended self, subtopics, linkages, reasonings, and intermediate conclusions drawn from texts and teachings (Pabongka, 1991). In both free association and analytical meditation, however, the practitioner evokes sequences of thoughts from his or her own perspective and experience within the respective scaffolding. EMDR's free association is therefore an analog of analytical meditation for processing traumatic material by exploring and integrating it with the personal web of connections.

Case Example Continued: Crucial Processing Episode

At this point Tina has processed many of the associations for this target and reduced her distress level to 3 out of 10; in EMDR we aim for 0 or 1.

DEBORAH: Bring up the memory of the accident. Notice a worst moment. What do you see?

TINA: (*With tears welling up*) She's gasping. I'm holding her and I don't know what to do.

DEBORAH: (*Gently but resolutely*) As you think of that moment, what's a thought about yourself that's not good, a negative belief about yourself?

TINA: It's my fault. I couldn't save her.

DEBORAH: (*Nodding in acknowledgment*) And so, as you see this image, what would you rather think about yourself?

TINA: (*Tentatively, vulnerably*) I am worthy?

DEBORAH: (*Gently*) That's OK. It may not feel very strong right now. On a scale of 1 to 7, how true do those words feel to you now?

TINA: Like a 3?

DEBORAH: As you think of this image, what feelings do you notice?

TINA: (*With tears rolling down her face*) I didn't want her to die. I was desperate. It was pure agony.

DEBORAH: Using the scale of 1 to 10, how big is the sense of agony and desperation to you now?

TINA: (*The tears continue*) A 6. [This new material comes with a spike in distress.]

DEBORAH: And where do you notice that in your body?

TINA: My eyes. My heart. My hands and arms.

DEBORAH: Put all those pieces together—the image of you holding her, the thought "it's my fault," the desperation and agony, those sensations in your eyes, heart, hands, and arms. Follow my fingers.

[We do a BLS set. Tina takes a deep breath.]

TINA: That's weird. It's amazing. My body, it feels gently rocked. Restful. Peaceful.

DEBORAH: Go with that. [Another BLS set.]

TINA: She was gasping for air. I held her close.

DEBORAH: Go with that. [Another BLS set.]

TINA: (*Tenderly*) Oh my, I just remembered something. I touched my hand to her cheek. I kissed her on her forehead and told her I loved her.

DEBORAH: (*Responding tenderly*) Yes. Go with that. [A longer BLS set.]

TINA: (*Coughs, yawns*) Even though the picture is in my head, it's not disturbing. No chills. I'm outside it for the first time in my life. Not in it. Stepped back. Like a movie. Could see me holding her. Not inside it, but outside it.

DEBORAH: Go with that. [Another BLS set.]

DEBORAH: How disturbing is it to you right now?

TINA: (*Speaking quietly*) It's just at 1 out of 10. I'm watching it. It was a terrible incident. I picture it. Good. (*Looks straight at me and smiles gently.*)

Insight and Realization

Tina rapidly moved from anguish to relief; from reexperiencing the trauma to witnessing it from the outside, a process and outcome called *disidentification (decentering, cognitive restructuring, defusion*; Vago & Silbersweig, 2012, p. 23; Shapiro, Carlson, Astin, & Freedman, 2006, pp. 77–78; Engle & Follette, Chapter 4, this volume); from stubborn, nonconceptual misapprehension to accurate insight. Her trauma became just a memory, integrated with all her other memories, rather than a disconnected, undigested experience that recurs unbidden with its original suffering. The sharp drop in distress and calm body while in contact with the traumatic memory confirmed that it was a positive, comprehensive shift, not avoidance or dissociation.

This kind of realization and far-reaching transformation lies at the heart of EMDR (Lee et al., 2006). EMDR therapists routinely report such insight, and the literature describes many of them, for example, Adler-Tapia and Settle (2008, pp. 176–191), Wachtel (2002, pp. 131–133), Parnell (1998), and van der Kolk (2002, pp. 73–77). Shapiro (2001, pp. 13, 42, 70) notes that "increase in self-efficacy, desensitization of negative affect, elicitation of insight, shifting of body tension, and a cognitive restructuring occur simultaneously as the dysfunctional information is processed." The client experiences many such realizations large and small, which drive the course of healing (Lee, 2008). Though there is not always a singular, dramatic breakthrough like Tina's, the major ones represent turning points that generalize and become platforms for further progress. This kind of event in EMDR corresponds at the psychological level with realizations in Buddhism, which can be large and small. And Buddhism's final attainment, enlightenment, is a decisive realization from one's depths, leading to a transformation of being and total and enduring relief from suffering (Gyatso, Hopkins & Napper, 2006, p. 223; Jinpa, 2000, p. 14). As we shall see, Tina's breakthrough indeed ended her reexperiencing and its direct traumatic suffering.

Tina's disidentification from the traumatic memory as she "stepped back" and placed the traumatic memory in proper context is a signature experience of EMDR (Parnell, 1998, p. 84; Parnell, 1996, pp. 139–141). *Disidentification* in Buddhism means no longer mistakenly identifying with the body and/or the mind as a permanent, independent self (Tsering, 2005, p. 46), which releases the practitioner from the fundamental misapprehension that maintains samsaric suffering (Aronson, 2006, pp. 78–79; McLeod, 2002, pp. 196–199; Bodhi, 1980). In EMDR, by contrast, the client disidentifies with his or her reexperiencing self and returns to his or her prior self, which, although no longer contaminated by the suffering of PTSD, is still perceived as permanent and independent and therefore still suffers in the samsaric sense.

EMDR and Psychological Mindfulness

How does EMDR compare with mindfulness-based systems of psychotherapy and behavioral medicine such as mindfulness-based stress reduction (MBSR), mindfulness-based cognitive therapy (MBCT), dialectical behavior therapy (DBT), and acceptance and commitment therapy (ACT), which we term *psychological mindfulness* (PM; Shapiro et al., 2006). Hölzel et al. (2011) reviewed empirically supported components of PM and consolidated them into: (1) attention regulation; (2) body awareness; (3) emotion regulation; (4) change in perspective on the self, described by different authors as disidentification from a static sense of self, *reperceiving, decentering,* and *observer perspective.* Because PM draws on only the initial stages of Buddhist practice, however, "studies do not describe the drastic change in the sense of self that highly experienced meditators have reported" (Hölzel et al., 2011, p. 548).

EMDR addresses all these components. Rather than formal meditation, however, EMDR's attention regulation is only an analog of meditative concentration. Nonetheless, EMDR's insight and disidentification experiences significantly, often dramatically, improve the functioning and quality of life of the client with PTSD. This supports the analogy model and the premise that EMDR is implicitly contemplative.

Insight and Sudden Gains

Psychology also studies insight in the form of "aha" experiences, sudden breakthroughs that solve a problem or produce new learning (Ash, Jee, & Wiley, 2012). This resonates with realization in both EMDR and Buddhist practice, particularly in the spontaneous nature of insight. Studies show that *sudden gains* in reducing PTSD symptoms from session to session occur in up to 50% of TF-CBT treatments (Aderka, Appelbaum-Namdar, Shafran, & Gilboa-Schechtman, 2011). Though there are no formal studies yet on sudden gains in EMDR, anecdotal evidence implies that they are at least as common. All this suggests that insight processes may be at work in other trauma therapies besides EMDR (Briere, Chapter 1, this volume), though in less obvious ways.

Bilateral Stimulation and Dual Attention

Though BLS has been questioned as perhaps extraneous, a recent metastudy (Lee & Cuijpers, 2012) on the additive effect of eye movements, correcting and updating an earlier metastudy (Davidson & Parker, 2001), found moderate effect size in therapeutic trials and large effect size in nontherapy studies. The merely moderate effect in therapy does not contradict EMDR's strong overall efficacy but reflects the fundamental structure of EMDR. BLS is not, as is widely misunderstood, the only or even the major therapeutic process in EMDR (Hyer & Brandsma, 1997). Rather, BLS is a *catalyst* that enhances the actual core process, information processing via mostly silent free association (Solomon & Shapiro, 2008, p. 321). Thus EMDR can indeed work without BLS, but it works better, often much better with BLS, which is consistent with the above metastudy results.

Studies on several hypothetical psychological and neurological mechanisms are suggestive but still inconclusive (Gunter & Bodner, 2009). To complement that work, we speculate about how BLS operates across the analogy with Buddhist practice, particularly the Vajrayana, the esoteric component of the Mahayana. Vajrayana is itself a kind of catalyst for Buddhist practice; it aims at the same goal as the Mahayana and also uses concentration and insight, but its techniques are said to be more potent and rapid (Tsering, 2012, pp. 9–10; Yeshe, 2001, p. 17).

The rhythmic character of BLS likely evokes the relaxation response (Lee et al., 2006, pp. 104–105) induced by numerous contemplative practices such as mantra recitation and visualization (Benson & Proctor, 2010, pp. 13–14, 24–25), both Vajrayana techniques. Repetitive attention in Vajrayana visualization is said to unblock mental energy (G. K. Gyatso, 2000, pp. 200–202), the psychological analog of which might be breaking up fixed cognitive and emotional patterns and increasing mental flexibility. BLS could thus help EMDR clients efficiently elicit and process linked memories, an often noted effect of EMDR (van der Kolk, 2002, pp. 72–78; Wachtel, 2002, pp. 131–133). Indeed, research has shown that eye movements improve recall and semantic flexibility (Kuiken, Bears, Miall, & Smith, 2001) and episodic memory (Propper & Christman, 2008). Also, BLS makes the client attend simultaneously to outer and inner events, an effect called *dual attention* (Lee et al., 2006, p. 98), which may subtly help juxtapose and integrate maladaptive inner traumatic experience with objective reality. The connection between inner and outer is an important theme of Vajrayana (G. K. Gyatso, 2000, p. 112; Yeshe, 2001, p. 3).

We may thus view BLS, like other aspects of EMDR, as an analog for individual trauma therapy of meditative methods. The BLS attention pattern is very simple compared to the almost unlimited intricacy of Vajrayana meditation, reflecting the asymmetry of the analogy. Because the therapist directly helps facilitate and maintain a meditative-like state, the client needs no training and only normal, not heightened, attentional control. Anchoring the client's attention outward and controlling the speed and duration of movement help regulate arousal and minimize inadvertent triggering of traumatic reactions from purely inward attention.

Toward a Metatheory:
Change in EMDR and Buddhist Practice

EMDR resolves traumatic material by juxtaposing it with contrasting material that integrates with and corrects the traumatic misapprehension (Solomon & Shapiro, 2008). In BLS sets, the client engages with traumatic material using relatively normal attention, and that is sufficient to effect change. The dissonant, corrective information then undermines specific misapprehensions, such as the here-and-nowness of the memory, the permanence of the suffering, or negative self-image.

There is an unlimited variety of such corrective information: experiential, cognitive, affective, somatic, relational, and reasoned material from past, present, and future, only a fraction of which involves direct exposure to the trauma target. Examples from the case study hint at the range: present safety augmented by safe place; other memories, perhaps altered by their own processing, such as the death of Tina's father; recovered information from the traumatic memory itself which enabled Tina to restore a sense of narrative and meaning in her breakthrough episode; and the attachment-based Socratic interweave. Particularly salient in EMDR is the use of corrective information with positive valence, an aspect of EMDR's positive pole, which generates sharper contrast than merely neutral material and therefore probably stronger and more effective realizations.

The client makes most of the connections on his or her own, using EMDR's capacity to efficiently uncover associations and forgotten material (van der Kolk, 2002, pp. 72–78), and does so with almost no theoretically based guidance. We may thus view EMDR as a metatherapy accommodating a variety of change processes, a framework to stimulate and assist the natural process of healing from trauma, with the client's association process determining the direction, content, and character of the trajectory.

The law of opposing states (Goleman, 2008, pp. 75–76) is a Buddhist metatheory of change that echoes trauma therapy's principle of juxtaposition with corrective information. This law says that "opposing families of mental states interact in a constant dynamic" and that contradictory states of mind "cannot coexist without one undermining the other"; for example, "hatred cannot exist in a moment of loving kindness" (Gyatso, 2005, pp. 145–150). It is a generalization at almost a philosophical level of various opposition–juxtaposition principles in modern psychology such as cognitive dissonance, reciprocal inhibition, conditioning, extinction, memory reconsolidation, desensitization, and habituation. This principle is said to underlie Buddhist practices for cultivating realizations and liberating insight by reasoning, introspective exploration, and other methods (J. Makransky, personal communication, January 6, 2013), as well as developing qualities such as compassion (Dodson-Lavelle et al., Chapter 22, this volume).

Two other principles support change in Buddhist practice and analogously in EMDR. The law of impermanence says that change is possible despite the apparent chronicity of suffering. The doctrine of Buddha Nature assures that success is attainable and that change tends toward realization and enlightenment or, at the psychological level, is biased toward healing and well-being. These manifest in numerous ways in EMDR's trauma processing. For example, the elements of the traumatic image and linking themes that come to the fore in free association are the "hottest," most in need of processing, and most likely to generate strong healing realizations. Tina evoked her father's death in free association presumably because it shared the traumatic theme of death of a loved one. The triggering effect thus promotes healing in the EMDR context rather than destructive reexperiencing, turning traumatic material into a force for its own demise. This resonates with use of contradiction in many Buddhist insight methods, which turns thought against itself to dissolve misapprehension and generate nonconceptual, liberating realization (Newland, 2009, p. 78; G. K. Gyatso, 1995, pp. 526–541). It may also be another reason for the efficient action of EMDR, requiring relatively little direct exposure.

Case Example Continued: The PC

Tina's reexperiencing and distress symptoms are now below clinical levels. We turn to remaining emotional issues, particularly her self-deprecation, by strengthening the PC, which has been in the background so far.

DEBORAH: As you think about the image you started with, the moment your friend died, is "I'm worthy" still the thought you would prefer about yourself?

TINA: I want to change it to "I'm a loving person."

DEBORAH: Good. On the scale from 1 to 7, how true is that thought?

TINA: Oh, I think a 5.

DEBORAH: What gets in the way of a 6 or 7?

TINA: I don't know if she heard me, felt my kiss; maybe I was too late.

DEBORAH: Go with that. [A BLS set.]

TINA: (*With tears running down her face*) Oh, I see, it doesn't work that way; it's about the love. I gave her what she needed the most. I told her I loved her. I *am* a loving person.

DEBORAH: (*Gently*) Yes. So, on the scale of 1 to 7, how true is that thought now?

TINA: A 7. I couldn't save her, but I did love her, do love her.

The PC and Future Ideal State

The PC shifted here from aspiration to explicit ideal future state. It thus corresponds, through the asymmetric analogy, with Vajrayana methods (Tsering, 2012, p. 3) in which the meditator visualizes him- or herself as already enlightened while still aware of ordinary, unenlightened reality. Those practices induce states of bliss and profound absorption, leading to faster realizations (Yeshe, 2001, pp. 79–80), which correspond in EMDR to the positive affect that helps the client stay in contact with traumatic material. By analogy, therefore, the PC is perhaps another reason that EMDR is effective with so little direct exposure. Unsurprisingly, recent research has shown that positive affect enhances insight and problem solving (Subramaniam, Kounios, Parrish, & Jung-Beeman, 2009).

Case Example: Conclusion

When I see Tina for the next session she reports that her reexperiencing symptoms are gone, along with the other emotional and somatic markers of PTSD. Six months later we check in by phone. Tina has remained asymptomatic, and her life is back on track. She thanks me again for helping her and exclaims that EMDR saved her life. I reply that it was an honor to witness her remarkable healing.

Conclusions

The model of correspondence between EMDR and Buddhist practice enables us to view principles of PTSD therapy through a contemplative lens. The asymmetry means that translating Buddhist practice into PTSD therapy requires careful analysis of both sides and their contrasts. The benefit of the asymmetry is that we can apply a much wider range of Buddhist practices and principles to trauma therapy than are usually considered. In particular, although even complete resolution of PTSD is clearly not the same as enlightenment in Buddhism, it is analogous in the psychological realm. Thus we can elucidate mechanisms of action in EMDR and PTSD therapy in general and open the way to new approaches and techniques by reference to the full range of Buddhist practices.

Here are some observations and speculations we can draw:

- Misapprehension and insight are underappreciated in trauma and may be useful for understanding many treatment models.
- Positive techniques can play an important role in PTSD treatment, especially when intimately woven into therapy.
- Stable, lucid attention is useful for PTSD therapy, but the client needs only sufficient concentration from calming and grounding to effect the required traumatic exposure.
- Moving as well as fixed attention has a role to play in therapy.
- Mahayana and Vajrayana Buddhism, as well as mindfulness approaches based on the Theravada, offer principles and techniques valuable for addressing PTSD.
- It is helpful to distinguish core therapeutic processes from supporting and catalytic techniques but not to minimize the latter, as they can be important to efficiency and even success.

Perhaps most important, just as Buddhism encompasses a wide range of theory and practice to suit the variety of humanity within its core principles, EMDR is an integrative framework, a metatherapy that accommodates the many ways that people naturally process distress, leveraging the creative capacity of the mind to right itself with insight. This principle is also reflected in the evolution of PE therapy to incorporate stress-inoculation and cognitive-behavioral methods, as well as the impetus toward mindfulness-based techniques and the growing role of self-compassion, both represented in this volume. Integrative approaches may thus be the way forward in trauma treatment.

References

Aderka, I. M., Appelbaum-Namdar, E., Shafran, N., & Gilboa-Schechtman, E. (2011). Sudden gains in prolonged exposure for children and adolescents with posttraumatic stress disorder. *Journal of Consulting and Clinical Psychology*, 79(4), 441–446.

Adler-Tapia, R., & Settle, C. (2008). *EMDR and the art of psychotherapy with children*. New York: Springer.

Aronson, H. (2006). Buddhist practice in relation to self-representation: A cross-cultural dialogue. In M. Unno (Ed.), *Buddhism and psychotherapy across cultures: Essays on theories and practices* (pp. 61–86). Somerville, MA: Wisdom.

Ash, I. K., Jee, B. D., & Wiley, J. (2012). Investigating insight as sudden learning. *Journal of Problem Solving*, 4(2), 1–27.

Benson, H., & Proctor, W. (2010). *Relaxation revolution: The science and genetics of mind–body healing*. New York: Simon & Schuster.

Bisson, J. I., Ehlers, A., Matthews, R., Pilling, S., Richards, D., & Turner, S. (2007). Psychological treatments for chronic post-traumatic stress disorder: Systematic review and meta-analysis. *British Journal of Psychiatry, 190*(2), 97–104.

Bodhi, B. (1980). *Transcendental dependent arising: A translation and exposition of the Upanisa Sutta.* Retrieved October 23, 2012, from *www.accesstoinsight.org/lib/authors/bodhi/wheel277.html.*

Bodhi, B. (2013). The Noble Eightfold Path: The way to end suffering. *Access to Insight.* Retrieved January 5, 2013, from *www.accesstoinsight.org/lib/authors/bodhi/waytoend.html.*

Brewin, C. R., Lanius, R. A., Novac, A., Schnyder, U., & Galea, S. (2009). Reformulating PTSD for DSM-V: Life after Criterion A. *Journal of Traumatic Stress, 22*(5), 366–373.

Davidson, P. R., & Parker, K. C. (2001). Eye movement desensitization and reprocessing (EMDR): A meta-analysis. *Journal of Consulting and Clinical Psychology, 69*(2), 305–316.

Ehlers, A. (2010). Understanding and treating unwanted trauma memories in post-traumatic stress disorder. *Journal of Psychology, 218*(2), 141–145.

Foa, E. B., Keane, T. M., Friedman, M. J., & Cohen, J. A. (Eds.). (2009). *Effective treatments for PTSD: Practice guidelines from the International Society for Traumatic Stress Studies.* New York: Guilford Press.

Freud, S. (1895). The psychotherapy of hysteria. In J. Breuer & S. Freud (Eds.), *Studies on hysteria* (pp. 253–306). New York: Basic Books.

Goleman, D. (2008). *Destructive emotions: A scientific dialogue with the Dalai Lama.* New York: Random House.

Greenwald, R. (2007). *EMDR within a phase model of trauma-informed treatment.* New York: Haworth Press.

Gunaratana, H. (2011). *Mindfulness in plain English: 20th anniversary edition.* Somerville, MA: Wisdom.

Gunter, R. W., & Bodner, G. E. (2009). EMDR works . . . but how?: Recent progress in the search for treatment mechanisms. *Journal of EMDR Practice and Research, 3*(3), 161–168.

Gyatso, G. K. (1995). *Joyful path of good fortune: The complete Buddhist path to enlightenment* (2nd ed.). Glen Spey, NY: Tharpa.

Gyatso, G. K. (2000). *Essence of Vajrayana: The highest yoga tantra practice of Heruka body mandala.* Glen Spey, NY: Tharpa.

Gyatso, T. (2005). *The universe in a single atom.* New York: Random House.

Gyatso, T., Hopkins, J. D., & Napper, E. (2006). *Kindness, clarity, and insight.* Ithaca, NY: Snow Lion.

Hanh, T. N. (2012). *Awakening of the heart: Essential Buddhist sutras and commentaries.* Berkeley, CA: Parallax Press.

Harvey, P. (2000). *An introduction to Buddhist ethics: Foundations, values and issues.* Cambridge, UK: Cambridge University Press.

Herbert, J. D., Lilienfeld, S. O., Lohr, J. M., Montgomery, R. W., O'Donohue, W. T., Rosen, G. M., et al. (2000). Science and pseudoscience in the development of eye movement desensitization and reprocessing: Implications for clinical psychology. *Clinical Psychology Review, 20*(8), 945–971.

Ho, M. S. K., & Lee, C. W. (2012). Cognitive behaviour therapy versus eye movement desensitization and reprocessing for post-traumatic disorder: Is it all in the homework then? *Revue Européenne de Psychologie Appliquée/European Review of Applied Psychology, 62*(4), 253–260.

Hölzel, B. K., Lazar, S. W., Gard, T., Schuman-Olivier, Z., Vago, D. R., & Ott, U. (2011). How does mindfulness meditation work?: Proposing mechanisms of action from a conceptual and neural perspective. *Perspectives on Psychological Science, 6*(6), 537–559.

Hyer, L., & Brandsma, J. M. (1997). EMDR minus eye movements equals good psychotherapy. *Journal of Traumatic Stress, 10*(3), 515–522.

Jinpa, G. T. (2000). The foundations of a Buddhist psychology. In G. Watson, S. Batchelor, & G. Claxton (Eds.), *The psychology of awakening: Buddhism, science, and our day-to-day lives* (pp. 10–22). York Beach, ME: Weiser.

Korn, D. L., & Leeds, A. M. (2002). Preliminary evidence of efficacy for EMDR resource development and installation in the stabilization phase of treatment of complex posttraumatic stress disorder. *Journal of Clinical Psychology, 58*(12), 1465–1487.

Kuiken, D., Bears, M., Miall, D., & Smith, L. (2001). Eye movement desensitization and reprocessing facilitates attentional orienting. *Imagination, Cognition, and Personality, 21*(1), 3–20.

Lee, C. W. (2008, May 4). Crucial processes in EMDR: More than imaginal exposure. *Journal of EMDR Practice and Research.*Retrieved from *http://researchrepository.murdoch.edu.au/1618.*

Lee, C. W., & Cuijpers, P. (2012). A meta-analysis of the contribution of eye movements in processing emotional memories. *Journal of Behavior Therapy and Experimental Psychiatry, 44*(2), 231–239.

Lee, C. W., Taylor, G., & Drummond, P. D. (2006). The active ingredient in EMDR: Is it traditional exposure or dual focus of attention? *Clinical Psychology and Psychotherapy, 107,* 97–107.

Leeds, A. M. (2009). *A guide to the standard EMDR protocols for clinicians, supervisors, and consultants.* New York: Springer.

Lipke, H. (2000). *EMDR and psychotherapy integration: Theoretical and clinical suggestions with focus on traumatic stress.* Boca Raton, FL: CRC Press.

Lutz, A., Slagter, H. A., Dunne, J. D., & Davidson, R. J. (2009). Attention regulation and monitoring in meditation. *Trends in Cognitive Science, 12*(4), 163–169.

Makransky, J. (2007). *Awakening through love: Unveiling your deepest goodness.* Somerville, MA: Wisdom.

McLeod, K. (2002). *Wake up to your life: Discovering the Buddhist path of attention.* New York: HarperCollins.

Michael, T., Ehlers, A., Halligan, S. L., & Clark, D. M. (2005). Unwanted memories of assault: What intrusion characteristics are associated with PTSD? *Behaviour Research and Therapy, 43*(5), 613–628.

Minton, K., Ogden, P., & Pain, C. (2006). *Trauma and the body: A sensorimotor approach to psychotherapy.* New York: Norton.

Newland, G. (2009). *Introduction to emptiness: As taught in Tsong-kha-pa's Great Treatise on the Stages of the Path.* Ithaca, NY: Snow Lion.

Pabongka, R. (1991). *Liberation in the palm of your hand: A concise discourse on the path to enlightenment.* Somerville, MA: Wisdom.

Parnell, L. (1996). Eye movement desensitization and reprocessing (EMDR) and spiritual unfolding. *Journal of Transpersonal Psychology, 28*(2), 129–153.

Parnell, L. (1998). *Transforming trauma: EMDR: The revolutionary new therapy for freeing the mind, clearing the body, and opening the heart.* New York: Norton.

Propper, R. E., & Christman, S. D. (2008). Interhemispheric interaction and saccadic horizontal eye movements: Implications for episodic memory, EMDR, and PTSD. *Journal of EMDR Practice and Research, 2*(4), 269–281.

Rauch, S., & Foa, E. B. (2006). Emotional processing theory (EPT) and exposure therapy for PTSD. *Journal of Contemporary Psychotherapy, 36*(2), 61–65.

Rimpoche, G. (2005). *Gom: A course in meditation.* Ann Arbor, MI: Jewel Heart.

Schubert, S. J., & Lee, C. W. (2009). Adult PTSD and its treatment with EMDR: A review of controversies, evidence, and theoretical knowledge. *Journal of EMDR Practice and Research, 3*(3), 117–132.

Shapiro, F. (2001). *Eye movement desensitization and reprocessing (EMDR): Basic principles, protocols, and procedures* (2nd ed.). New York: Guilford Press.

Shapiro, F. (Ed.). (2002). *EMDR as an integrative psychotherapy approach: Experts of diverse orientations explore the paradigm prism.* Washington, DC: American Psychological Association.

Shapiro, F., & Maxfield, L. (2003). EMDR and information processing in psychotherapy treatment: Personal development and global implications. In M. F. Solomon & D. J. Siegel (Eds.), *Healing trauma: Attachment, mind, body, and brain* (pp. 196–220). New York: Norton.

Shapiro, S. L., Carlson, L. E., Astin, J. A., & Freedman, B. (2006). *Mechanisms of Mindfulness, 62*(3), 373–386.

Smyth, N. J., & Poole, D. (2002). EMDR and cognitive-behavior therapy: Exploring convergence and divergence. In F. Shapiro (Ed.), *EMDR as an integrative psychotherapy approach: Experts of diverse orientations explore the paradigm prism* (pp. 151–180). Washington, DC: American Psychological Association.

Solomon, R. M., & Shapiro, F. (2008). EMDR and the adaptive information processing model: Potential mechanisms of change. *Journal of EMDR Practice and Research, 2*(4), 315–325.

Spates, C. R., Koch, E., Cusack, K., Pagoto, S., & Waller, S. (2009). Eye movement desensitization and reprocessing. In E. B. Foa, T. M. Keane, M. J. Friedman, & J. A. Cohen (Eds.), *Effective treatments for PTSD: Practice guidelines from the International Society for Traumatic Stress Studies* (2nd ed., pp. 279–305). New York: Guilford Press.

Stickgold, R. (2008). Sleep-dependent memory processing and EMDR action. *Journal of EMDR Practice and Research, 2*(4), 289–299.

Subramaniam, K., Kounios, J., Parrish, T. B., & Jung-Beeman, M. (2009). A brain mechanism for facilitation of insight by positive affect. *Journal of Cognitive Neuroscience, 21*(3), 415–32.

Thompson, B. L., & Waltz, J. (2010). Mindfulness and experiential avoidance as predictors of posttraumatic stress disorder avoidance symptom severity. *Journal of Anxiety Disorders, 24*(4), 409–415.

Tsering, G. T. (2005). *The Four Noble Truths.* Somerville, MA: Wisdom.

Tsering, G. T. (2012). *Tantra: The foundation of Buddhist thought.* Somerville, MA: Wisdom.

Vago, D. R., & Silbersweig, D. A. (2012). Self-awareness, self-regulation, and self-transcendence (S-ART): A framework for understanding the neurobiological mechanisms of mindfulness. *Frontiers in Human Neuroscience, 6,* 296.

van der Kolk, B. A. (1994). The body keeps the score: Memory and the evolving psychobiology of posttraumatic stress. *Harvard Review of Psychiatry, 1*(5), 253–265.

van der Kolk, B. A. (2002). Beyond the talking cure: Somatic experience and subcortical imprints in the treatment of trauma. In F. Shapiro (Ed.), *EMDR as an integrative psychotherapy approach: Experts of diverse orientations explore the paradigm prism* (pp. 10–20). Washington DC: American Psychological Association.

van der Kolk, B. A., & McFarlane, A. C. (1996). The black hole of trauma. In B. A. van der Kolk, A. C. McFarlane, & L. Weisath (Eds.), *Traumatic stress: The effects of overwhelming experience on mind, body, and society* (pp. 3–23). New York: Guilford Press.

van der Kolk, B. A., McFarlane, A. C., & van der Hart, O. (1996). A general approach to treatment of posttraumatic stress disorder. In B. A. van der Kolk, A. C. McFarlane, & L. Waisaeth (Eds.), *Traumatic stress: The effects of overwhelming experience on mind, body, and society* (pp. 417–440). New York: Guilford Press.

Wachtel, P. L. (2002). EMDR and psychoanalysis. In F. Shapiro (Ed.), *EMDR as an integrative psychotherapy approach: Experts of diverse orientations explore the paradigm prism* (pp. 123–150). Washington, DC: American Psychological Association.

Wallace, B. A. (2006). *The attention revolution: Unlocking the power of the focused mind.* Somerville, MA: Wisdom.

Yeshe, T. (2001). *Introduction to tantra: The transformation of desire* (3rd ed.). Somerville, MA: Wisdom.

8

The Internal Family Systems Model in Trauma Treatment

Parallels with Mahayana Buddhist Theory and Practice

Richard C. Schwartz and Flint Sparks

The internal family systems (IFS) model of psychotherapy has been embraced by trauma therapists because it offers several solutions to the complex challenges of treating complex trauma. The model itself and its application to trauma have been described more extensively elsewhere (Schwartz, 1995; Goulding & Schwartz, 1995). IFS represents a synthesis of three paradigms. One of these is called the *normal multiplicity of the mind*—the idea that we all contain many different subminds. The second is known as *systems thinking*, including family systems theory and practice. The third has been called many things by different therapies and spiritual traditions (e.g., the spirit, Buddha Nature, or soul) but here is called *Self leadership*. In this chapter, we briefly introduce the basic principles of IFS and then draw on some of the core elements of IFS work with trauma to discuss how the model relates to some aspects of Buddhist philosophy and practice, specifically those of the Mahayana tradition.

IFS is an established approach with training programs throughout the United States, six European countries, and Israel. Since 2000, the trainings have been coordinated by the Center for Self Leadership (*selfleadership. org*), which sets standards for certification and organizes an annual international professional conference.

Multiplicity of the Mind

IFS views the mind as a dynamic system composed of many subminds, called parts. Freud (1923/1961) opened the door for exploration of multiplicity with his descriptions of the id, ego, and superego. Various post-Freudian theorists have moved beyond his tripartite model and discussed a range of inner entities. Perhaps the most influential of these is object relations theory, which, since Melanie Klein in the 1940s, has asserted that our internal experience is shaped by introjected "objects," representations of significant people in our lives (Klein, 1948; Gunthrip, 1971).

Jung (1935/1968, 1963, 1968, 1969), in his discussion of archetypes and complexes, took the notion that we contain many minds a step further, because he considered them as more than just introjects. In 1935, Jung (1935/1968) described a complex as having the

> tendency to form a little personality of itself. It has a sort of body, a certain amount of its own physiology. It can upset the stomach, it upsets the breathing, it disturbs the heart—in short, it behaves like a partial personality. . . . I hold that our personal unconscious . . . consists of an indefinite, because unknown, number of complexes or fragmentary personalities. (pp. 80–81)

Jung's younger contemporary Roberto Assagioli (1973, 1965/1975; Ferrucci, 1982) also posited that we are a collection of subpersonalities. Since Assagioli, a number of theorists have pointed to a natural multiplicity; in exploring this territory, they have made observations that are remarkably similar to one another. Rowan (1990) and Carter (2008) offer a more detailed history of work on the multiplicity of the mind.

Regardless of orientation, most theorists who have explored intrapsychic process have described the mind as having some degree of multiplicity. Scanning the currently influential psychotherapies, we find that object relations describes internal objects (Klein, 1948; Gunthrip, 1971; Fairbairn, 1952; Kernberg, 1976; Winnicott, 1958, 1971); self psychology speaks of grandiose selves versus idealizing selves (Kohut, 1971, 1977); and cognitive-behavioral therapists describe a variety of schemas and possible selves (Markus & Nurius, 1987; Dryden & Golden, 1986; Young, Klosko, & Weishaar, 2003). Although these theories vary regarding the degree to which the inner entities are viewed as autonomous and possessing a full complement of emotions and cognitions—as opposed to being interdependent, unidimensional, specialized mental units—they all suggest that the mind is far from unitary.

Theories of psychological trauma that undergird the literature on dissociative identity disorder (DID) view them as fragments of a potentially unitary personality. Experts on DID recognize the multiplicity of their clients; however, they view these personalities as the result of early trauma and abuse, which forced the person to split off many "alter" personalities (Kluft, 1985; Bliss, 1986; Putnam, 1989, Nijenhuis, Van der Hart, & Steele, 2002).

Regardless of the theorized source of inner entities (learning, trauma, introjection, the collective unconscious, or the mind's natural state), some of these theorists view them as complete personalities. They share a belief that these internal entities are more than clusters of thoughts or feelings, or mere states of mind. Instead, they are seen as distinct personalities, of different ages, temperaments, talents, and even genders, and each with a full range of emotion and desire. The DID theorists hold this view, although they limit it to highly traumatized people. Jung's later writing describes archetypes and complexes in ways that approach full-personality multiplicity, as does a Jungian derivative called voice dialogue (Stone & Winkelman, 1985). In addition, ego state therapy, developed by hypnotherapists John and Helen Watkins (Watkins, 1978; Watkins & Johnson, 1982; Watkins & Watkins, 1979), and Assagioli's psychosynthesis subscribe to full-personality multiplicity.

Many trauma therapies propose that the existence of subpersonalities is a sign of pathology—a consequence of the fragmentation of the psyche by traumatic experiences. In contrast, like Jung, psychosynthesis, ego state therapy, and voice dialogue, the IFS model sees all parts as innately valuable components of a healthy mind. In fact, according to IFS, a fully functioning inner system requires these subminds, each with its different perspectives, talents, and resources, to function well. Trauma does not create these parts but instead forces many of them out of their naturally valuable functions and healthy states into protective and/or extreme roles. The goal of therapy, then, becomes not to eliminate parts but instead to help them relax into the knowledge that they no longer have to be so protective. The client is guided to help him or her realize that he or she is no longer under the same level of threat and that there exists a natural inner leader whom he or she can trust. In this way, IFS brings family systems thinking to this internal family, understanding distressed parts in their context, just as family therapists do with problem children, and restoring inner leadership in a way that parallels the creation of secure attachments between parents and children.

Case Example

We now turn to a clinical example that illustrates central IFS concepts and methods. We also draw parallels from the teachings of Mahayana Buddhism throughout this chapter.

Lois was a delightfully lively and adventurous child until the night her drunken father entered her bedroom and molested her for the first time when she was 7. Until that night she had been full of curiosity and joyful innocence. Her unfettered parts found everything interesting and exciting. Those naturally emerging parts were stunned by her father's behavior and felt dirty and ashamed, assuming that she must have done something to provoke him. No longer curious and excited, some parts began to carry the physical and emotional pain of the episode and became frozen in time around this incident.

Other parts of Lois who had enjoyed learning in school now shifted their roles and became keepers of the secret and watchers of her father's mood. They transformed into inner critics, admonishing her for her mistakes and reminding her that she was bad. She became hypervigilant and extremely sensitive to the shifting moods and behaviors of the people around her. In later years, Lois's mother confessed that she had noticed a sudden change in Lois's temperament at about that age. Her little pistol of a daughter had suddenly become withdrawn, cautious, and perfectionistic.

This foundational assumption—that all parts are inherently valuable but can be distorted by the extreme emotions and beliefs taken on as a result of destructive or terrifying experiences (called "burdens" in IFS)—makes a big difference in how therapists encourage trauma survivors to relate to their inner worlds. It also parallels the view of Tibetan Buddhism, which says that everything that arises within an individual's mind has an "enlightened" aspect and can be brought to the path of liberation and away from suffering. Instead of trying to challenge, ignore, extinguish, or replace their irrational thoughts and feelings, IFS clients are encouraged to turn toward these inner parts with curiosity and compassion and listen to their painful stories about how they are attempting to help. In this way the trauma survivor learns directly from her or his protective parts why and how they took on their protective roles. The traumatized parts are also able to show the survivor what happened to them in the past when they took on the burdens they now carry. When clients hear and feel directly from their parts, it is a more intense, visceral, and somatic experience than thinking about what happened to them or about why they are highly defended. Parts want their experience to be fully witnessed by the client, not simply thought about.

With this crucial shift, the painful inner world and the relationships among the parts begin to make sense to the client. The client can then go beyond merely witnessing the distressing events and can engage his or her parts intimately to let them know they are now understood and cared for. The client can actually enter the old scenes in order to form new, loving relationships with these exiled parts stuck in the past. With a clearer understanding and concern for the hurt or shame they carry, the client can bring these vulnerable parts to new places inside their minds that are more safe and nourishing. This combination of compassionate witnessing and retrieval of hurt or protective parts from the past allows them to unburden—to release the extreme emotions and beliefs they carry—which in turn often produces an immediate shift not only in the parts themselves but also in the entire internal system as well. The parts begin to transform back into their valuable essences and once again function with more freedom and vitality.

Healing Engagement

Lois had always vaguely remembered that her father had done some sexual things to her in her bedroom one night when she was young, but she had kept that memory in the recesses of her mind and had never dwelled on it. In doing so, protective parts had locked away the formerly trusting, lively parts of her ("exiles" in IFS) that had been so shocked and hurt by her father's actions. She had become dominated by hypervigilant, perfectionistic critics ("protectors" in IFS) who were determined to keep this terrible thing from happening to her again.

The IFS therapist gently invited Lois to focus on the critical voice in her head that was constantly telling her that she was bad. In this process of warm engagement and inner dialogue, she was able to ask this critical part what it feared would happen if it stopped saying these harsh and threatening things to her all the time. She immediately heard the answer, "You would be hurt again." Lois first expressed appreciation to the critic for trying to keep her safe all these years. She then asked the critic a crucial question: If she could safely access and heal the exiled parts that were trapped in places where she was originally hurt in the past, would the critic then feel compelled to attack her so much? The critic replied that it would not need to do this, and, in fact, if it was freed up from this extreme role, it could instead begin to advise her about who was trustworthy and who was not.

With the critic's permission, Lois then focused on the vague but persistent emotional pain she felt in her chest and immediately saw an image of herself as that 7-year-old. Lois was able to express her love and care for that 7-year-old and asked if the little girl would show her what happened to her in the past. After fully and compassionately witnessing what her father had done that night, Lois entered the scene and took the girl in her arms, telling her that she had done nothing to provoke him—that what happened was completely about him and not her. She then took the girl to the beach and helped her release the long-held beliefs about her badness and unburden the old sensations of shock that had been held in her body. The 7-year-old immediately felt much lighter and spontaneously wanted to play. Upon seeing this change in the 7-year-old, the critic also began to unburden the heavy responsibility for protection and gladly took on its new and more appropriate role as social advisor. This witnessing process, in which a part is finally able, as the client accesses wise and healing qualities including mindfulness, loving kindness, and compassion, to be known with respect to what happened and how bad it felt without being totally overwhelmed, is one of the primarily healing mechanisms in IFS.

The Self and Mindfulness

When a therapist is truly respectful of a trauma client's inner protectors and deeply confident regarding the client's ability to heal her or his exiles, often core traumatic material can be reached relatively quickly, as was true with Lois. To do this, however, Lois had to access an internal state in which she could clearly observe these parts rather than being merged with them. This process of helping a client separate from her parts is similar to helping her become mindful of, rather than immersed in, her thoughts and feelings, as is practiced in many Buddhist meditations. Without being triggered or overwhelmed by parts, she had the space and steadiness to become curious about and, later, compassionate toward them. Because of its potency and efficacy in focusing attention and expanding awareness in clinical work, contemporary psychotherapists from many schools are embracing mindfulness as a useful tool (Germer, Siegel, & Fulton, 2005; Siegel, 2010). Some therapists teach mindfulness skills to their clients and encourage the regular practice of mindfulness meditation in order to support this capacity for witnessing awareness. Because of the difficult histories of trauma survivors and because of the habitual and embodied nature of the traumatic impact on their inner systems, trauma survivors are thought to need considerable practice of mindfulness skills before they can achieve the kind of differentiation from their extreme emotions that Lois, in the context of an IFS intervention, displayed rather rapidly.

In contrast to the generally held belief that qualities such as mindfulness, loving-kindness, and compassion are mental capacities that need to be cultivated or strengthened through practice, like developing a muscle through exercise, we find that trauma clients often can access those qualities in early sessions. IFS posits the inherent existence of a spacious essence in each person that, when accessed spontaneously, manifests leadership qualities that include mindfulness, loving-kindness, and compassion. This essence is also characterized by a profound sense of calm, confidence, clarity, connectedness, and creativity. IFS calls this essence the *Self*. This Self does not need to be developed or cultivated and, especially relevant to this chapter, is not damaged by trauma. Most people, and particularly trauma clients, have little access to the Self in their daily lives because it is obscured by the protective parts that dominate them. When their parts trust that it is safe to allow the Self to manifest, clients will immediately display many of those qualities without having meditated or practiced any particular skills.

From this perspective, then, mindfulness meditation is very valuable, not to cultivate these inherent qualities, but to help clients access these qualities—or the Self—and to remind protective parts that when they release their grip and let the Self lead in daily life, many things are better. In other words, from the perspective of IFS, meditations can be viewed as practice sessions for helping parts become familiar with and trust Self leadership.

In some Buddhist traditions and mindfulness-based psychotherapies, a person is taught to witness his or her thoughts and emotions from a place of acceptance but not necessarily to actively engage with them (see Schwartz, 2011; Sparks, 2011). The following is an example of this kind of instruction:

> Recognize fear when it arises, observe the feeling of it in your body, watch it try to convince you that you should be alarmed, see it change and move on . . . . Notice how the awareness which contains fear is itself never fearful. Keep separating from the fear; settle back into the vast space of awareness through which fear passes like a cloud. (Hanson, 2009, pp. 89, 90)

Our experience is that when clients access Self, not only do they stop identifying with their parts, but they are also able to witness their parts and begin illuminating inner conversations with them. As they get to know these parts, they naturally begin to convey love and appreciation to them, even to parts they had hated or dreaded much of their lives. In this way, in the language of IFS, Self becomes an active, attuned leader of the internal family system of a trauma client—a loving, secure inner attachment figure for terrified and hurt parts.

Through years of experimenting, Schwartz (1995) developed ways to help clients, even those with severe trauma histories, to quickly access the Self and, within this larger perspective, begin to heal. Clients are encouraged to simply ask the protective parts that ordinarily run their lives to either relax or separate from themselves inside. Once these parts begin to separate or allow space for the Self, clients will suddenly and spontaneously shift from such states as fear, rage, or disgust and naturally become more curious, compassionate, or calm. For example, when Lois first focused on her protective self-critic, the therapist asked her how she felt toward the critic. This is the key question in IFS that allows the client to separate from a part and begin to access her or his Self. Lois responded to this question by reporting that she felt rage toward the critic. The therapist then had her ask the rage (viewed as another part that was blended with her awareness) if it was willing to relax or step back to allow more internal space. She sensed the anger dissipating. When Lois was then asked how she felt toward the critic, she replied, "I'm just interested in why it's calling me those names." The moment the rage relaxed, Lois spontaneously displayed several of the qualities of Self: curiosity (offered in her words), calm (heard in her voice), and confidence (shown in her overall demeanor).

From this more stable and resourceful perspective of Self, clients can begin highly productive inner dialogues with their parts. These mindfully engaged inner dialogues often lead quickly to the manifestation of other qualities of Self, such as compassion, clarity, appreciation, and gratitude. Clients can then extend these qualities to their parts. When parts sense this level of acceptance and love from the client's Self, they begin to reveal their vulnerabilities, which ultimately leads to further healing and transformation.

This conviction alone—that trauma does not touch one's essence and that one does not have to meditate or practice mindfulness skills for years to begin to experience liberation from suffering—is tremendously empowering for many trauma survivors. Very often, these clients hold the belief that they have been so damaged that they will never heal and that their very essence is tarnished. A second important IFS conviction—that parts are not what they seem and that by turning toward them with compassionate curiosity rather than trying to get rid of or decommissioning them, they transform into valuable qualities—is equally empowering and often very surprising to trauma survivors. Parts want to be met with mature leadership, and they long to be liberated from their extreme roles and released to their valuable functions within the internal system. This is not to suggest that isolated trauma clients will suddenly know how to operate effectively in the outer world without learning some life skills. We do posit, however, that the ability for self-regulation and self-compassion in the inner world is innate and can be accessed more quickly than many trauma approaches have recognized. Curiously, these same convictions are at the heart of the Buddha's teachings, and these same healing capacities are expressions of the practices he taught.

IFS and the Buddha's Wisdom

As Buddhism began to take shape in Northern India in the years following the life of Gautama Siddhartha, different groups of followers expressed what they thought were the true essence of his teachings. One of those groups later developed into a school now known as the Mahayana (the Great Vehicle) that was a departure from the traditional lineage in several important ways and is strikingly similar to the convictions of IFS in treating trauma. Central to the Mahayana perspective is the ideal of the bodhisattva. A bodhisattva is a person committed to delaying his or her own freedom from the endless cycles of suffering in order to help all other beings become so liberated. Whether or not one believes ontologically in such an ideal, the towering gifts of Mahayana Buddhism are how it holds compassion for others and dedication to their liberation as its primary goal.

The early Mahayanan teachers believed that true freedom was what we already are, not what we create through practice. They called this truth our "Buddha Nature," and it was this vast mind and infinitely warm heart that they pointed to as our "True Nature" (Chodron, 2005; Leighton, 2012; Makransky, 2007; McDonald, 1984). From this perspective we do not need to cultivate or develop Buddha Nature because it is who and what we already are and have always been. Likewise, these teachings suggest that we cannot destroy our Buddha Nature, because it is not subject to the arising and passing away of changing conditions. It is the vast space in which all conditions arise and pass away, and when functioning freely it is characterized by four primary qualities: loving-kindness (unconditional friendliness), compassion (the capacity to meet suffering without turning away and unconditional motivation to relieve others' suffering), equanimity (calm and stable abiding, even in the face of suffering), and sympathetic joy (joy in the happiness of others). In this crucial turn from a focus on self-liberation to focusing on the liberation of others, and in the firm conviction that our nature is that of a Buddha (freedom and wakefulness), we discover the parallels to the beliefs and methods of the IFS model of treating trauma.

What is described as Self in IFS can be seen as one's Buddha Nature.[1] If there is an unbound space and radiant quality in every person that is untouched by traumatic events and is immediately available as a compassionate and healing presence, then IFS is a skillful means of helping clients awaken to and lead from their True Nature (for another account of IFS as a skillful means of this kind, see Engler & Fulton, 2012, pp. 182–188). One's "inner Buddha or bodhisattva" is then revealed to be the prime healing resource for all conditioned or damaged parts that long for help. Self is then seen not as another part in this internal system. It is not the "free or good part" as opposed to the "damaged or bad parts." Self is the spacious heart and mind in which all parts arise and function, and it is also, then, the source and energy of liberation from unnecessary suffering.

Self and the Bodhisattva Way

There is a vow derived from the Mahayana that expresses this shared reality of IFS and Buddhist practice. The *bodhisattva vow* lays out the basic

---

[1] "Buddha Nature" is a subtle idea in Mahayana Buddhism that does not, although it is sometimes interpreted as doing so, contradict the equally central Buddhist concepts of "no self" (*anatta*) and the "emptiness" (of inherent existence) of all phenomena, including objects and beings. In one sense, as noted by Engler and Fulton (2012), the IFS concept of *Self* corresponds to the Buddhist notion of no-self (anatta); in another sense, it is akin to the Hindu notion of *atman*, the primordial transpersonal soul (often translated into English as "Self").

framework for a life grounded in one's Buddha Nature and dedicated to serving others. Here is one traditional translation:

> Beings are numberless, I vow to free them;
> Delusions are inexhaustible, I vow to end them;
> Dharma-gates[2] are boundless, I vow to enter them;
> Buddha's Way is unsurpassable, I vow to become it.

This formulation is an expression of unbound care for any being who suffers, and if one considers the mind to be populated by inner personalities, then it is not a huge stretch to consider bringing similar levels of compassion and care to the suffering and vulnerable inhabitants of the inner world of a client with a trauma. In their fullness, the vows are impossibly large. But, read more practically, they become a commitment to taking up a particular way of life. The bodhisattva takes up the practice path of helping others to be free from suffering. The bodhisattva is committed to helping all beings not only to become aware of their conditioning but to help them release the limitations of their conditioning. They use every event as an opportunity to turn life toward freedom and to find ways to fully embody the Buddha's teachings. Translated from the IFS perspective, the client's Self, or inner bodhisattva, is committed to the liberation of all parts from their respective suffering.

This view is consistent with current conceptions of healing in the fields of psychological trauma and neuroscience, in which encountering one's traumatic memories and conditioning in the context of safety and connection with a therapist is said to foster processes of extinction learning and memory reconsolidation, which liberate clients from conditioned fear, shame, addiction, and other habitual and suffering-inducing responses to trauma triggers (e.g., Maren, 2011; Schiller et al., 2010). With IFS, however, the modus operandi is accessing one's own healing capacities—including mindfulness, compassion, calm, and connectedness—and using them to explore, understand, and *transform* parts of oneself that have been gripped by an endless cycle of posttraumatic suffering. As noted by Engler and Fulton (2012), this aspect of IFS mirrors the understandings and practices of tantric Tibetan Buddhism, also within the Mahayana tradition, in which "all mind states are valuable energies that can be transformed into wholesome qualities" (2012, p. 184).

With this understanding in mind, we can translate the bodhisattva vow in IFS terms as follows:

---

[2] "Dharma-gates" are the everyday challenges in life experience that become opportunities to learn and grow.

Parts are numerous; I take up the practice of freeing them from their extreme roles.

Burdens (extreme beliefs and emotions) are numerous and create distortion and delusion; I take up the practice unburdening, which leads to the clarity of Self leadership.

Experiences on my path endlessly trigger parts that need healing; I take up the practice of using those "trailheads" to identify and heal all those suffering parts.

Self leadership is unsurpassable; I take up the practice of embodying Self energy.

The Self of the Therapist

Of course, this vow is not just for clients. When a therapist can embody Buddha Nature or Self, clients immediately sense the safety, acceptance, and compassion of the therapist's presence. Their protective parts relax and uncover the Self. If the therapist remains calm, caring, and confident in the face of the client's parts that feel desperately hopeless, suicidal, or shameful, the client will begin relating to her or his parts in this way as well. Parts then have the freedom to drop their guards and reveal their truth. In doing so they can be seen more clearly for the roles they have played, they are revealed to be something different from what they have always seemed, and it becomes clear that they simply want to be loved and enabled to express their goodness.

These qualities are particularly important when working with trauma clients because their inner systems are often highly distrusting, hypervigilant, and reactive. Inevitably the therapist's protective parts will be triggered (traditionally known as countertransference), which can potentially lead to subtle shifts away from the Self of the therapist. This, in turn, will threaten the client's protectors, which can lead to damaging polarizations within the client's system.

To be optimally effective in the treatment of trauma, the IFS therapist is encouraged to engage is several key practices:

1. Being mindful in sessions, so as to remain aware when one's protectors take over.
2. Asking his or her own protector parts to separate in the moment of being triggered, in order to allow for a return to Self leadership.
3. If Self leadership is not restored immediately, repairing with the client by admitting that a part had taken over and apologizing for the loss of Self leadership.
4. Working between sessions with any parts of one's own that were interfering or triggered.

Regular mindfulness practices and compassion meditations will support a therapist's intention to engage in all four of these IFS practices. In doing so the therapist not only becomes increasingly sensitive to the ways his or her own parts manifest in his or her body and mind but is also better able to notice when he or she loses Self leadership in the therapeutic relationship and to compassionately accept that reality and return to Self leadership.

Self-to-Self Connectedness

We are convinced that an essential aspect of healing for trauma clients lies in the sacred connectedness that develops between the Self of the client and the Self of the therapist. The more the client feels met by Self, the more emboldened she or he feels to enter the terrifying inner worlds, knowing she or he is not alone. Additionally, she or he can begin to take more risks in the outside world, trusting the energetic connection to the therapist even when they are not together.

Toward the end of his career Carl Rogers put it beautifully:

> I find that when I am closest to my inner, intuitive self, when I am somehow in touch with the unknown in me . . . whatever I do seems to be full of healing. Then, simply my presence is releasing and helpful to the other. There is nothing I can do to force this experience, but when I can relax and be close to the transcendental core of me . . . it seems my inner spirit has reached out and touched the inner spirit of the other. Our relationship transcends itself and becomes part of something larger. Profound growth and energy are present. (as cited in Prendergast, Fenner, & Krystal, 2003, p. 93)

Self to Self, Buddha Nature to Buddha Nature, soul to soul, inner spirit to inner spirit—regardless of what this experience is called, those who have tasted it know its healing power and long to rest in it. When this profound connection opens and is stabilized between a trauma client and a therapist, the client then has a vibrant model to help her or him form parallel connections between her or his own Self and its parts.

Returning to our example, when Lois felt this gentle, reassuring, Self-to-Self connection with her therapist, it allowed her to have an open mind toward her inner critic, as well as an open heart to her fearful 7-year-old. These parts finally felt witnessed and warmly met by her Self. No longer isolated and polarized, the parts realized that they belonged to something larger and could relax into this loving embrace. In this spacious opening she awakened her own bodhisattva energy that could then extend compassionate care to all her parts. In doing so she was enacting the vow to relieve the suffering of all beings within herself. Not only were these parts freed from the suffering of the past, but her loving presence also helped them release their burdens, all of which had prevented her from having full access to the Self found at the heart of each part. This realization and release allowed each part to function more freely in accord with Buddha Nature.

Conclusion

In the IFS method, clients suffering from the effects of trauma are invited to turn toward the parts of themselves that they habitually avoid or hate and, instead, find that these parts long to be met by the client's Self, who is ready and willing to provide a healing embrace. The tangle of internal parts, the layers of protection, and the pain of exiled parts can seem daunting at first, but clients are often surprised at the power and efficiency of this engaged, mindful, and loving practice when they meet the confidence, calm, and connectedness—the free flow of Self—of a well-trained IFS therapist who is aware of his or her own parts.

In parallel to the contemplative tradition of Mahayana Buddhism, by accessing what is called Self leadership in IFS, therapists embody the bodhisattva vow in service to their clients, and clients become bodhisattvas to their own suffering inner parts. In this view, even severely traumatized clients are not separated from their Buddha Nature, which abides just beneath the surface of their protective parts and which will emerge fully developed and undamaged when those parts trust that it is safe to relax and open to the spacious presence inside. The more the protectors separate from the automatic tangles of conditioning, the more qualities such as curiosity, confidence, courage, compassion, creativity, calm, clarity, and connectedness manifest in the client's awareness and presence. These qualities emerge spontaneously and naturally, and meditation can remind parts to trust them and let them remain.

This emergence of Self in trauma clients can seem unbelievable—too miraculous to be possible—until we see that this transformational capacity is actually grounded in human nature, as described by the centuries-old tradition of Mahayana Buddhism and the bodhisattva way. The IFS model is an approach to treating trauma with underlying assumptions that mirror those of Mahayana Buddhism.

References

Assagioli, R. (1973). *The act of will.* New York: Penguin Books.

Assagioli, R. (1975). *Psychosynthesis: A manual of principles and techniques.* London: Turnstone Press. (Original work published 1965)

Bliss, E. L. (1986). *Multiple personality, allied disorders, and hypnosis.* New York: Oxford University Press.

Carter, R. (2008). *Multiplicity: The new science of personality, identity, and the self.* Boston: Little, Brown.

Chodron, P. (2005). *No time to lose: A timeless guide to the way of the Bodhisattva.* Boston: Shambhala.

Dryden, W., & Golden, W. (Eds.). (1986). *Cognitive–behavioral approaches to psychotherapy.* London: Harper & Row.

Engler, J., & Fulton, P. R. (2012). Self and no-self in psychotherapy. In C. K. Germer & R. D. Siegal (Eds.), *Wisdom and compassion in psychotherapy: Deepening mindfulness in clinical practice* (pp. 176–188). New York: Guilford Press.

Fairbairn, W. R. (1952). *An object relations theory of the personality.* London: Tavistock.

Ferrucci, P. (1982). *What we may be.* Los Angeles: Tarcher.

Freud, S. (1961). The ego and the id. In J. Strachey (Ed. & Trans.), *The standard edition of the complete psychological works of Sigmund Freud* (Vol. 19, pp. 3–66). London: Hogarth Press. (Original work published 1923)

Germer, C., Siegel, R., & Fulton, P. (2005). *Mindfulness and psychotherapy.* New York: Guilford Press.

Goulding, R., & Schwartz, R. C. (1995). *Mosaic mind: Empowering the tormented selves of child abuse survivors.* New York: Norton.

Gunthrip, H. (1971) *Psychoanalytic theory, therapy and the self.* New York: Basic Books.

Hanson, R. (2009). *Buddha's brain.* Oakland, CA: New Harbinger.

Jung, C. G. (1956). *Two essays on analytical psychology.* New York: Meridian.

Jung, C. G. (1963). *Memories, dreams, reflections* (A. Jaffe, Ed.; R. Winston & C. Winston, Trans.). New York: Pantheon Books.

Jung, C. G. (1968). *Analytical psychology: Its theory and practice: The Tavistock lectures.* London: Routledge & Kegan Paul. (Original work published 1935)

Jung, C. G. (1968). *The collected works of C. G. Jung: Vol. 9, Part I. The archetypes and the collective unconscious* (2nd ed.; H. Read, M. Fordham, & G. Adler, Eds.; R. F. C. Hull, Trans.). Princeton, NJ: Princeton University Press.

Jung, C. G. (1969). *The collected works of C. G. Jung: Vol. 8. The structure and dynamics of the psyche* (2nd ed.; H. Read, M. Fordham, & G. Adler, Eds.; R. F. C. Hull, Trans.). Princeton, NJ: Princeton University Press.

Kernberg, O. (1976). *Object relations theory and clinical psychoanalysis.* New York: Aronson.

Klein, M. (1948). *Contributions to psychoanalysis.* London: Hogarth Press.

Kluft, R. P. (Ed.). (1985). *Childhood antecedents of multiple personality disorder.* Washington, DC: American Psychiatric Press.

Kohut, H. (1971). *The analysis of the self.* New York: International Universities Press.

Kohut, H. (1977). *The restoration of the self.* New York: International Universities Press.

Leighton, D. (2012). *Faces of compassion: Classic Bodhisattva archetypes and their modern expression: An introduction to Mahayana Buddhism.* Somerville, MA: Wisdom.

Makransky, J. (2007). *Awakening through love: Unveiling your deepest goodness.* Somerville, MA: Wisdom.

Maren, S. (2011). Seeking a spotless mind: Extinction, deconsolidation, and erasure of fear memory. *Neuron, 70,* 830–845.

Markus, H., & Nurius, P. (1987). Possible selves: The interface between motivation and the self-concept. In K. Yardley & T. Honess (Eds.), *Self and identity: Psychosocial perspectives.* Chichester, UK: Wiley.

McDonald, K. (1984). *How to meditate: A practical guide.* Somerville, MA: Wisdom.

Nijenhuis, E. R. S., Van der Hart, O., & Steele, K. (2002). The emerging psychobiology of trauma-related dissociation and dissociative disorders. In H. D'Haenen, J. A. Den Boer, H. Westenberg, & P. Willner (Eds.), *Textbook of biological psychiatry* (pp. 1079–1098). London: Wiley.

Prendergast, J., Fenner, P., & Krystal, S. (2003). *Sacred mirror: Nondual wisdom and psychotherapy.* St. Paul, MN: Paragon House.

Putnam, F. W. (1989). *Diagnosis and treatment of multiple personality disorder.* New York: Guilford Press.

Rowan, J. (1990). *Subpersonalities: The people inside us.* London: Routledge.

Schiller, D., Monfils, M.-H., Raio, C. M., Johnson, D. C., LeDoux, J. E., & Phelps, E. A. (2010). Preventing the return of fear memories in humans using reconsolidation update mechanisms. *Nature, 463,* 49–53.

Schwartz, R. (2011, September/October). When meditation isn't enough. *Psychotherapy Networker,* p. 35.

Schwartz, R. C. (1995). *Internal family systems therapy.* New York: Guilford Press.

Siegel, D. (2010). *The mindful therapist: A clinician's guide to mindsight and neural integration.* New York: Norton.

Sparks, F. (2011, September/October). The shadow side of meditation: Getting stuck in the present moment. *Psychotherapy Networker,* p. 39.

Stone, H., & Winkelman, S. (1985). *Embracing ourselves.* Marina del Rey, CA: Devross.

Watkins, J. (1978). *The therapeutic self.* New York: Human Sciences Press.

Watkins, J., & Johnson, R. J. (1982). *We, the divided self.* New York: Irvington.

Watkins, J., & Watkins, H. (1979). Ego states and hidden observers. *Journal of Altered States of Consciousness, 5,* 3–18.

Winnicott, D. W. (1958). *Collected papers.* New York: Basic Books.

Winnicott, D. W. (1965). *The maturational processes and the facilitating environment.* New York: International Universities Press.

Winnicott, D. W. (1971). *Playing and reality.* London: Routledge.

Young, J. E., Klosko, J. S., & Weishaar, M. (2003). *Schema therapy: A practitioner's guide.* New York: Guilford Press.

9

Teaching Mindfulness-Based Stress Reduction and Mindfulness to Women with Complex Trauma

Trish Magyari

Childhood sexual abuse affects up to 16% of men and 3–27% of adult women in nationally representative samples across the United States (Molnar et al., 2001). Survivors of childhood sexual abuse may suffer symptoms across the trauma spectrum and be at 1.5–10.2 times the risk for most major mental disorders, including depression and posttraumatic stress disorder (PTSD; Molnar et al., 2001). Repeated trauma or the accumulation of multiple traumas may result in clusters of symptoms known as *complex trauma* that include anxiety, substance abuse, self-efficacy and sleep issues, and somatic complaints (Kimbrough et al., 2010; Briere & Spinazzola 2009).

This chapter reviews the results of several pertinent research studies from our group, theoretical considerations regarding the mechanisms of action of mindfulness-based stress reduction (MBSR)/mindfulness intervention for those with PTSD, and, most important, guidelines and recommendations for teaching "trauma-sensitive" MBSR specifically and the component mindfulness skills more generally. Our experience has led us to advocate for a trauma-informed approach to teaching the full MBSR curriculum of mindfulness exercises that allows the greatest chance of mastery,

---

Dedicated to the memory of Lisa Kimbrough, PhD.

healing, and success by anticipating and creating empowering solutions through skilled attention to the known challenges of working with this population. It is important to note that the components of the MBSR curriculum related to self-compassion training are especially relevant and valuable for those with complex trauma.

These guidelines are intended to be helpful not only to MBSR and mindfulness teachers but also to psychotherapists who are introducing their clients to these practices in session or whose clients are concurrently participating in an MBSR/mindfulness-based cognitive therapy (MBCT) group. Although there are a number of challenges to using mindfulness-based interventions for those persons with complex trauma (described later) and a number of issues to be sensitive to, our research data and clinical experience show that this is a well-accepted and extremely effective approach to addressing complex trauma. The combination of training to be present in *this moment* of one's life, combined with very specific and concrete instructions on how to "welcome" one's own experiences in a way that is healing rather than retraumatizing, triggering, or otherwise self-injuring, is the value of mindfulness training in general and MBSR in particular.

Background

MBSR is a semistructured, secular mindfulness curriculum that involves didactic teaching, experiential practices, as well as ample time for integration of learning. It is generally offered in an 8-week group format, with a retreat in the latter weeks of the series. Sessions are 2½ hours long, with the exception of the first and last sessions, which are 3 hours long. Retreats vary from 4 to 6 hours. The curriculum involves three main types of activities: (1) *formal meditations,* including sitting meditation (anchoring one's awareness on breath, sound, body, emotions, thoughts, and choiceless awareness), body scan, walking meditation, and mindful yoga (2 routines), and loving-kindness meditation; (2) *informal practices,* involving bringing mindfulness to activities of daily life while eating, talking, listening, and walking, as well as during stressful events; and (3) *mindful inquiry,* training in noticing and "being with" our own subjective experiences as they are happening, in a friendly way. This involves asking "What is happening right now?" and "Can I be with my experience in a friendly way?" Sessions also include time for integration/processing of the at-home practices since the previous session; didactic information about the stress cycle, stress reactivity, and the stress response (and its relationship to PTSD); and specific exercises to apply the material to everyday life experiences, including how to stay present with experiences that are emotionally distressing or that generate strong negative emotion.

Theoretical Considerations

DSM-5 places PTSD symptoms into four categories:

1. Intrusion symptoms, including triggers, flashbacks, nightmares;
2. Avoidance, including dissociation, avoiding people/places/things, as well as both emotional and memory numbing;
3. Arousal/reactivity, in which fight-or-flight reactivity is overworking, coupled with difficulty calming down; and
4. Negative mood and cognitions, such as rumination over negative events.

The changes from DSM-IV to DSM-5 leave intact the overall list of PTSD symptoms. The new diagnostic criteria are not expected to significantly alter the rate of PTSD diagnoses (Calhoun, 2012).

MBSR is an intervention that specifically and systematically addresses all of these symptom domains. Intrusion symptoms are addressed by teaching skills to stay present and work with intrusive memories and triggers as with any other phenomena—by teaching clients not to react to reflexive inner reactivity. Clients are coached to *move toward* what they are experiencing with a friendly attitude to themselves, even when they don't like their experience, thus decreasing avoidance symptoms. Arousal/reactivity symptoms decrease through the calming effect that mindfulness practices have on the nervous system, specifically by activating a parasympathetic response. Additionally, mindfulness of current surroundings can be used to notice safety when it is present. We work with negative mood and cognition by disrupting the downward spiral of depressive rumination, and with self-loathing by learning not to react to it but instead to identify thoughts simply as thoughts. Additionally, clients learn how to respond to self-critical thoughts in a kind way, creating a more positive relationship with themselves. MBSR also involves training to identify and stay with positive experiences that are often overlooked or rejected in persons with negative mood states.

According to a theoretical framework put forth by John Briere, trauma potentially affects the domains of identity, relationship problems, and affect regulation (Briere & Rickards, 2007; Briere & Spinazzola, 2010). Each of these is described more fully below, including how MBSR/mindfulness addresses the following issues.

1. Identity issues, including reduced access to oneself and being other-directed, are addressed through increasing inner-directed awareness and developing self-knowledge.
2. Relationship problems, including difficulty separating past from present in interpersonal relationships, are addressed by increasing

the ability to identify and stay with present-moment experiences, decreasing reflexive reactivity, and teaching specific mindful communication skills such as listening and speaking.

3. Affect regulation, including a reduced ability to self-regulate moods, thoughts, and feelings, is addressed by increasing self-calming skills; self-compassion; and learning to respond rather than react, especially to inner reactivity and negative emotional or cognitive states.

Research Evidence

This chapter focuses on MBSR research specifically for the complex trauma population at the University of Maryland Center for Integrative Medicine, funded by the Mental Insight Foundation. Between 2006 and 2010 we conducted MBSR with participants in three research studies for persons with PTSD from childhood sexual trauma: (1) a pilot study, MICAS (Mindfulness Intervention for Child Abuse Survivors), that included men and women (three cohorts); (2) a randomized clinical trial, AMWELL (Acupuncture and Meditation for Wellness), for women only (seven cohorts); and (3) a follow-up study, MICAS II, of participants in the pilot study to collect long-term data on our outcome assessments, additional descriptive data, and also qualitative information regarding the original intervention. In the MICAS study, we excluded those with bipolar disorder, dissociative identity disorder (DID), or psychosis, and those with active addiction or who had been in recovery for less than 6 months. In the AMWELL study, we included bipolar disorder, and we had many participants with this diagnosis, as well as at least one participant who met all criteria for DID. MICAS participants were also required to be in ongoing concurrent psychotherapy; due to the paucity of adverse events in the pilot study, we did not require concurrent psychotherapy for the AMWELL study. Adverse events were limited to a few cases of transient distress between the first and second sessions.

The results of the previously published MICAS study showed lasting decreases in all of the major outcome variables, as well as PTSD symptoms (Kimbrough, 2010). Specifically, there were significant decreases in anxiety, depression, and PTSD symptoms ($p < .0001$) as measured at 4 weeks, 8 weeks, and 24 weeks from baseline. Concurrently, mindfulness as measured on the Mindful Attention Awareness Scale (MAAS) increased compared with baseline and remained significantly increased at the 4-, 8-, and 24-week measures. When PTSD symptoms were analyzed by symptom cluster, declines were significant for all three symptom clusters at the 4-, 8-, and 24-week measurements; decreases were greatest in the "avoidance" symptom cluster. This is an important point, as many clinicians feel that the avoidant symptoms are the most debilitating for those with complex trauma and provide the greatest challenges to treatment.

Qualitative data were also collected by written questionnaire at week 4 and at week 8, immediately following the intervention. The following comments illustrate MBSR's ability to address PTSD symptomatology and to have personal meaning for the participants (comments have been disguised to preserve study participant's confidentiality without altering meaning):

PARTICIPANT A'S WORDS

- Week 4: "At last I can let go of the shame and anger. Now I can stay with those thoughts without panicking or trying to avoid them."
- Week 8: "In this group I've learned that I am not my crazy thoughts and it's OK to feel scared, sad, or angry. It doesn't mean that I am falling apart. The most important part was learning not to bury my thoughts. That's at the core of my being able to forgive myself."

PARTICIPANT B'S WORDS

- Week 4: "Before this class, I was stuck. This class is on growing and healing. It's really useful to learn not to be so judgmental of myself."
- Week 8: "To be in this moment, present, and not dwell on the past. I've learned that I have the strength to heal myself and to be a friend to myself. It's like I've been awakened. It felt good to be reintroduced to myself."

PARTICIPANT C'S WORDS

- Week 4: "This class has given me a tool that will help me to handle my life better. The most useful tool for me is the body scan."
- Week 8: "In this group I've been formally introduced to myself. I feel like I am finding myself after being lost for a very long time, and I am feeling more secure about who I am during this period of my life. I am also more willing to reach out to people rather than withdraw from everyone. The body scan helped me to get in touch with the places where I hold all the pain, in addition to all the normal aches and pains. I found myself again."

Participant C was also interviewed 2¾ years after the MBSR course as part of the MICAS II study. Some of the behavioral changes that she reports since the MBSR course include:

- Recognizing how "stressed" she was in her former job and finding a new, more fulfilling job that she has been in for the last 2½ years.

- Stopping smoking after many previous failed attempts; now smoke-free for more than 2 years.
- Getting married after a lengthy engagement. "Finally felt safe enough"; feeling happy in marriage.
- Taking up running. She now runs a 5-mile race on a regular basis.

These behavior changes illustrate increased self-awareness, increased relationality, decreased reliance on an addictive substance for coping, and increased healthy behaviors. Such changes were echoed in other participants' follow-up reports.

Most important, MBSR is an intervention that is highly valued, accepted, and appreciated by the participants. Although many participants had unstable living conditions, compliance was very high, with a mean attendance at seven of nine sessions, including those who did not participate in the intervention at all after randomization. Self-report journals and subjective experiences reported in the group revealed a high compliance with practice and only mild adverse events during the research. Notable was the lack of distressing events during the silent, eyes-closed mindfulness meditations or lying-down yoga routines, two activities often considered to be too emotionally challenging for those with complex trauma. We concluded that therapeutic approaches prescribing the opposite of avoidance, that is, acceptance or exposure, may be most successful for treating complex trauma and that MBSR may a potent therapeutic adjunct to traditional psychotherapy. MBSR is a widely available, cost-effective way for clients to gain skills that may help them to be able to process the intense emotional experiences that often occur in trauma-focused therapy. Therefore, MBSR could also act synergistically with individual or group psychotherapy to increase effectiveness.

MICAS participants were brought back again 2–3 years from baseline and roughly 1½–2½ years following the 24-week assessment. All written assessments were readministered and new data were collected regarding trauma and mental health history, as well as feedback on the course itself. The most consistent feedback on the course was that participants liked and valued the fact that they didn't need to "tell their trauma story" to the group and that the MBSR curriculum focused on their lives now and on moving forward. Analysis of the outcome measures shows a continued significant reduction in depression, anxiety, and PTSD symptoms from baseline (M. Chesney, personal communication, April 9, 2012).

Clinical Considerations

The following guidelines come from (1) my clinical experience of leading the MBSR groups for the MICAS and AMWELL studies; (2) facilitating over

50 additional MBSR groups for a variety of chronic pain and/or chronic illness populations; (3) recommendations gleaned from participants during follow-up interviews for the MICAS II study; and (4) Char Wilkins, MSW, with whom I have co-led two workshops on this subject at the University of Massachusetts annual MBSR conference.

Clinical Challenges in Providing MBSR/Mindfulness Interventions to Complex Trauma Survivors

The clinical challenges of teaching mindfulness/MBSR arise primarily from the PTSD symptoms of *avoidance, reexperiencing,* and *reactivity.* Rather than seeing these challenges as limiting factors, we have developed methods of addressing them that features one of the core mindfulness tenets of "responding" rather than "reacting" to a participant's emotional reactivity. Of greatest importance when considering these challenges is how to evoke a sense of mastery of the MBSR material so as not to perpetuate the cycle of failure so familiar to those with complex trauma. Specific challenges experienced by survivors of complex trauma include:

- A decreased ability to experience and/or stay with physical sensations, leading to physical numbing and/or dissociation;
- A decreased ability to experience and/or stay with emotions, leading to emotional numbing and/or emotional reactivity;
- A decreased ability to stay with present moment, leading to dissociation;
- An increased identification with and attachment to a negative story line and memories, leading to flashbacks and ruminating;
- Increased self-judgment and unworthiness, leading to thoughts that they are not doing it right or good enough or that that they are bad;
- Fear that PTSD symptoms (e.g., worry, avoidance) will be triggered if they become present to their own experiences;
- Feelings of hopelessness, failure (e.g., self-doubt, unworthiness);
- A feeling of being unsafe at home, leading to inability to practice at home;
- A tendency to start with the most challenging practices rather than the easiest.

The approach to MBSR and mindfulness-based therapy described here responds to these clinical challenges while also maintaining the integrity of the MBSR intervention.

Appropriate Candidates for MBSR/Mindfulness Groups

The experience of clients in our program supports the belief that MBSR/ mindfulness is an appropriate intervention for many individuals who are healing from complex PTSD. However, attention to timing is important to ensure the maximum therapeutic benefit from MBSR. Some clients are best served initially by having individual therapeutic work on their trauma histories *prior* to entering a group situation—in particular, those in the immediate crisis phase of their trauma healing, those with ongoing physical safety concerns, and those who are not yet stable on medications indicated for co-occurring conditions. Contraindications for group MBSR include being actively suicidal, in an active addiction process, or actively psychotic. During this preliminary individual work, it is helpful to put in place basic tools for staying present that will allow the client to focus on the didactic material in the future group setting without dissociating or falling asleep when others are talking. Lastly, although "believing" in the efficacy of the mindfulness approach is *not* a prerequisite to being helped by it, the client does need to be open to an approach that requires personal time and effort (weekly class attendance, at-home practice) and also must be able to organize life on a practical level to attend regular weekly sessions.

Teacher/Therapist Characteristics

Teaching MBSR to groups of people with PTSD requires an advanced level of mindfulness training, practice, and embodiment, as well as a deep understanding of the traumatized psyche. The most important characteristic for the MBSR teacher/therapist is to be advanced enough in the practice of mindfulness him- or herself so that he or she is not reacting in an outer way to a client's inner or outer reactivity. The therapist models the desired response to reactivity by nonjudgmentally naming the cognitive, physical, and emotional experiences that the client reports experiencing. It is natural for the MBSR participant to react in habituated ways to new experiences that may be frightening to her; this reaction primarily stems from negative cognitive patterns being activated by sensory experiences. A therapist who lacks experience in mindfulness approaches might prematurely conclude that "the client can't do it" or that "this isn't right for them" when clients encounter predictable challenges (such as noticing that they can't "feel" parts of their body during the body scan or getting anxious when their minds are quiet) in the first few weeks of the MBSR class. Our experience has shown that clients are able to work through temporary challenges brought on by mindfulness practice with clarification of the instructions and an eye to working with negative self-judgment.

Instead of encouraging avoidance, the mindful therapist gently guides the client through concrete inquiry with questions such as "What is happening right now in your body?" "What are your feelings?" "Can you be with them in a friendly way?" When negative cognitions arise, and they will, it is important to name them as thoughts and to go back to staying with the sensory experiences. Other helpful characteristics include exuding confidence both in mindfulness as a modality and in the client's potential for recovery and ability to learn mindfulness skills. A sense of humor about trauma reactivity is also helpful. Above all, the teacher is a mindfulness practitioner and embodies the practices in class.

It can be invaluable for individual therapy to continue during the group MBSR experience so that material can be integrated with a known and trusted helper. The following guidelines for the referring therapist increase the chances of a positive clinical outcome.

1. Encourage the client to have an individual face-to-face meeting with the MBSR teacher prior to the course beginning. This will allow the teacher to get to know the client's point of entry and, more important, to build trust before the group begins.
2. Reassure the client that she will not have to share her trauma story in the group; however, it is not "taboo" if such sharing is relevant to present-moment experiences. Many of our participants said that the MBSR approach of "moving forward" rather than reviewing the past was what they appreciated most.
3. Help clients integrate new experiences by remaining present with challenging ones.
4. Sign appropriate consents so that the therapist and the MBSR teacher can consult, if needed.
5. Encourage the client to call the MBSR teacher if she develops distress at home while doing the practices. Most issues are resolved by clarifying instructions.
6. Give positive feedback for any movement toward the mindfulness goals of increased presence, awareness of the client's own subjective experience, naming of experiences, not reacting to cognitive reactivity, self-soothing following self-judging, recognizing challenges versus distress and responding appropriately to these situations.

Sensitivities to Trauma to Incorporate into Standard MBSR and Other Mindfulness Interventions

Many of the suggestions for "trauma-sensitive MBSR" stem from adhering to good teaching practices; paying special attention to clarity, safety, trust, and boundaries; and, above all, being aware of how to handle known and expected challenges. Each of these sensitivities may also be useful for therapists introducing mindfulness approaches into individual sessions.

Safety Concerns

The room should be a private one, with any public window openings covered during the group. The teacher sits in a chair from which he or she can watch the door; very often latecomers to the group will enter during the opening meditation. The teacher verbalizes who is entering the room: for example, "Sally is taking off her coat now and joining the circle." Confidentiality is particularly important; although the MBSR teacher may know much about participants' trauma history, the level of sharing is left up to group members. Confidentiality guidelines are discussed and decided upon in the first session. The MBSR teacher ensures group members' feeling of safety with a question such as, "Is there anything else you'd like to ask for to feel safe in this group?"

Giving Choice/Control to Participants

The language of mindfulness instructions is very important. Use language that involves "invitations": asking permission, emphasizing choice, and giving people time to go at their own pace. For example: "When you're ready, I invite you to open your eyes and rejoin the group." Helping the clients to maintain a sense of control over the process of the intervention is empowering and helpful to recovery.

Introducing Mindfulness in a Concrete Fashion/Titrating Silent Practice

"Mindfulness" is often equated with a silent meditation on the breath. Although persons with complex trauma histories or PTSD may benefit over time from extended silent periods of breath meditation, they often benefit from other, more concrete guided mindfulness practices as a first introduction. We introduce clients to mindfulness meditation using an "arriving" practice that guides them through an exploration of the different domains of present-moment experience (sensory, physical, emotional, cognitive) with only short periods (two to three breath cycles of silence) between concrete instructions. Many clients surprise themselves with their ability to discern and name their subjective experiences without evoking distress, thus building a sense of mastery and confidence in both the practices and their ability to learn them. Meditation on the breath and the body scan are both introduced later in the same initial MBSR session using concrete language and instruction for continuous inner "noting" of experience.

The Therapist's Treatment of Client Reactivity

Listen carefully for self-judgments, such as "I can't do this," "I'm not doing it right." These are natural responses to beginning mindfulness practice that often cause a great deal of distress. It is important to reframe these cognitions as examples of self-judgment that can be acknowledged and responded to appropriately: becoming aware, naming (i.e., "judging"), noticing how one experiences self-judging on a somatic level, and responding in a kind way to any reactivity that has already occurred following the self-judgment (more on this later).

Normalizing PTSD Coping Strategies and Honoring Their Role in the Past

It is important to tell the client, "We aren't trying to 'get rid' of anything" (Wilkins, 2014). Use of MBSR removes the self-blame clients may feel for avoidant behavior or an inability to control reactivity to flashbacks or triggering experiences; there is no need to further blame maladaptive coping strategies such as perfectionism or dissociation. It is helpful to explicitly state early on in the group that the "hurt little girl was doing the best she could at the time" and is to be honored for keeping the client alive until adulthood, and that "now we are learning another way" to respond to past traumas that will permit a fuller way of living (Wilkins, 2014).

Being Explicit with Clients about How to Stay within the Therapeutic Window during Class and at Home

This should be done before any meditation practice. It is of utmost importance to give a number of explicit directions and guidelines before doing any extended formal practice, such as differentiating between the constructive challenge of staying present with unpleasant experiences and the unproductive "staying with" once a client has lost mindfulness and is living within a distressing experience or "in the distress zone." The therapist should give examples of how to recognize each and what to do if clients find themselves in the distress zone, especially when at home: Stop the exercise, open your eyes, stand, use your senses to notice you are safe, get water, and/or do something self-soothing; then name the experience: "distress," "dissociating," "flashback," and so forth. When the ability to be mindful has returned, the client is guided to restart the meditation. In later sessions we discuss how to know whether one is entering the distress zone, seeing clearly the cognitions that take one there, and using present-moment experiences to stay out of or exit the distress zone once in it. We give explicit words to track and note inner reactivity ("judging," "adding-on," "telling stories," "spinning"). Because participants are apt to swamp themselves by taking on too much in the beginning, we guide them to "Pick up the 5-pound weight, not the 50-pound weight." In practical terms this means not doing extended silent practice without guidance from a CD or teacher until skills to constructively use the meditation time are developed, generally after the first two or three weekly sessions.

Balancing Teaching of Awareness and Compassion

Awareness is generally stronger in the beginning, so teach compassion from the beginning in order to balance both mindfulness tenets. We believe it is ethical practice to increase awareness in distressed individuals only when compassion is in place to hold that awareness, and until participants can allow a compassionate acceptance of mindfulness experiences, the therapist should support them in this process. Therefore, active compassion (kindness and friendliness to one's own experience) is woven throughout the MBSR series in implicit and explicit ways. Most important, knowing how to be kind toward the self-judging cognitive habit is essential to MBSR success. In addition, the formal loving-kindness meditation is introduced early in the series, at the end of the second session, beginning with instruction on how to send messages of goodwill to oneself.

Giving Instructions on How to Transcend the Cycle of Self-Loathing

It is important to respond instead of react to cognitive self-judgments. Because self-loathing and self-judging cognitive habits are generally very strong in this group, it is important to give explicit instructions for working with this habit in order to break the downward spiral that comes from feeling bad about oneself for having such a habit. If mindfulness is strong and there is no inner reaction stemming from "believing" these self-judgments, the client may note, "judging," and keep going. However, more often there *is* an inner reaction—some sense of feeling bad or wrong or defective stemming from the self-judgment. In this case, it is helpful for the client to respond to the reaction before continuing. Responding in this way sets up a new, more healing habit. The response may be nonverbal—clients may put their own hands on their own cheeks or over their own hearts when they feel the reaction to self-judging—or it may be verbal. When reacting to self-judgment, the client may say to herself, "It's OK," "It's all right," "Let it go," "Let it be," "I'm OK just as I am," or even simply "forgiven." Therapists teach a menu of options, and clients are occasionally asked to share the method of self-soothing that is working the best for them.

Emphasis on Naming the "Habits of the Mind"

From the first session, the teacher discusses the therapeutic value of getting to know the habits of the mind. Cognitive neuroscience is helpful in this regard; clients may understand the concept of "neural grooves" and the value of noticing and naming cognitive habits as just that—habits or "grooves" that may or may not be relevant to the present moment.

I challenge participants to notice and acknowledge their most common habits—planning, worrying, analyzing, judging, spinning stories, fantasizing, or "spacing out."

Adaptations to Standard MBSR

As mentioned previously, in our program we use the full MBSR curriculum, as developed at the University of Massachusetts and described in Jon Kabat-Zinn's (2013) book *Full Catastrophe Living*. However, there are adaptations in class size, format, and structure that may also be useful for therapists introducing these practices into therapeutic groups. In general, what makes trauma-sensitive teaching is in the "how" of it, rather than the "what" of it.

Smaller Group Size and Longer Sessions

For a group designed for clients with complex PTSD, six to eight people is an ideal group size if there is only one leader. The ideal MBSR format for a dedicated PTSD group is 10–12 weeks of 2-hour sessions (as contrasted to 8 weeks for general MBSR) and a 4- to 6-hour retreat, followed by 3–6 months of monthly 2-hour sessions to reinforce and stabilize gains. For participants in mixed community MBSR groups, I recommend contracting ahead of time for one to two individual sessions midcourse and monthly individual sessions after the group is over to integrate and stabilize mindfulness skills. Becoming part of an ongoing mindfulness practice group in the community is also very helpful.

Use of an Enrollment Interview

Participants benefit greatly from a face-to-face meeting with the MBSR teacher before the first session. If this is not logistically possible, an individual meeting should be held sometime in the first 2 weeks. During this meeting the point is not to elicit the full trauma "story" but rather to ask about current symptoms, triggers, what has helped so far, supports, and any special request. The teacher should specifically tell the client that it is the normal progression of things to experience more symptoms during the first few weeks of mindfulness practice and that this is generally temporary; participants are urged to contact the teacher between sessions if they encounter distress.

Predictable Class Structure

Participants benefit from having a reliable structure to the class, which can be consciously and slowly made flexible (if needed) as the group progresses.

We begin with an opening meditation of previously learned material; a check-in practicing the naming of raw experiences rather than "story"; dyad sharing regarding at-home practices, using a mindful listening–speaking format to stay present to one's own experience; questions and answers; new material; check-in; review of pertinent notebook pages; assignment of at-home practices; and a ritualized ending involving holding hands while standing in a circle, emphasizing connection to self (body/breath), group members, and the earth.

Increased Process Time

After every meditation, a go-round mindful inquiry for "one or two words of your current experience: physical, emotional or mental," with attention paid to the degree of presence, provides additional opportunity to process experiences. Teachers must watch for signs of distress and help them to be named. Discussion time should be increased to stay within the therapeutic window and address avoidance.

Additional Practice Staying in Contact with the Self during Dyads

Dyads are a great format in which to practice mindful listening and mindful speaking on a weekly basis, as well as to process at-home experiences. Even with mindfulness in place, participants can be pulled out of themselves through the process of relating to others; we practice coming back to ourselves through the "three breaths break" between dyad questions. While participants stay with their experience of three breath cycles, the therapist reinforces that they are moving from outer to inner, from "doing" to "being," and invites participants to notice what this is like.

Positive Psychology Enhancements

Class material is taught in a manner designed to emphasize the positive psychology tenets of mastery, cultivating gratitude, acknowledging one's efforts, savoring positive experiences, connection, noticing what works, coping effectiveness training, and honoring one's own inner wisdom.

Body Scan Sensitivities and Adaptations as an Example

We have encountered many questions about introducing the body scan to those with sexual abuse histories, and I offer here some guidelines. Spending unstructured silent time focusing on bodily sensations (or lack of sensations) may be distressing to some participants in the beginning; on the other hand, increasing one's ability to "be with" physical experiences is very helpful to healing from trauma. Therefore, our overall approach is to give much anticipatory guidance before the practice so that there is the highest chance of having an affirming experience. This includes normalizing the typical experiences of physical numbing and/or distress at encountering physical sensations. It is important also to guide the practice such that the teacher cues to concrete bodily sensations as these areas are encountered during the normal feet-to-head scan; for example, sensations of contact with the floor, of one's heartbeat, of the sensations of breathing. As clients often fill the silence in the beginning with unproductive cognitive habits, the teacher must keep things moving along, encouraging them to be curious about their own experiences: Where am I the coolest? Warmest? The most relaxed? The most tense? Is my in-breath cooler or warmer than my out-breath? Additionally, clients will have already explored their physical state briefly during the "arriving" meditation and can build on that experience of learning to identify and note their bodily sensations in a friendly way to a more sustained and detailed meditation.

Before the body scan, we offer not only a discussion about what we are doing and the purpose of it but also anticipatory guidance regarding staying within the therapeutic window. We define the difference between an experience being challenging but still mindful and being outright distressing, such that the client is emotionally and/or cognitively swamped and has lost mindfulness altogether. From our perspective, there is nothing to be gained when total beginners who have PTSD are in the distress zone. It is preferable for clients to use their awareness to notice this and make wise choices regarding self-care and mindfully finding their way out of distress. Prior to beginning the body scan, we also invite participants to invoke a "safe place" or "loving presence" as a resource. This could be visualization as part of the preparation, or it might be a concrete photo or talisman kept nearby. Beginning in the second group session, we invite participants to invoke a mindful quality that they already have inside them to accompany them during their practice time. Part of the body scan homework in the first session is to locate a "home base" within the body—that place where they can maintain their awareness in relative comfort. This may not be the most "comfortable" place in the body but the place that they can reliably find and hold in mindful awareness. This will be a topic for discussion in session 2.

Participants who say they can't "feel anything" after the body scan are led in inquiry. We ask whether they can feel their feet on the floor and their bodies in the chairs, right now. Generally, they will say "yes" to this question. This helps clarify that this is a case of their thought habits telling them they cannot do it, not that in fact they cannot feel their bodies at all. This understanding is then used as an invitation to practice self-compassion in response to self-judging. It is important to emphasize the acknowledgment of what participants *can* feel and being patient and compassionate about the fact that it may take a while for more complete awareness of sensation to occur.

Conclusion

In this chapter, I have reviewed the theoretical and research evidence indicating that mindfulness practices in general, and MBSR in particular, may be useful therapeutic modalities for persons with complex trauma histories and specifically for women healing from childhood sexual abuse. Mindfulness interventions have been shown to significantly reduce PTSD symptoms, including avoidance symptoms, and are designed to generate less reactive ways to relate to events that generate negative moods and cognitions. Although there are a variety of clinical challenges for this population, clients with complex PTSD will benefit most from mindfulness interventions that include trauma-sensitive titrated instruction, thoughtful adaptations, and helpful collaboration between the referring therapist and the mindfulness provider. With attention to these factors, MBSR and other mindfulness interventions may allow individuals to free themselves from the sequelae of past traumatic life events and move forward with renewed mental health.

Acknowledgments

The following people have contributed ideas to the development of this approach: Char Wilkins, Tara Brach, Jack Kornfield, John Makransky, Sharon Salzberg, Larry Rosenberg, Jon Kabat-Zinn, Margaret Chesney, John Briere, Marsha Linehan, and Bill O'Hanlon. Many thanks to Michele Calder Carras for expert help in editing an early draft of the manuscript and a special acknowledgment to Lisa Kimbrough Pradham for her research dedication to this population.

With deep gratitude to all of the men and women who have entrusted their suffering to our care and whose lives are blossoming—moment by moment. *May they be well. May they be safe. May they be happy and free.*

References

Briere, J., & Rickards, S. (2007). Self-awareness, affect regulation, and relatedness: Differential sequels of childhood versus adult victimization experiences. *Journal of Nervous and Mental Disease, 195*(6), 497–503.

Briere, J., & Spinazzola, J. (2009). Assessment of the sequelae of complex trauma: Evidence-based measures. In C. A. Courtois & J. D. Ford (Eds.), *Treating complex traumatic stress disorders: Scientific foundations and therapeutic models* (pp. 104–123). New York: Guilford Press.

Calhoun, P. S., Hertzberg, J. S., Kirby, A. C., Dennis, M. F., Hair. L. P., Dedert, E. A., et al. (2012). The effect of draft DSM-V criteria on posttraumatic stress disorder prevalence. *Depression and Anxiety, 29*(12), 1032–1042.

Kabat-Zinn, J. (2013). *Full catastrophe living, revised edition.* New York: Bantam Books.

Kimbrough, E., Magyari, T., Langenberg, C., Chesney, M., & Berman, B. (2010). Mindfulness intervention for child abuse survivors. *Journal of Clinical Psychology, 66*(1), 17–33.

Molnar, B. E., Buka, S. L., & Kessler, R. C. (2001). Child sexual abuse and subsequent psychopathology: Results from the National Comorbidity Survey. *American Journal of Public Health, 91*(5), 753–760.

Wilkins, C. (2014). Mindulness, women and child abuse—Turning toward what's difficult. *Social Work Today, 14*(2), 10.

10

Focusing-Oriented Psychotherapy

A Contemplative Approach to Healing Trauma

Doralee Grindler Katonah

Even when one is overcome by the impact of a traumatic event, the *wholeness* of the person continues and holds the potential to integrate the trauma in a transformative way. The healing of trauma is expressed when life becomes *more* meaningful, alive, and purposeful. A strengthening of character, a deepening of faith, a grounding in one's inherent goodness, and the feeling of empowerment to express one's deepest desires are the fruits (Levine, 2010). Contemplative approaches to work with trauma aim to create a connection with this *wholeness* and release the resources already available within each person.

I believe that even when faced with trauma one can find direct access to this *wholeness* through interacting with the *felt sense,* which opens the pathway to integration (Gendlin, 1997). Survivors of unresolved trauma experience a deep loneliness and require the compassionate presence of another person who is able to resonate with this bodily level of experiencing.

The focusing-oriented approach (Gendlin, 1996) to psychotherapy is an embodied contemplative practice that posits a living body that is an undivided whole that knows what is needed next for development. This "living-body" approach draws upon mindfulness, neurobiology, relational connection, and spiritual potential as a unified process. It values directing our nonjudgmental attention to the *felt sense,* the bodily source of a more integrated kind of knowing—a knowing that carries forward the well-being and growth of the whole person (Gendlin, 1969). This chapter introduces this contemplative therapeutic method through a detailed presentation and commentary on a series of verbatim clinical exchanges demonstrating a focusing-oriented approach to working with a childhood rape trauma. I hope to define and demonstrate elements of the focusing process that enable the integration of past trauma and that restore a person's connection to her or his deepest purpose in present living. Specific process interventions are illustrated and explained with an emphasis on their impact on personal and spiritual transformation.

Context

Research shows that talk therapy alone does not access the wisdom of the body (Ogden, Minton, & Pain, 2006; van der Kolk, 2006). Neuroscience research finds that after situations of extreme stress and trauma, when there is a reminder of the events, only certain regions of the brain are activated. Intense emotions, accompanied by physical arousal, activate the limbic system while deactivating the areas of the brain that integrate sensory experience with motor responses, that modulate physiological arousal, and that generate language and flexible assessment of one's current situation (van der Kolk, 1996). Discussing the results of his positron emission tomography (PET) scan study of people with posttraumatic stress disorder (PTSD) who are exposed to trauma-related stimuli, van der Kolk (1996) reports:

> There is an increase in perfusion of the areas in the right hemisphere associated with emotional states and autonomic arousal. Moreover, there is a simultaneous decrease in oxygen utilization in Broca's area— the region in the left inferior frontal cortex responsible for generating words to attach to internal experience. These findings may account for the observation that trauma may lead to "speechless terror," which in some individuals interferes with the ability to put feelings into words, leaving emotions to be mutely expressed by dysfunction of the body. (p. 193)

This biological adaptation to an inescapable situation interferes with one's ability to integrate the reality of a past trauma, to formulate the meanings of the experience that promote growth and vitality in one's present living.

The focusing-oriented approach guides the client to a *felt sense* of the situation, which isn't the same as emotions per se. Tapping into the *felt sense* automatically increases physical relaxation. This allows the formation of a more subtle sense of the whole of the situation, directly felt but without words or symbols. The *felt sense* carries dimensions of the experience that have not been able to be symbolized meaningfully. As clients are able to "be with the *felt sense*," rather than just reexperiencing a traumatic aspect, words, images, gestures, and sounds form that express meaning. Each emergent symbolization is then checked back with the *felt sense* until it (word, image, gesture, etc.) resonates exactly with this bodily knowing. Thus the focusing-oriented approach works exactly at the felt edge of a bodily sense of the trauma and moves back and forth between the *felt sense* and the fresh symbolizations. This back-and-forth process enables an unworded body sense to become known through meaningful symbols that continue to resonate with the body, opening the whole organism to the possibility of integrated growth in the present.

Spirituality is now recognized as a significant dimension of human meaning (Pargament, 2007). Measures of spiritual and religious beliefs and practices are positively correlated with mental and physical health (Saunders, Miller, & Bright, 2010). Our natural religious desire is to reach out, beyond ourselves, to seek larger sources of healing and perspective on the significance of our lives. When suffering cannot be explained or easily relieved, people are more likely to pray, to speak to a spiritual advisor, and to return to or seek out a religious or spiritual community (Pargament, 1997). At the same time, under situations of trauma, people are more vulnerable to a crisis of faith, in which past religious beliefs and resources are questioned and people may feel abandoned or betrayed by God. Spiritually sensitive care responds to the client's own search, questioning, and desire for a relationship to the transcendent (Pargament, 2007).

William James provides an understanding of the dynamics of spiritual transformation when facing a life-changing crisis (James, 1961). He believed that forms of religious life are developed in response to direct experiences of the Divine that are felt to be deeply personal. He makes a distinction between the religiosity of the once-born and that of the twice-born. Each typology reflects a pattern of how one relates to suffering and evil that grows out of such spiritual experiences.

The once-born is grounded in the experience of God as near, and the joy of this presence permeates all experience "whose soul is of this sky-blue tint, whose affinities are rather with flowers and birds and all enchanting innocences than with dark human passions" (James, 1961, p. 79). To live the once-born pattern, suffering and injustice are dealt with by turning away from the suffering and concentrating one's mind on the good (James, 1961, p. 86).

However, according to James, this "sky blue" spirituality is precarious. What happens when suffering is so great that it can't be turned away from? James found an example in Leo Tolstoy. Around age 50, Tolstoy was struck with a sudden loss of a sense of vitality and purpose to his life (Tolstoy, 2010). He was beset with the question, Why? Tolstoy wrote: "I felt that something had broken within me on which my life had always rested, that I had nothing left to hold on to, and that morally my life had stopped"

(James, 1961, p. 130). As James says, "the sense that life had any meaning whatsoever was for a time wholly withdrawn" (James, 1961, p. 131).

The process of facing the question of human suffering transforms current beliefs toward wider meaning. The twice-born faces suffering and death and through this process finds that suffering and death are not victorious over a faith that arises and proclaims the preciousness of life. This potential for spiritual transformation can be accessed through the *felt sense* (Grindler Katonah, 2006).

Theory

Focusing-oriented psychotherapy is an emerging family of psychotherapies inspired by Gendlin's discovery of focusing as a predictor of successful personality change (Gendlin, Beebe, Cassens, Klein, & Oberlander, 1968) and by Rogerian psychotherapy (Rogers, 1961) and refined by focusing-oriented psychotherapy outcome research reported in a review of more than 80 studies (Hendricks, 2001). Further studies investigate *clearing a space,* the first step of focusing (Grindler Katonah, 2010, 2012).

The roots of focusing-oriented psychotherapy are in Gendlin's philosophy of the implicit (1996, 1997), which illuminates *how it is possible* for the process of living to form something new that brings change in the direction of further development. It is the body sensing itself living and functioning to further the life of the whole organism. "An organism is an environmental interaction that continuously regenerates itself. It does not follow from the past, but it does take account of it. We can show that the regenerating is a kind of precision. We call it 'implicit precision'" (Gendlin, 2012). If you pay attention to your body, the *felt sense* forms from this implicit precision and becomes known and explicated. Thus a *felt sense* is not just perception, not just feeling, not just sensation, not just cognition; rather, all come together as a felt intricacy that knows more than what we can say in the usual way about what is needed to further life now. Speaking directly from what is felt draws upon language and concepts in new ways, unique to the person, while remaining connected to the *felt sense* of what needs to emerge next.

Focusing-oriented psychotherapy (Gendlin, 1996) engages the *felt senses* that form in response to one's situation, felt in the body just below the normal level of consciousness. The term *felt sense* refers to this "bodily felt whole" of one's situation. When first accessed, the *felt sense* is concretely felt but conceptually vague. It is a bodily sense that is an undivided whole, including unfinished potential meanings that further development felt as an undifferentiated mesh.

The therapist invites the client to *pause* and bring her or his attention to the body. The client learns to cultivate a manner of attention that includes qualities of nonjudgment, gentleness, and curiosity. This *pausing and attending* helps the person to develop the "right distance" from the problem, creating the ability to *be with* what is felt rather than inside the problem. Direct access to this felt level is precisely what a trauma survivor needs to regain the ability to symbolize his or her experience in a titrated fashion.

After *pausing and attending* and allowing a *felt sense* to form, information emerges freshly from different avenues of expression, such as images, words, gestures, art, and behaviors. When the *felt sense* is connected to trauma memories that cannot be verbalized, descriptions of the qualities of the felt sensations or sounds and body gestures function as explicit symbolizations that move the process forward. The new symbolizations are checked back with the body for accuracy and are confirmed through a bodily resonating. This process of symbolizing and checking is what moves the whole organism forward into further action or expression of meaning. New meaning is lived, not just known, thus freeing the person from fixed action patterns that constrict one's current living. Physiological release (deeper breathing, easing of tension) and increased confidence and hope accompany this shift. In the therapeutic encounter the process moves back and forth between sensing and symbolizing, checking and waiting.

The *felt sense* is inherently *relational. Felt senses* form within both client and therapist, mediated through their relationship as it lives in each session. This relational mesh includes the client's experience of nonjudgmental presence communicated by the therapist. It also includes difficulties that arise within the therapeutic relationship that may also express the meaning of the relational difficulties experienced by the client. However, each *felt sense* also includes a sense of something wanting to emerge fresh, beyond the problem. Many therapeutic models emphasize relational difficulties as they are recreated in the interaction between client and therapist. In the focusing-oriented therapeutic model, the therapist is attending to his or her *felt sense* of what wants to grow or develop within the client. Often this "growth direction" is expressed by the client as a "still, small voice," whereas what is problematic carries more intensity. The therapist registers this communication from the "still, small voice" in the body and speaks *from* her or his sense of this forward direction (Gendlin, 2004). The therapist learns to *attend, pause,* and *notice* fresh symbolizations within him- or herself and communicates their emergence with the invitation to the client to check for resonance. If accurate, this communication from the therapist resonates with the implied step of change within the client. Thus the therapist's *felt sense response* carries forward growth directions in the client. When the therapist pays attention in this way, something distinctive emerges that he or she was not previously aware of or likely to think about. Through this process a deep trust grows in this level of bodily implying that pulls both people toward further development. Both the therapist and the client discover something new that brings further aliveness. This therapeutic process is constituted by this larger interactive process that moves beyond our individual knowing.

Focusing has directionality. The *felt sense* always implies the next step of living. *Steps of change* that emerge from the *felt sense* are unique to the person and cannot be derived from a protocol, nor a culturally constructed meaning, nor a theoretical perspective per se. Rather, they express an intricacy of meaning that moves the person's particular purposeful aliveness forward. The small *steps of change* bring the person back to the present with greater capacity to fully engage in his or her present life with renewed meaning and purpose.

Case Example

Introduction to the Case

Mary (pseudonym) obtained my name from her insurance company and spoke over the phone in an agitated tone. She had recently experienced a panic attack and was given a prescription by her physician. She related her symptoms to what she had experienced a year previously after a relative died in a car accident, leaving behind her husband and daughter. Through our phone conversation she recognized that her symptoms might be expressing unresolved grief, and she scheduled an appointment.

At our first session, I saw a woman of medium build who appeared burdened by sadness and fear. She was 30 years old and reported a happy marriage. She was a teacher who seemed popular among friends and within her church community. She described her grief reaction, saying: "Why wasn't it me? Why did God do this?"

I learned that this sudden loss was not the only trauma Mary was facing. Since the death of her relative, she began having flashbacks to a childhood rape at age 11. She had been visiting a family member at a lake resort and was walking home at dusk from a park when she noticed a boy, whom she had met earlier, following her. She felt some uneasiness when he approached her, but nothing in her imagination could have prepared her for the violent rape that occurred. Currently she experienced sleep disturbance related to the resurgence of rape flashbacks that would haunt her at night.

By the third session, she revealed that she had suffered a miscarriage. She feared she would never become pregnant and raise a family. This loss of a lifelong dream to become a mother, along with the death of her relative and the remembrance of the childhood rape, created a complex trauma picture, which included a loss of faith.

She was raised in a Christian family. She recalls that she went to church and always "loved God." She delighted in God and believed God wanted her to make everyone happy. Her faith had been strong and unquestioned until now. She feared she was turning away from God.

The therapy progressed over the course of 1 year. I worked to create a safe space through my listening presence and communication of unconditional regard. With my guidance, through attending to a *felt sense* of her grief in the moment, Mary became open to a broad range of emotions. Gradually, she developed a capacity to be with her experience in a focusing-oriented way through cultivating an interested curiosity, an ability to hold an experience at a little distance while remaining relatively calm, and to approach difficult memories and emotions with compassion rather than judgment. Also, during this time, I emphasized inviting her to sense what she needed for her self-care. Rather than prescribing a particular practice or behavior, I asked her to sense what was needed and to listen carefully to the symbolizations that emerged and resonated. She recalled always wanting a dog as a child, but her parents had never responded to this desire. She actually found a puppy, and the bodily connection that was generated with this animal gave her a sense of safety she hadn't experienced before. Because she found what "fit" or "resonated" for her, it became easy for her to regularly attend a yoga class. The regular body practice and the increased sense of inner safety helped her develop a capacity to be with a *felt sense* of a difficult memory without falling into intense affect and repetitive thoughts. Thus aspects of the trauma were felt, reflected upon, and released in a gradual manner.

Still, she continued to express hopelessness about becoming a mother and trusting in life again. The injustices of the untimely death of her relative and of her rape led to a crisis of faith: Where was God when she needed Him?

The following series of therapeutic interactions demonstrate how a focusing-oriented approach furthers integrative processing. Each vignette segment is followed by a commentary to highlight the steps of the process.

After this first year, Mary suffered another panic attack, and she came to this session agitated. She looked pale and sad. She reported that just prior to the panic attack, she was spending the day with her best friend, who had just heard that her niece had been raped.

I noticed that as she was talking she stroked her neck and her voice had a labored quality to it. I invited her to bring her attention to her body and notice what was there.

CLIENT: I feel all this tension; a kind of tightness here in my neck. . . .

THERAPIST: So, let's make some space to notice all of that in your neck. Take a moment to let it be as it is.

CLIENT: (*Deep breaths . . . legs uncross . . . eases into the chair . . .*)

By making space to notice the body sensations, I am supporting the developing mindful relationship *within* the client—her ability to be with what is occurring in her body with attitudes of nonjudgment, compassion, and curiosity. This ability allows a connection to what is felt without falling into it or distancing too much. New information now can emerge in a titrated way.

THERAPIST: You may want to notice how your body responds to your words . . . tension/tightness. . . . As you say them again to yourself . . . is there a sense of "fit," resonating in your body?

Recall that the focusing approach works in a back-and-forth fashion. When a "content" such as a word or image emerges from the body, one does not automatically accept this symbolization as an accurate fit with what the body knows. Rather, the therapist invites the client to "pause" and check the words back with the body to see if the body resonates. If there is not a "fit," then the therapist invites the client to try another word, gesture, or image. This is an important step in the process because, when there is not this fit and the client continues to talk, the body process shuts down.

CLIENT: (*silence, inner checking*) . . . Well, that isn't quite right. It's more like: "I can't breathe." (*Takes a deep breath, head nods slightly, noting the bodily response to the "fit."*)
THERAPIST: "I can't breathe. . . . " (*Repeats the client's language to resonate with the body.*)

Notice that through checking, the first symbolization didn't resonate. A more accurate symbolization emerges, and the body confirms the fit through such responses as a deeper breath, head nodding spontaneously, and so forth. Mary also notices the resonance as this awareness further allows the bodily process to continue.

CLIENT: (*quiet for a while*) Oh, I felt like I couldn't breathe. . . . His hands grabbed my throat. . . . I wanted to scream but I couldn't. . . . I thought I was going to die. . . .
THERAPIST: Take a moment to allow your body to sense all of that . . . how much you wanted to scream . . . but you couldn't. You thought you were going to die.

When a new meaning unit emerges, it is important to give the body time to integrate what happened. This is a form of titration. If you move too quickly to more language, often the person comes out of a body process.

CLIENT: (*Takes another deep breath.*) I don't know why I didn't run away as soon as he approached me. I wish I had just run away . . . it's like I just couldn't for some reason . . . like I was supposed to be nice . . . yet, I didn't know that what was happening was even possible. . . .

THERAPIST: So even now you sense how you wished you could have run away . . . wished you could have done something . . . then maybe this wouldn't have happened. (*Pause.*) I am wondering . . . how would you say this the way your body is carrying it right now? You may even want to move your body to express this.

CLIENT: (*Slowly stands up.*) . . . (*Pushes out with her hands.*) . . . (*Shouts.*) I'm not going with you! . . . (*Turns body and starts to cry.*)

THERAPIST: Let's just make room for what emerged. You took a big step just now . . . expressing how you wished you could have acted . . . sense how that feels to move like that. . . . (*Again, the pausing and attending supports the integration.*)

CLIENT: I hardly ever cry. My throat isn't as tight. I feel more alive now. (*Sitting down, deeply breathing.*)

This step of change includes a body movement with a verbal communication. An important aspect of integrative processing is to access how the body "knew" how to act if the circumstances had allowed it. This expression into behavioral action now restores her capacity to act on her own behalf.

Acting on Her Own Behalf in the Present

During the next several sessions Mary talked about a colleague in her current life who had made sexual advances toward her. In the prior session she had found a *felt sense* of how she wished she could have acted on her own behalf when facing a sexual violation. Now a similar issue in her current life surfaced. At first, she was anxious about this. She talked about this encounter and realized she could no longer ignore that she did not want to be solicited in this way.

THERAPIST: I want to invite you to sense how it would feel in your body if this situation went differently, the way that would feel best for you.

CLIENT: (*pausing while sensing inside*) . . . Strong, tall . . . and safe . . . like I can protect myself.

THERAPIST: "Strong, tall . . . and safe . . . like I can protect myself." (*Said with same pacing and voice tone as client.*)

From the wholeness of our being we already know what it would feel like in our bodies *if* we could live from a sense of what is best for us or in alignment of our fullness of being. Here Mary found a *felt sense* of this new way of being. After this, her behavior changed, and she began to take stands on her own behalf. She was able to speak strong words to set a boundary with the colleague.

The Explicit Functioning of the Inner Relationship

Through this careful processing of the traumatic memories, Mary was able to develop an inner relationship of compassion with the "young girl" in her who was raped. She began to talk about this young girl inside who "died back then." Not only had she lost her "carefree innocence," but she was also "stuck in time," unable to grow up.

THERAPIST: I invite you to bring your attention inside with a quality of compassion and interest. . . . How do you sense that young girl now? The girl in you that was traumatized and no one was there to comfort her. . . . How is it inside now when you notice her?

CLIENT: I can sense how scared she was. . . . It's like I'm saying to her. . . . It's OK to feel scared. . . . Mmmm. That feels good . . . to talk to her like that. It's like I feel young again . . . there is a little energy there . . . like I'm coming alive a little.

THERAPIST: So there is a new sense of feeling young again. . . . Maybe it fits to say: "I'm coming alive a little. . . . " Check inside.

CLIENT: Mmmmmm . . . I'm coming alive a little! (*deep breaths, shy smile*)

Remember that the bodily process continues in relationship to the exact fit of the symbolization. Therefore, it is crucial that the intended empathic responses do not go even a bit ahead of the person's symbolization. To say "I'm coming alive a little . . . " is staying right with the tentativeness of what is emerging and nothing more. It can be seen in her next response that her body responded to my response with more openness.

CLIENT: Yes, she's smiling, looking up at me.

The next week Mary reported that she took the step of sharing her rape experience with a friend. This is an example of an experiential step. From the bodily experience of "coming alive a little," she had found what was needed to carry this aliveness forward in her present life. The young girl part of her who was stuck in time made a genuine connection with a friend that week. Now this trauma was more integrated with her present life, as she no longer had to hide her childhood trauma.

Spiritual Transformation

Several sessions later, Mary brought up again that she didn't want to have children anymore. She had looked into *in vitro* fertilization, but "it probably wouldn't work," she said. I listened to how the death of her relative, the uncertainty of life and death, frightened her. She also was afraid to risk renewing her faith by turning toward God and bringing her deepest longing to God.

Suddenly, I felt a strange sensation, like a warm wind blowing through me. As I attended to this new *felt sense* arising in me, the biblical story of Elizabeth and Zechariah popped into my awareness. The appearance had a decentering quality, as though it came from a different realm. . . . I don't usually quote scripture. However, I felt compelled to tell her this story in the Gospel of Luke I:8–14 (Revised Standard Version), about how an angel came to Zechariah and told him that his wife was with child and that, after years of barrenness, she would give birth. I noticed that her eyes widened and she listened intently.

I wondered with her whether her faith could be a resource now.

This is an example of how the therapist attends to her own emergent symbolizations and is able to sense from a "larger knowing." The implied growth step in the client interacts with the therapist's *felt sense* such that, if the therapist is listening in this way, something beyond the therapist's personal knowing is able to arise into symbolization in the moment that, when shared, carries forward the client's potential for living out her deeply felt purpose.

Mary reported to me the next week that she went to Church that Sunday and that this same scriptural passage was read. This convergence of hearing this story both from me and her minister touched her deeply, and she felt her bitterness releasing. She reported feeling a connection to her longing to have a child and a sense of hope. I invited her to check inside with her *felt sense*. What she found was a desire to pray to Mother Mary.

Several weeks later she announced that she and her husband had decided to pursue *in vitro* fertilization. She expressed confidence that she was in a different place now. She spoke about her prayers to Mother Mary and the aliveness of her faith.

The egg retrieval occurred without any complications. She reports this dream: She saw a mother with child sitting at the feet of a statue of Mary and a light reflected all around. The next day a viable zygote was implanted. Her pregnancy occurred without complication. She gave birth to a healthy girl.

An amazing spiritual event occurred that grew out of a deeply integrative process. Through listening deeply to bodily formed meanings, she integrated the significant aspects of her life experience so far: the death of her relative, the childhood rape, her longing to become a mother, and her loss of faith. Her "twice-born" faith deepened through facing her trauma. Her body became open to creating a child, and her marriage achieved a deeper level of intimacy. A transformation occurred as she actualized her deepest desires.

Conclusion

Even when faced with trauma, the wholeness of the person continues. Focusing-oriented psychotherapy fosters a connection to this wholeness by cultivating a nonjudgmental and interested attention to a whole sense of "something" felt in the body, that is, the *felt sense.* Words, images, and gestures further symbolize the experience. Symbols are checked back with the body to resonate with the *felt sense.* With this contemplative approach one allows what is arising from the body to form and thereby gains access to a larger wisdom, directing the whole person toward integrative growth. As the trauma is integrated, specific steps of change in the client's present life are generated naturally from within the person, restoring the capacity to live fully in the present with authentic purpose. The therapist communicates an empathic resonance with the trauma survivor to create the safety for this integration and to nurture the capacity for further growth. In a manner consistent with the research in neurobiology, the focusing-oriented approach integrates mindfulness, relational connection, and spiritual potential in a unified process that brings symbolic expression to previously mute traumatic experience and frees the client to live more fully and authentically.

Focusing-oriented psychotherapy is known as a contemplative approach to trauma work. It is also applied to clinical areas such as work with children; depression and anxiety; adaptation to living with AIDS and cancer; pain management; short-term psychotherapy; and cross-cultural models of community wellness, including teaching focusing to nongovernmental organizations in Afghanistan, barrios in Ecuador, and the bush in South Africa. For information on training and further resources, see *www. focusing.org.*

References

Gendlin, E. T. (1969). Focusing. *Psychotherapy: Theory, Research, and Practice,* 6, 4–15.

Gendlin, E. T. (1996). *Focusing-oriented psychotherapy: A manual of the experiential method.* New York: Guilford Press.

Gendlin, E. T. (1997). *A process model*. Retrieved from *www.focusing.org/process.html*.

Gendlin, E. T. (2004). The new phenomenology of carrying forward. *Continental Philosophy Review, 37*(1), 127–151.

Gendlin, E. T. (2012). Implicit precision. In Z. Radman (Ed.), *Knowing without thinking: The theory of the background in philosophy of mind* (pp. 141–166). Basingstoke, UK: Palgrave Macmillan.

Gendlin, E. T., Beebe, J., III, Cassens, M. J., Klein, M., & Oberlander, M. (1968). Focusing ability in psychotherapy, personality, and creativity. In J. M. Shlien (Ed.), *Research in psychotherapy* (Vol. 3, pp. 217–241). Washington, DC: American Psychological Association.

Grindler Katonah, D. (2006). The *felt sense* as avenue of human experiencing for integrative growth. In L. T. Hoshmand (Ed.), *Culture, psychotherapy, and counseling: Critical and integrative perspectives* (pp. 65–91). Thousand Oaks, CA: Sage.

Grindler Katonah, D. (2010). Direct engagement with the cleared space in psychotherapy. *Person-Centered and Experiential Psychotherapies, 9*(2), 157–168.

Grindler Katonah, D. (2012). Research on clearing a space. *Folio: A Journal for Focusing and Experiential Therapy, 23*(1), 138–154.

Hendricks, M. (2001). Focusing-oriented/experiential psychotherapy. In D. Cain & J. Seeman (Eds.), *Humanistic psychotherapy: Handbook of research and practice* (pp. 221–251). Washington, DC: American Psychological Association.

James, W. (1961). *The varieties of religious experience*. New York: Collier Books.

Levine, P. (2010). *In an unspoken voice: How the body releases trauma and restores goodness*. Berkeley, CA: North Atlantic Books.

Ogden, P., Minton, K., & Pain, C. (2006). *Trauma and the body: A sensorimotor approach to psychotherapy*. New York: Norton.

Pargament, K. I. (1997). *The psychology of religion and coping: Theory, research, practice*. New York: Guilford Press.

Pargament, K. I. (2007). *Spiritually integrated psychotherapy: Understanding and addressing the sacred*. New York: Guilford Press.

Rogers, C. (1961). *On becoming a person*. Boston: Houghton Mifflin.

Saunders, S. M., Miller, M. L., & Bright, M. M. (2010, September 6). Spiritually conscious psychological care. *Professional Psychology: Research and Practice, 41*(5), 355–362.

Tolstoy, L. (2010). *A confession*. Whitefish, MT: Kessinger.

van der Kolk, B. (1996). The complexity of adaptation to trauma: Self-regulation, stimulus discrimination, and characterological development. In B. A. van der Kolk, A. C. McFarlane, & L. Weisaeth (Eds.), *Traumatic stress: The effects of overwhelming experience on mind, body, and society* (pp. 182–213). New York: Guilford Press.

van der Kolk, B. (2006). Clinical implications of neuroscience research in PTSD. *Annals of the New York Academy of Sciences, 1071*, 277–293.

11

Yoga for Complex Trauma

David Emerson and Elizabeth K. Hopper

Stretching back millennia and originating in the geographic area now known as India and Pakistan, humans have engaged in a variety of practices that we collectively refer to as *yoga* (Feuerstein, 2001). Surveying the many styles and vast intricacies of yoga is beyond the scope of this chapter, which instead will focus narrowly on what is commonly referred to as hatha yoga. This is a gentle style of yoga that promotes balance in mind and body through the use of breathing, meditation, and, particularly important for our purposes, physical postures, or "asanas." Hatha yoga became popular in the Western countries in the late 20th century as a form of physical exercise and relaxation; this modern iteration emphasizes the physical postures. According to a 2012 study conducted for the *Yoga Journal* by Sports Marketing Surveys USA, there are about 20 million adults in the United States practicing some form of yoga, mostly a variety of hatha yoga. Over the past several years studies have emerged that demonstrate the potential benefit of this ancient practice with regard to many physical and mental health conditions that people struggle with today (Salmon, Lush, Jablonski, & Sephton, 2009; van der Kolk, 2006). For example, studies have shown the benefits of hatha yoga for those suffering from symptoms of insomnia, anxiety, and depression (Khalsa, 2004; Khalsa, Shorter, Cope, Wyshak, & Sklar, 2009; Pilkington, Kirkwood, Rampes, & Richardson, 2005).

At the Trauma Center at the Justice Resource Institute (JRI) in Brookline, Massachusetts, we are engaged in research and clinical work utilizing our own unique variation of hatha yoga, which we call *trauma-sensitive yoga*, as a complementary intervention for complex posttraumatic stress disorder (PTSD). We found that a 10-week course of trauma-sensitive yoga was associated with a significant decrease in PTSD symptoms in trauma survivors with complex, treatment-resistant PTSD. Women who received this yoga-based intervention also reported significant decreases in affect dysregulation and increases in tension-reduction activities (van der Kolk et al., 2014). There is also evidence that hatha yoga can alter neurotransmitter levels (i.e, gamma-aminobutyric acid, or GABA) associated with PTSD (Streeter et al., 2007). Although mindfulness (a close cousin that focuses mostly on the attentional aspects of yoga) has been studied in the empirical arena over the past two decades and has recently received significant attention from both clinicians and scientists, we may be on the cusp of a much deeper understanding of the clinical benefits of moving and breathing in organized, purposeful ways—practices at the heart of hatha yoga.

We have learned, mostly through feedback from our students[1] over the years, that hatha yoga, as it is taught in most settings, must be modified in order to be tolerable and effective for trauma survivors. The modifications we have made to hatha yoga have led us, as noted previously, to coin a new term, *trauma-sensitive yoga*. Trauma-sensitive yoga is focused mostly on the body and is centered on the subjective, felt experience of one's own moving and breathing. In our sessions, we invite students to notice what it feels like to intentionally reach their arms high overhead and take a few deep breaths; what sensations they are aware of as they purposefully use the big muscles in their legs and at their core (abdominal) to support themselves in a strong, Standing Warrior posture; what they feel as their feet make contact with the ground; and what it feels like to purposefully exert some control and agency with regard to how they move and breathe. In other words, we are inviting our students, through the use of our modified hatha yoga, to explore what it feels like to have a body and to move and breathe in an intentional and organized way. In this chapter, we explain some of our reasons for using yoga in the context of trauma treatment, outline some of our trauma-sensitive modifications, and use case examples to illustrate our approach.

Trauma-Sensitive Yoga in the Context of Treatment

Trauma survivors are reexperiencing the trauma within their bodies on a daily basis. In that sense, the body has become the enemy (van der Kolk, 1994; Ogden & Minton, 2000). Our clients at the Trauma Center at JRI often feel that their bodies betrayed them in the past and continue to betray them in the present. Conditioned somatic responses such as hyperarousal or dissociation are often brought about by triggers—external stimuli or internal emotional or physiological reactions that elicit traumatic memories

---

[1]We generally refer to people in our yoga classes as "students" and, more specifically, to persons doing yoga in the therapy office as "clients."

or symptoms (Sexual Assault Centre, University of Alberta, 2008). Smelling a metallic scent can usher in a "video reel" of vivid memories of early abuse. Experiencing a physical sensation such as the muscles contracting around the throat can lead to a cascade of emotional, somatic, and cognitive reactions. Although one can attempt to cognitively understand the origins of these reactions, that intellectual process often does not stop the trigger from taking over one's body. The heart races, the hands clench, the gut wrenches. There is a sense of being overwhelmed, over and over again, by one's bodily sensations and the experience of being trapped in a body that is out of control—these are the sources of much of the suffering associated with trauma and PTSD. So we begin with the assumption that most of the people we work with are suffering greatly in relation to their bodies. This suffering can be understood from a somatic perspective (e.g., "I feel constant pain in my abdomen" or "I cannot feel my legs at all"); from an interpersonal perspective (e.g., "I cannot tolerate my children touching me. It is too much of a reminder of my trauma"); or from a neurobiological perspective (e.g., structural and functional brain changes detectable with magnetic resonance imaging; van der Kolk, 2006; Lanius, Vermetten, & Pain, 2010). In any case, the suffering involves, at best, a sense of being disconnected from one's body or, at worst, a deep visceral hatred for one's "failed," "damaged," or "broken" organism.

Our first step with trauma-sensitive yoga is to help people simply *tolerate* having a body (Emerson & Hopper, 2011). We do not ask them to *like* having a body, just to experiment in a safe way with being embodied. The way we do this is by directing attention to simple motor processes; for example, "When you are ready, bring your feet flat to the floor" or "If you like, experiment with lifting your hands up to about shoulder height." We frame our cues as *invitations* rather than *commands* and consider this one of our key trauma-sensitive modifications to hatha yoga. These kinds of invitations give our students opportunities to do something purposeful with their bodies without having to make any meaning out of it. At this stage, we do not ask people to interact with their experiences or make meaning out of them. Rather, we invite them to just "do" something with their bodies that is not harmful and is relatively neutral. Readers might imagine other suitable examples: "If you like, lengthen up through the top of your head"; "When you are ready, experiment with turning your head from left to right"; or, if you are sitting in a therapy office, "If you like, experiment with standing up."

The only purely physical parameter is that the action you are inviting your client to engage in should be physically possible for him or her. For example, if you are working with someone who is a multiple amputee and in a wheelchair or hospital bed, be sure to pick actions that are possible for the person. If you are unsure about what kinds of movements are possible for a client, we encourage you to collaborate with your client in experimentation. This may be a way to begin encouraging your clients to listen to their bodies and to work within a comfortable range of experience. As you begin to invite your clients to purposefully move their bodies, you are helping them to "have a body," and this experience is a critical starting point in trauma-sensitive yoga as we define it. We are neither asking people to experience their bodies through thinking about them (e.g., whereas in traditional talk therapy a therapist might work with a client to gain insight into the reasons why he or she cannot feel his or her legs, we just ask the client to begin to use his or her leg muscles in a purposeful way), nor are we inviting them to experiment with "feeling" or "sensing" their bodies yet. We are just inviting them to do something physical. In fact, when the practice of "having a body" involves a simple movement such as bringing one's feet flat onto the floor, we need not attempt to convince anyone that they have a body, because they can start to experience that for themselves.

To date, we have developed two models for trauma-sensitive yoga: as an integrated part of individual therapy and as stand-alone practice for individuals or small groups. To understand how a client might use both, consider the following case example.

Michelle[2] came into the Trauma Center at JRI seeking body-based therapy. She had tried a number of traditional talk therapies in the past but noted that she still felt "stuck." She identified a tension in herself between wanting to get help and "get better" while at the same time being terrified of dealing with anything that was really important. She reflected that there was a part of her that tended to intellectualize and to talk circles around a lot of therapists; when this happened, although she was sometimes proud of her ability to prevent the therapist from "analyzing" her, she also felt that she was wasting her time by avoiding what was really going on. Michelle said that she often appeared to be a "good patient" on the outside and wanted her therapist to be pleased with her. Although cognitive-behavioral therapy can be helpful for some traumatized people, this was not the case for Michelle. She described how, despite faithfully completing her homework and using the language to show that she could identify her "cognitive distortions" and shift her thinking, deep down she felt no different. Indeed, she reported feeling more and more depressed and hopeless about not being seen or understood by her therapist.

Michelle described a little of her early history to her new therapist. She grew up in a home with an absent mother and a father who was emotionally very volatile and suffered from chronic mental illness. Her father had periods of severe depression in which he abused alcohol and prescription medications and passed out on the couch in a completely unresponsive state. During these times, he would often lock himself in his room for days on end, and Michelle could hear her father sobbing behind the door. She described several times

---

[2]All of our case examples are composites in order to protect identity.

when an ambulance came to her house and her father was taken to the hospital for days or sometimes weeks. At other times, her father would become rageful, verbally attacking Michelle and her older sister Janine. Michelle also witnessed her father physically attacking Janine and seeing her sister with welts and bruises all over her body. When Michelle was 10, her father committed suicide, and Janine took over parenting responsibilities. Michelle described Janine as being resentful of having to take care of Michelle and repeating her father's pattern of rage and verbally abusive behavior.

Michelle described her childhood as a "nightmare" that, for the most part, she doesn't remember. She coped by becoming "spacey" and emotionally disconnected very early in life. She didn't have any close relationships during childhood and had never had an emotionally intimate relationship. She had dated a man for 4 years just after college but never felt anything for him, just pretending to care about him. She noted sarcastically that he never noticed because she continued to have sex with him and that that was probably all he wanted anyway. She had had numerous sexual partners but did not enjoy sex; she did not understand why she felt compelled to have sex with any man that she dated. Michelle was unable to feel her body. She occasionally felt extreme fear and panic, but this feeling was always followed immediately by a floating sensation and a sense of "emotional deadness."

Michelle had tried going to several yoga classes because she had read about body-oriented interventions for trauma. However, she tended to push herself to keep up with the instructor and usually ended up feeling even more spacey and numb afterward. She had not attended a yoga class for 6 months because she had injured herself at the last class she had attended. Michelle wanted to try the "trauma-sensitive" yoga classes offered by the Trauma Center and also wanted to try body-oriented intervention using yoga.

Michelle's therapist initially worked with Michelle on noticing her body. Their goal was for Michelle to acknowledge sensations in her body and to bring awareness to her discomfort without attempting to change it. They worked on establishing a Seated Mountain Form (an organized way of sitting in which the practitioner focuses on feeling her or his stabile foundation and also on creating some length in her or his spine) as a home base, and then tried a centering experiment in which the therapist guided Michelle to gently move her torso forward and backward, side to side, and in circles, focusing in on her center and bringing attention to her "core." As she brought attention to her body in this way, Michelle was able to identify a sensation of tension as her muscles clenched up, followed by a feeling of panic. Almost immediately, she described feeling light-headed and spacey, and then feeling a sense of "shutting down" and numbness throughout her body. Because Michelle had become triggered by attending to her body and did not have body-oriented resources established, the therapist used a "top-down" psychoeducational approach to help Michelle ground herself. As part of this process, the therapist described the window of tolerance, drew a picture of it, and described how she and Michelle would work together to help her to stay within her window of tolerance while doing the experiments, slowly increasing what Michelle could tolerate. The frame for success was shifted from "the most intense" to "finding what is right for you." Experimentation, with a curious and mindful stance, and regulation were established as key factors very early in the therapeutic process. The role of the therapist as coregulator was also established through this early intervention.

Because attention to her core seemed to be particularly triggering for Michelle, the body-based work shifted to an initial focus on her extremities. She was able to practice grounding exercises, such as feeling her feet on the floor. She was also able to do experiments that focused on using her body as a resource. For instance, she was able to tolerate doing seated leg lifts, noticing the tension in her quadriceps muscles and the muscles in her abdomen that help to support her leg and keep it lifted. She was also able to notice strength-based emotions that were associated with certain movements, such as the power she felt when moving from Seated Mountain to Standing Mountain. Although her upper extremities and chest were initially difficult for her, as Michelle built her tolerance for noticing body sensations, she was gradually able to notice the tension in her upper body—without panicking or "spacing out"—as she practiced neck rolls and shoulder rolls.

In the trauma-sensitive yoga class, Michelle was struggling with being triggered and dissociating. She enjoyed strength-based postures such as Standing Warrior, a powerful form in which both feet are on the ground, with the front leg bent to about a 90-degree angle so the big muscles on top of the thigh are highly activated and the back leg extended back, straight and strong. In Standing Warrior, practitioners may also extend their arms front to back, which creates more stability by engaging muscles in the upper body and which gives the practitioner a chance to experiment with taking up space. Michelle enjoyed feeling empowered by these exercises. However, she had difficulty in the class with postures in which she felt more vulnerable or exposed. In particular, she struggled with Downward Dog and forward bends. Michelle used therapy to talk about these experiences, to practice coping responses (such as using grounding skills when she noticed herself begin to become light-headed), and to develop a plan for using her coping skills in class. She practiced a seated forward fold in the therapy office, controlling the length of time that she was in the fold, in order to practice positive self-talk and to increase her ability to tolerate the distress that came up while in this posture. She also identified "safe" postures that she could return to if she felt triggered in class, such as Child's Posture or Seated Mountain.

Breathing was also a challenge for Michelle, as she tended to breathe shallowly through her mouth and experienced dissociation if she attempted to slow her breathing. After several months of focusing on larger body movements, Michelle felt ready to bring some attention to her breath. She initially just allowed her breath to flow as it typically did, noticing it without trying to change it. After some time, to help provide some structure and to hold her attention while she deepened her breath, she used body-oriented tools (alternating nostril breathing) and cognitive tools (ratio breathing, in which counting is used to make the out-breath twice as long as the in-breath, which also increases parasympathetic relative to sympathetic nervous system activation). As she built trust in her therapist, Michelle was more able to use the relationship as a guide and a reflection of her own experience. She slowly began to increase her eye contact during yoga-based interventions. She and her therapist began to experiment with what it felt like to be the "leader" or "follower" in body movements, such as Sun Breaths, and what it felt like to move in rhythm with another person.

After 6 months, Michelle had still not focused on her early trauma history in therapy, beyond what she had discussed during the intake. She shared with her therapist how different the therapeutic process had been so far. In other therapies, she had felt overwhelmed with talking about her past and had shut down. In this experience, she was able to slowly experience feeling her body in a more positive way and to learn to tolerate some more uncomfortable sensations and emotions without having to shut them down. She reflected that she had been less dissociative in her day-to-day life and had started to open up a little to other people in a way that she hadn't felt able to do before. Although the body-based exercises were foreign and often difficult for her, she felt like she was making real change in her life.

This case provides an example of a number of the principles of yoga-based intervention for trauma. As in most types of trauma therapy, there is an emphasis on building self-awareness and regulatory skills. As Michelle became more comfortable with noticing her body, tolerating its sensations, and regulating her emotions, she did not need to rely as much on dissociation as her primary coping strategy and began to spend more time "having a body" and being "in the moment." These changes started to have positive ripple effects on the rest of her life, including her relationships, her perception of herself, and her ability to participate more fully in life.

As a clinical issue, we know that many trauma survivors, like Michelle, experience their bodies as sources of pain, fear, and helplessness. These feelings can lead survivors to reject or deny their bodies and begin to live their lives either "in their heads" or in dissociated states. If these coping mechanisms become very ingrained, traditional Western, verbally oriented therapies may not be sufficient. Trauma-sensitive yoga can be used, in the therapeutic milieu, as a body-oriented intervention that can help survivors directly alter their relationships to their bodies and, therefore, to themselves. Yoga is helpful because, instead of just thinking and talking about the body, experiential exercises are used, with the guidance of the therapist, to bring the focus to present somatic experiences. In the clinical realm, mindfulness and reflection can be used as well to bring awareness to body processes that are occurring when using yoga. Attention to targeted sensations and to micromovements can be used as regulatory strategies to focus on building successful experiences with distress tolerance and self-awareness.

Adding Complexity
to the Trauma-Sensitive Yoga Experience

Many of the people that we work with report numbing in some part or parts of their bodies—they just cannot feel their legs, for example. Rather than trying to convince them, through talking, that they have legs, we can invite them to stand up and to experiment with noticing what that feels like. This leads us to another step in the therapeutic process associated with trauma-sensitive yoga. Once a client has started to practice purposeful action and begins to feel safe within his or her body, then we move on to inviting him or her to *notice* what is happening, to *feel* what he or she is doing, to *interact with* his or her body. We call this practice of noticing and interacting with one's body "befriending your body," because we believe that if one starts to become curious about and interested in what his or her body is doing, he or she begins to develop a sense of openness and friendliness toward it, and this deepens the process of healing trauma.

To build curiosity, to get to a place at which something—anything—happening in one's body is interesting instead of triggering, is one of the important aspects of the kind of therapeutic intervention that trauma-sensitive yoga offers. When introducing a practice of befriending the body, our cue would be something like, "When you are ready, bring your feet flat to the floor and *feel your feet making contact with the floor.*" Now we are asking people to *feel*. This may be followed by "There may be some things you can do to help you feel your feet on the floor, like tap your heels or your toes." So we continue to invite our clients to investigate the visceral, felt sense of their feet on the ground. Notice that we are still not asking them to enjoy it or to make any kind of meaning out of it whatsoever. This is important because, in many public yoga classes, a teacher may say something like "Notice how great it feels to have your feet on the ground." This would not be a trauma-sensitive prompt. We do not assume that feeling one's feet on the ground is "great"; in fact, one of our clients felt great sadness when she felt her feet on the ground for the first time in 20 years. That is OK. We stick to the sensation, just the physical feeling, and if that feeling becomes overwhelming, we can move on to another feeling practice. Or we can shift focus to stretching or strengthening muscles and feeling what that's like. The bottom line is that we help our clients tolerate and investigate body-based experience, and we support them in this investigation, but we leave the interpretation of the experience up to them.

Self-Regulation in Trauma-Sensitive Yoga

Finally, once folks have developed a capacity to willfully move and breathe and to experience some sort of curiosity around sensory awareness, we invite them to experiment with using their yoga practice to manage the way they feel, that is, self-regulation. We call this practice "body as a resource." Which postures are regulating is totally subjective; what works for some might not work for others. This is one reason that we don't prescribe postures so much as make yoga available in a safe way so that trauma survivors can experiment and discover for themselves. For some of our students, standing in a strong form and using big muscle groups on purpose is very empowering, but for others it is a trigger and destabilizing. For some, allowing muscles to stretch and attending to how that feels is very calming, whereas for others that experience makes them feel too vulnerable and exposed.

Following are two more short case examples that illustrate how trauma-sensitive yoga can help people develop and experience their bodies as a resource. Both of the examples described are amalgamations of people we have seen at the clinic over the years.

Caroline found that at certain times of the day, alone in her house, she would become overwhelmed with a sense of fear and powerlessness, a sense that someone bad was nearby and was going to harm her. She felt it in her body. Her chest would feel compressed; her breath was cut off; her hands would clench; her heart would pound. Through the yoga practice that she had been engaged in for several months at the Trauma Center, she had discovered that the Standing Warrior posture helped her to feel and use the big muscles in her legs, making her feel powerful. She could feel her leg muscles engaged. When she extended her arms she could breathe a little deeper than normal, and she liked the feeling of breathing in the form. One day, when that feeling of being overwhelmed was creeping in, she decided to try her Standing Warrior form. Up until that point, the yoga stayed in the yoga classroom, and she had not, in a sense, taken it with her out into the world. For some reason, on this day, it occurred to her that yoga was something she could use, not just something she did. What she discovered, just as her body was reacting to fear and powerlessness, was that by focusing on feeling her leg muscles being strong and engaged, extending her arms into the space around her and taking a few full breaths, the feeling of terror and impending harm was significantly diminished. The change was clear and relieving enough that she showed her therapist her Standing Mountain posture right in the office during their next meeting, and together they were able to practice a little yoga during the therapy hour.

Another example of yoga becoming a self-regulation tool is described next. In this example, a young man named Andy practices the handstand posture with his trauma-sensitive yoga teacher.

Andy, a 17-year-old who was in residential treatment for assaulting a teacher at the public school, had a significant trauma history. Abandoned by his biological father at age 2, Andy was raised by his mother, who suffered from both her own debilitating trauma history and chronic drug addiction. As a result, Andy experienced chronic emotional and physical neglect from his mother and was also repeatedly physically abused by several of his mother's boyfriends right up until he left the home. By the time he was 12 or 13, though, Andy was fighting back, and, because he was a big, strong kid, one of his mother's boyfriends ended up in the hospital with a concussion and a broken arm. No matter what else was happening for Andy, he was learning to use his body in this way. In therapy, at the residential treatment program, Andy would talk, with his chest puffed out and his spine tall, about how proud he was of his strength and his ability to protect himself. However, Andy was also afraid of the lack of control he felt over his body. As he became more comfortable with his therapist, he began talking, with his shoulders slumped and his back rounded and his eyes down, about his fear of the strength he felt in his own body: "What if I lose control and kill somebody someday?" With tears in his eyes, he reflected, "I don't want to hurt people." Along with his regular therapy, Andy started doing trauma-sensitive yoga. Early on, he and the yoga teacher agreed that they would focus on a strong posture and that they would make a project out of it. They would take the school year to practice a posture called Crane (a handstand in which the student, with both hands on the ground, places his knees on his triceps and, using a lot of upper body strength, experiments with balancing on his hands). In order to get to the form, Andy's yoga teacher suggested that they try some warm ups–simple neck and shoulder rolls, gentle self-massage around neck and shoulders, and sun breaths. Andy was beginning to experiment with using his body in new ways. More specifically, he was finding new ways of using his strength. The experiment was not meant to take away Andy's strength but to help him use it for something new, in which no one would be hurt and no one would be going to the hospital or jail.

In these examples, one could imagine both Caroline and Andy in an office, with a therapist, talking. Caroline might say, "At around 2 in the afternoon, when I am home alone, I am overcome with terror. I can barely breathe. I am sure someone is coming for me, to hurt me." This might lead to some conversation about feeling safe and *thinking* about ways to be safe. With the Standing Warrior form, Caroline found a way to *feel* safe. It was not theoretical. It was not her brain trying to convince her body to "stop freaking out" (an exercise that might lead to more shame and suffering because the body keeps "freaking out" anyway).

Andy might say to his therapist, "I feel my muscles tense up, and I think I am going to kill somebody," and this might lead to a conversation around body control and how, as Andy gets older, he will have more control over his impulses. With the Crane form, Andy could practice using his muscles and strength without hurting someone else. Another person doesn't have to try to convince Andy of this. He can experience it for himself; he goes to yoga, he uses his muscles, the yoga teacher says, with a smile, "see you next week," and Andy goes back to class. There is no intellectual meaning-making required.

Now, this is not to say that both Caroline and Andy don't benefit tremendously from being able to verbally express their thoughts and feelings, to cognitively understand their reactions, and to make meaning of their experiences. But because trauma is held in the body, the ability to have a new, positive somatic experience is an incredible asset for many trauma survivors. This is the beginning of a path toward regaining a part of the self that was taken away. Because of this, we believe that clinicians need to bring many more body- and experience-oriented treatments into the healing process; trauma-sensitive yoga is one such method.

A Word of Advice and Caution

Because trauma-sensitive yoga can occur both within the context of the therapy office and outside of it, we encourage people to work within the range of their professional competence. That is, if you are a yoga teacher working in the context of trauma treatment, we suggest keeping your focus on the yoga practice and staying clear of processing trauma content. If you are a clinician who is not trained as a yoga teacher, we recommend adding little bits of yoga with which you feel comfortable but not getting too far into complex ranges of movement and challenging dynamics (for additional support, see Emerson, 2015). Also, therapists may do a little more processing with their clients regarding their experiences with the forms, and this processing may move into trauma content.

In either case, for both yoga teachers and therapists, sometimes students or clients will be triggered during these experiences. Again, we have general advice for both yoga teachers and therapists. For yoga teachers, we have found that it is most important not to overreact; know that your students are triggered all of the time and that they have survived. You are, however, giving them new ways to respond to triggers. For example, instead of falling into an automatic reaction such as dissociating, they can deliberately try to experiment with a variety of yoga forms. If your student is triggered in one form, you might invite him or her to try something else. As a therapist, you can fall back on your training when a client is triggered. You may decide to shift out of yoga altogether, for example, and focus instead on a more cognitive approach. The bottom line is: Whether you are a therapist or a yoga teacher, use the skills you have been trained to use and are most comfortable with and join in the experiments with your clients or students as you help them to interact with triggered reactions instead of being overwhelmed by them. This experimental approach, learning by doing, is very much in line with the spirit of trauma-sensitive yoga.

References

Emerson, D. (2015). *Trauma-sensitive yoga in therapy: Bringing the body into treatment*. New York: W. W. Norton.

Emerson, D., & Hopper, E. (2011). *Overcoming trauma through yoga*. Berkeley, CA: North Atlantic Books.

Feuerstein, G. (2001). *The yoga tradition*. Prescott, AZ: Hohm Press.

Khalsa, S. B. (2004). Treatment of chronic insomnia with yoga: A preliminary study with sleep–wake diaries. *Applied Psychophysiology and Biofeedback, 29,* 269–278.

Khalsa, S. B., Shorter, S. M., Cope, S., Wyshak, G., & Sklar, E. (2009). Yoga ameliorates performance anxiety and mood disturbance in young professional musicians. *Applied Psychophysiology and Biofeedback, 34,* 279–289.

Lanius, R., Vermetten, E., & Pain, C. (2010). *The impact of early life trauma on health and disease: The hidden epidemic*. Cambridge, UK: Cambridge University Press.

Ogden, P., & Minton, K. (2000). Sensorimotor psychotherapy: One method for processing traumatic memory. *Traumatology, 6*(3), 149–173.

Pilkington, K., Kirkwood, G., Rampes, H., & Richardson, J. (2005). Yoga for depression: The research evidence. *Journal of Affective Disorders, 89,* 13–24.

Salmon, P., Lush, E., Jablonski, M., & Sephton, S. E. (2009). Yoga and mindfulness: Clinical aspects of an ancient mind/body practice. *Cognitive and Behavioral Practice, 16,* 59–72.

Sexual Assault Centre, University of Alberta. (2008). *What is a trigger?* Retrieved November 9, 2012, from *http://psychcentral.com/lib/2008/what-is-a-trigger*.

Streeter, C. C., Jensen, J. E., Perlmutter, R. M., Cabral, H. J., Tian, H., Terhune, D. B., et al. (2007). Yoga asana sessions increase brain GABA levels: A pilot study. *Journal of Alternative and Complimentary Medicine, 13*(4), 419–426.

van der Kolk, B. A. (1994). The body keeps the score: Memory and the emerging psychobiology of post traumatic stress. *Harvard Review of Psychiatry, 1,* 253–265.

van der Kolk, B. A. (2006) Clinical implications of neuroscience research in PTSD. *Annals of the New York Academy of Sciences, 1071,* 277–293.

van der Kolk, B. A., Stone, L., West, J., Rhodes, A., Emerson, D., Suvak, M., et al. (2014). Yoga as an adjunctive treatment for posttraumatic stress disorder: A randomized controlled trial. *Journal of Clinical Psychiatry, 75*(6), 559–565.

Part III

NEUROBIOLOGICAL/ SOMATIC ISSUES AND APPROACHES

12

Harnessing the Seeking, Satisfaction, and Embodiment Circuitries in Contemplative Approaches to Trauma

James W. Hopper

This chapter offers an understanding of some key brain and psychological processes involved in trauma, in suffering and healing, and in potentially transformative contemplative practices—especially those for cultivating mindfulness, love, kindness, and compassion. This understanding is structured by a framework that draws on knowledge from many scientific, clinical, and contemplative traditions and necessarily goes beyond scientific data to provide an integrative vision. The framework highlights and clarifies how the brain circuitries of seeking, satisfaction, and embodiment can be harnessed to cultivate healing, freedom, and happiness. (A "circuitry" is a collection of brain areas that work together to perform certain tasks.) As explained in this chapter with references to neuroscience research, like the brain circuitry of fear, the circuitries of seeking, satisfaction, and embodiment are among the best established brain circuitries in neuroscience. In addition, the framework presented here is consistent with well-established ways of understanding and treating trauma, as well as the emerging contemplative approaches featured in this book.

The framework is a way of understanding human suffering, healing, and happiness in terms of (1) four key brain circuitries and (2) cycles of suffering and cycles of healing that entail particular relationships among the four circuitries. ("Cycle" here means a set of experiences and actions that unfold repeatedly, in the same order, and typically in a self-perpetuating way.) In this chapter the framework is introduced and explained in four steps. First, the brain circuitries of fear, seeking, satisfaction, and embodiment are described. Because the brain's seeking circuitry has been neglected in psychological trauma theory, research, and treatment—which have been dominated by attention to the fear circuitry—a central goal of this chapter, and a requirement for understanding and making use of this framework, is focusing more attention on the seeking circuitry. Second, what are referred to within the framework as fundamental "cycles of suffering," which involve relationships among the framework's key brain circuitries, are explained and briefly illustrated with examples familiar to clinicians working with traumatized clients. Third, I explain and illustrate fundamental "cycles of healing" specified by the framework and roles of the key circuitries in those cycles. Finally, I offer the framework's explanation of how the seeking, satisfaction, and embodiment circuitries can be harnessed by interventions with contemplative aspects and by contemplative practices—especially those that cultivate mindfulness, love, kindness, and compassion—to transform posttraumatic suffering and bring genuine happiness.

The framework offered here can be used by clinicians to understand—and to help their clients understand—posttraumatic symptoms and suffering, including addictions and emotion-regulation deficits associated with complex trauma. The framework can also be used to understand and explain potential pathways to healing, including how therapeutic interventions and contemplative practices can harness key brain circuitries to bring healing and happiness. Once familiar and conversant with the framework (especially when understanding is grounded in mindfully attending to moment-to-moment experience), clinicians and clients can easily see how the circuitries of fear, seeking, satisfaction, and embodiment are key drivers of their thoughts, feelings, and behaviors. This includes insight into the ongoing causes of symptoms; habitual ways of attempting to regulate emotional and physiological states; values, hopes, and life goals; and moment-to-moment reactions to what is pleasant and unpleasant, feared and wanted, and satisfying and fulfilling. In short, the framework is offered as a set of clarifying conceptual tools for exploring experience and behavior, for understanding suffering and healing, and for choosing and getting the most from clinical interventions and from the contemplative methods for treating trauma found in this book.

Fear Circuitry

The brain's fear circuitry includes the amygdala, a structure now commonly mentioned in the media and popular culture, as well as the hypothalamus and periaqueductal gray. It is one of the best known and most studied circuitries in the brain (LeDoux, 2000, 2012; Panksepp & Biven, 2012) and a major focus of research on psychological trauma and post-traumatic stress disorder, or PTSD (e.g., Shin & Handwerger, 2009). It is not uncommon for therapists to refer to the amygdala as a source of their clients' symptoms and suffering, which makes sense because the fear circuitry of which the amygdala is part triggers common fear responses such as a pounding heart, shallow breathing, freezing, and "spacing out" (LeDoux, 2012).

Two important points: First, the fear circuitry is not only involved in what terrifies us. It is triggered by *anything* we find unpleasant and want to avoid. Indeed, Joseph LeDoux's (2000, 2012) pioneering and ongoing research on rats uses relatively mild but aversive foot shocks, not terrifying or traumatic experiences, to elicit fear behaviors and study the mammalian fear circuitry. Second, all but the most reflexive efforts to avoid or escape unwanted experiences that have triggered the fear circuitry invariably recruit the brain's *seeking* circuitry (described next). Our brains are constantly, automatically—mostly without our awareness—"tagging" some things as unpleasant and unwanted, and thus things to *avoid* and *escape* (e.g., Belova, Patton, Morrison, & Salzman, 2007; Lin & Nicolelis, 2008). When feared and unwanted emotions such as sadness, loneliness, or shame are triggered—however much we notice or not—our brains may seek to escape into addictive experiences (Khantzian, 1999, 2003). And for some who have been hurt in important relationships, especially as children, even "positive" experiences with other people, such as being offered genuine affection, caring, or love, can be unwanted and cause fear and attempts to escape (Gilbert, McEwan, Matos, & Rivis, 2010).

Seeking Circuitry

The brain's seeking circuitry is part of the brain's "reward circuitry" and plays a central role in addiction (Alcaro & Panksepp, 2011). Like the fear circuitry, the seeking circuitry is one of neuroscience's most studied and best established circuitries, including in humans, thanks to decades of research funded by the National Institute on Drug Abuse. Brain researchers have given different names to this circuitry, based on different overall understandings of brain functioning and of this circuitry's roles in behavior and emotion. The term *seeking* was coined by Jaak Panksepp, an influential neuroscientist who has written a widely used textbook on affective neuroscience (Panksepp, 1998) and who views humans' and animals' brains as inherently caused, by this circuitry, to reach out and actively engage with the world. As the amygdala plays a central role in the fear circuitry, the nucleus accumbens plays a central role in the seeking circuitry. However, detailed knowledge of the brain areas that make up the seeking circuitry is not necessary to appreciate the roles it may play in trauma and healing.

Researchers have found that the seeking circuitry is what enables us to want and seek *anything* (e.g., Alcaro & Panksepp, 2011; Olsen, 2011). It could be a new dress, pair of shoes or watch, or a new technology toy that one seeks. It could be an affectionate comment from a girlfriend, boyfriend, spouse, or partner, praise from a coworker or supervisor, or accomplishing a life goal. It could be the next pain pill, the next drink of alcohol, the next hit of crack or porn video. As discussed later, when we strive to fulfill our highest moral, religious, and spiritual values and goals, this circuitry helps us do it.

For people struggling with trauma-related suffering, their seeking can become overly focused on—even enslaved to—quick fixes. These fixes can be intoxicated states brought on by alcohol or drugs, but most important, they are *any experiences that are sought to escape from suffering.* Such fixes may be self-harming behaviors such as cutting or burning to reduce inner turmoil or berating someone with an angry tirade to escape feeling power- less. They also include habitual "defense mechanisms" such as rumination, mindless distraction, or dissociative spacing out, which harm us, less obvi- ously, by disconnecting us from current experience (and therefore from our potential to respond to suffering and other unwanted experiences in healthy ways). The many ways we may ignore or deny what's actually happening around and within us all can be understood as *brief escapes or quick fixes that involve the seeking circuitry.* Such escapes tend to be not only brief, but also addictive, and unfulfilling in any lasting way—ultimately causing more problems than they solve.

The Pleasure of Seeking

The seeking circuitry is involved in the pleasures of seeking and expect- ing what we want and the excitement of both (Panksepp, 1998; Alcaro & Panksepp, 2011). But the "anticipatory pleasure" of seeking is only one kind of pleasure; it is different from the pleasure of satisfaction that comes from getting what we have sought, a distinction long recognized in ethol- ogy and psychology (e.g., Sherrington, 1906; Klein, 1987; Depue & Col- lins, 1999; Gilbert & Wilson, 2000; Kahneman & Snell, 1992). There is a difference between the pleasure of anticipating eating a hot fudge sundae and the pleasure of actually eating it. The same is true of any addictive sub- stance or behavior. (However, some substances, such as cocaine and meth- amphetamine, can be addictive precisely because they increase the pleasure of seeking itself.)

Seeking Imaginary Rewards

When we are not focused on a particular task, our minds tend to wander. This wandering includes running through plans or scenarios in our heads and imagining things we want to happen and do not want to happen. Brain researchers now call this the "default mode" of the human brain. It is what our brains do whenever we are "resting" or simply not fully absorbed in anything else, and the brain's "default mode network" (or circuitry) has been mapped (e.g., Gusnard & Raichle, 2001; Fransson, 2005; McKiernan, D'Angelo, Kaufman, & Binder, 2006). There are technical obstacles to measuring small bouts of seeking-circuitry activity during mind wandering, and the default mode and seeking circuitries are not identical. But research has shown their connection (Greicius, Krasnow, Reiss, & Menon, 2003), and if we step back and observe our own and our clients' daydreams, memories, and plans, we can see what they often revolve around: seeking hoped-for and imaginary rewards—of either getting or keeping things we want or, when fear drives our default-mode seeking, escaping from things we don't want or wish hadn't already happened. Default mode activity is even more dominated by fears and imagined escapes in states of negative affect and depression (Farrin, Hull, Unwin, Wykes, & David, 2003; Smallwood, Fitzgerald, Miles, & Phillips, 2009; Smallwood, O'Connor, Sudbery, & Obonsawin, 2007).

In short, the seeking circuitry is constantly active, often in response to the fear circuitry being triggered. It is constantly driving thoughts, feelings, and behaviors. For millennia the central role of seeking in human experience and behavior, and the importance of taking responsibility for what one seeks and focusing one's seeking on what promotes human flourishing, have been pointed out by contemplatives from major philosophical and religious traditions (e.g., Plato, Aristotle, Stoics, Jewish and Christian mysticism, Sufism, Buddhism, Confucianism, and Taoism).

Satisfaction Circuitry

Just as important as the seeking circuitry, in the framework advanced here, is what I refer to as the *satisfaction circuitry*. It is well established that opioid brain chemicals and receptors are involved in feelings of satisfaction, contentment, and connection with others (e.g., Akil et al., 1998; Depue & Morrone-Strupinsky, 2005; Machin & Dunbar, 2011; Nelson & Panksepp, 1998). As Panksepp and Biven (2012) have written, activated mu opioid receptors not only take away feelings of pain but "send messages of pleasant satisfaction in the brain" (p. 25). This opioid circuitry can give us deeply fulfilling pleasures of feeling happy and loved, and any time we feel *contented*, this circuitry is involved. Such experiences, of course, are minimal or missing in the lives of many traumatized people.

Again, one need not know every brain chemical, receptor type, and region involved in satisfaction (although there is substantial and growing research). But it is helpful to know that a central role in this circuitry is played by opioids, both because it is true and because most clinicians and many therapy clients have heard of opioids and their association with experiences of pleasure and satisfaction, thanks to media reports that opioids produced by the brain (i.e., "endogenous opioids") account for "runner's high" and to the high prevalence of opioid pain medication abuse and dependence in many communities. Indeed, like the brain's endogenous opiates, those from *outside* the body—whether snorted, injected, or ingested via pain pills—act directly on this satisfaction circuitry. That is why such opiate-induced highs involve intense (if short-lived) feelings of great satisfaction and well-being, even bliss.

Embodiment Circuitry

The framework offered here refers to another well-established brain circuitry, which I refer to as the *embodiment circuitry*, though it has been given other names that typically include "interoception" (e.g., Craig, 2002; Singer, Critchley, & Preuschoff, 2009). *Embodiment circuitry* includes the construct of interoception (i.e., the sense of the physiological condition of the entire body), but also denotes that this circuitry allows us to know *what it feels like to be in our bodies*. A key part of the embodiment circuitry is the insular cortex or insula, the one cortical region that brings together *all* information coming from the body (e.g., sensations of movement, touch, tension, pressure, pain, pleasure, etc.; Craig, 2002; Singer et al., 2009; Satpute, Shu, Weber, Roy, & Ochsner, 2013). For clinicians the construct of embodiment is important and helpful, because particular clients have differing degrees of awareness of body sensations, including those that go with emotions. A significant portion of traumatized people suffer from emotional numbing or dissociation, which can be understood as being relatively not embodied, and corresponds to less insula activity in response to trauma reminders (Hopper, Frewen, van der Kolk, & Lanius, 2007; Lanius et al., 2010).

Body Sensations Trigger Fear and Seeking (to Escape)

Information from the body includes unpleasant and unwanted sensations—such as those of pain, fear, anxiety, sadness, or withdrawal from an addictive substance. Information from the body also includes pleasant and wanted sensations, including those associated with substance intoxication and behaviors people find addicting. Such sensations, processed by the embodiment circuitry, can be strong drivers of craving, whether for addictive substances, food, or behaviors including gambling, shopping, and sex (Naqvi & Bechara, 2010). For example, researchers found that when people addicted to cigarettes suffered brain damage, it was much more likely that those with damage to the insula than to other brain areas abruptly quit smoking—suddenly, completely, and *without even trying*. Asked why, those with damage to this key part of the embodiment circuitry said such things as "My body forgot the urge to smoke" (Naqvi, Rudrauf, Damasio, & Bechara, 2007). As discussed later, pleasant body sensations, especially of satisfying and loving experiences, can be powerful antidotes to fear and the craving to escape.

Cycles of Suffering

Traumatized people are often caught in self-perpetuating cycles of suffering. It can be helpful to understand these cycles as unhealthy relationships among the circuitries of fear, seeking, satisfaction, and embodiment.[1]

What makes cycles of suffering self-perpetuating? Seeking is focused on escaping suffering in ways that do not really address one's pain and problems (let alone bring genuine and lasting satisfaction or happiness) but instead keep them going and make them worse. Cycles of suffering are both caused and partly *constituted* by the seeking of escapes that only perpetuate suffering. Cycles of suffering are often cycles of addiction, with addiction defined here broadly to include all habitual behaviors used repeatedly to seek escape from suffering, including such habitual mental behaviors as obsessing and ruminating. All of these cycles of suffering—however addictive they are, and however negative their immediate and long-term consequences—involve pursuit of quick fixes that bring no more satisfaction or "reward" than this: brief and partial escape from an unwanted experience.

In the framework advanced here, different cycles of suffering involve distinct unhealthy relationships among the circuitries of fear, seeking, satisfaction, and embodiment. For those struggling with trauma, the framework specifies two common cycles of suffering—one revolving around fear and anxiety, the other around depression, defeat, and demoralization. These two common suffering cycles and the corresponding activity of the brain circuitries of fear, seeking, and satisfaction are depicted in Figure 12.1.

In the *fear/anxiety cycle*, seeking is focused on avoiding things one is afraid of or anxious about and/or avoiding fear and anxiety themselves. Thus the seeking circuitry is driven primarily by the fear circuitry, not by pursuit of what is truly satisfying or fulfilling. When the escape ends, the suffering from which one sought to escape returns, and may be intensified because the way one sought escape itself causes or increases one's fear and anxiety (e.g., a person gets drunk to escape fears and anxieties and then feels fearful and anxious about the effects of their drunken behavior on

---

[1]Buddhist psychology and meditation practice are important sources of this framework, including their focus on fear/aversion and seeking/craving, which, along with ignorance, are known as the "three poisons," or three root causes of suffering (see also Grabovac, Lau, & Willets, 2011).

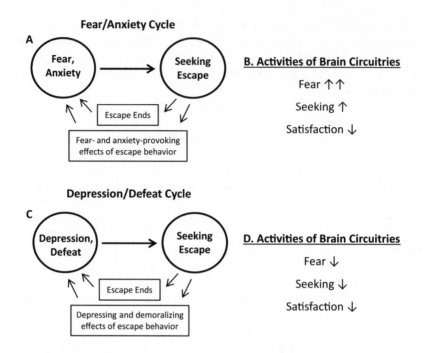

FIGURE 12.1. Suffering cycles and hypothesized activities of key brain circuitries. In the fear/anxiety cycle (A), seeking escape from what's feared and from fear and anxiety lead to more fear and anxiety, and (B) high fear-circuitry activity drives the seeking circuitry in the presence of little or no satisfaction-circuitry activity. The depression/defeat cycle entails (C) more sporadic seeking of escape from depression and defeat and (D) suppressed seeking-circuitry activity in the presence of little or no fear and satisfaction circuitry activity. In both cycles the embodiment circuitry is occupied to the extent that it processes bodily information with unpleasant sensations.

a loved one and his or her perceptions of them). In this cycle the embodiment circuitry is occupied with sensations of fear and anxiety, and with sensations of craving for escape from sensations of fear, anxiety, and craving. There is little activation of the satisfaction circuitry anywhere in the cycle, with the possible exception of briefly while experiencing escape (e.g., intoxication, sexual pleasure).

In this framework's *depression/defeat cycle*, a person feels stuck in and overwhelmed by something bad that has *already* happened. The fear circuitry is relatively inactive, because something that may have been feared has already come to pass. The embodiment circuitry is occupied by sensations that go with feeling heavy, slow, tired, low-energy, bad about oneself, and unmoved by things that should be motivating or enjoyable. The seeking circuitry is actually *suppressed*, so we do not expect good things to happen nor have much motivation for their pursuit (Treadway & Zald, 2011). To the extent that the seeking circuitry *is* active—whether sporadically in a burst, such as getting off the couch to go out and drink (or shop or have sex), or at an ongoing low level, as in someone motivated to smoke pot and watch TV all day—it focuses on escaping the bad feelings and sensations of depression and defeat. (This is true even when someone is engaged in the experiential avoidance of embodied emotional experience by ruminating on negative, pessimistic, and/or self-denigrating thoughts, memories, and fantasies.) As with the fear/anxiety cycle, when the escape behavior ends, the suffering of depression and defeat return, sometimes even worse than before, because the escape behavior (or the substance used to escape or the effects of withdrawing from the substance) is a cause of depression and feelings of defeat. And of course states of depression involve little or no activity of the satisfaction circuitry. Finally, the suppression and misdirection of the seeking circuitry in the absence of satisfaction—especially with one's own actions or lack thereof—contributes to *demoralization*.

Of course, sometimes people can be fearful or anxious *and* depressed, and may seek escape from other unwanted experiences too, for example of emotional numbness or dissociation. So long as one's seeking circuitry is suppressed or is focused almost entirely on escaping pain and suffering—rather than on seeking what is truly satisfying and fulfilling—one is caught in cycles of suffering.

Cycles of Healing and Recovery, Freedom and Happiness

Just as the framework specifies cycles of suffering, it describes cycles of healing. And just as the fear circuitry has been the focus of psychological trauma theory, research and therapy, the seeking circuitry has been neglected. A key contribution of the framework offered here is to focus attention on the seeking circuitry, including its potential roles in trauma-related suffering and, as addressed in this section, in healing from trauma and finding true happiness and fulfillment in life.

In the view advanced here, two keys to recovery and healing—and spiritual transformation—are focusing one's seeking circuitry on pursuing things that are (1) genuinely healing, not merely brief escapes from suffering (which can be confused with healing), and (2) truly satisfying and fulfilling, not merely fleeting pleasures. Therefore, the framework specifies two fundamental cycles of healing: *seeking to engage and transform suffering*, and *seeking true goods*. These cycles are seen as supporting each other and potentially simultaneous, but it is helpful to consider them separately—particularly with respect to how each is postulated to change relationships among the circuitries of seeking, fear, satisfaction, and embodiment.

Healing Cycle: Seeking to Engage and Transform Suffering

According to the framework, this brain-based healing cycle entails seeking to know, tolerate, understand, and make positive use of pain and suffering (see Figure 12.2). What it means to seek to engage and transform suffering will differ from one person to another. For some, seeking to know and understand their suffering means lots of work with a therapist or counselor. Others seek to engage with and transform their suffering through sharing with family and friends, with members of their religious or spiritual community, or members of a support group for those struggling with similar forms of suffering. For others, it means writing about their experiences of suffering or expressing them artistically. And for more and more people, as discussed later, it involves engaging in meditation or other contemplative practices that cultivate mindful and loving embodiment, which fosters mindful and loving thoughts and actions.

Whatever works for a particular person, the *seeking to engage and transform suffering* healing cycle entails just that: seeking to *engage* with pain, suffering, and unwanted experiences, and doing so *in healthy and healing ways* that decrease trauma and *break cycles of suffering*. For example, a client might seek to experience feelings of shame associated with a sexual abuse experience, in order to better understand the origins of those feelings and reduce their intensity and frequency, but this will only be healing if she first accesses feelings of safety in her body and compassion toward herself.

Whatever path someone takes, however, engaging the embodiment circuitry, which registers and allows awareness of one's suffering, is understood here to be critical and cannot be neglected. For many traumatized people, attending to bodily aspects of suffering can be very difficult and "triggering." For everyone, this healing cycle requires strong motivation, because it can be quite unpleasant to engage with our suffering, which we typically attempt to avoid. To sustain that seeking and to find success in engaging suffering, traumatized clients require *support*, often from a therapist, counselor, and/or spiritual teacher. Indeed, as shown in Figure 12.2, this healing cycle can involve seeking a variety of resources that enable engagement with suffering and its transformation, including not only healing-promoting support from others, but also self-regulation and other skills; knowledge of and insights into trauma and healing in general and in oneself as a unique individual; healing attitudes, including compassion and kindness toward one's suffering; and cultivating new habits to replace old habits of responding to suffering in ways that only exacerbate it. (Many of these capacities depend on the brain's prefrontal cortex, a circuitry beyond the scope of this chapter.)

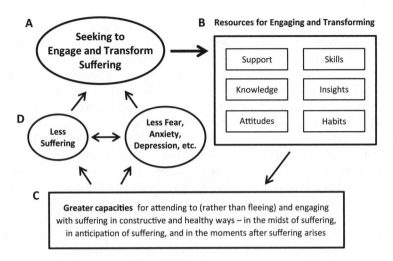

FIGURE 12.2. Healing cycle: Seeking to engage and transform suffering. In this cycle there is still suffering, but rather than seeking escape from suffering, (A) seeking is focused on acquiring (B) resources that allow (C) engaging with suffering (especially as bodily experiences processed by the embodiment circuitry) in constructive and healthy ways that transform suffering experiences into vehicles of (D) recovery and healing. The seeking circuitry is no longer driven by fear of suffering, but instead by motivations to know, understand, heal, and transform one's suffering.

True, engaging in this healing cycle is difficult and sometimes painful. But the payoff is huge. Traumatized people can come to live in much less fear. They can have more compassion for themselves, no matter what they're going through. They can find courage and strength inside that they never realized were there. In this framework's terms, they can free up their seeking circuitry to pursue much more satisfying and fulfilling things in life, which will bring more happiness and healthiness than they ever imagined possible.

Healing Cycle: Seeking True Goods

Fortunately, recovery and healing are not all about seeking to deal more effectively with pain and suffering. If that is all a clinician ever focuses on with a client, the work of therapy and healing is not so appealing, and definitely not inspiring, for the client or the clinician.

In the framework's second key healing cycle, *seeking true goods*, one is harnessing the brain circuitry of seeking—that always-active and powerful driver of our thoughts and behaviors—to seeking out the truly "good things in life." These true goods include love, peace, playfulness, and joy.

In this healing cycle one seeks and experiences the kind of happiness and satisfaction that come from being a good friend, a good spouse or partner, a good parent, or a successful worker or contributor to one's community.[2]

All traumatized people need to sort out, for themselves, what truly makes them happy. What they find to be the greatest goods in life, the things they most deeply value and find most satisfying to experience. This process of exploration and discovery may take some time, especially if they have had little experience with true goods and genuine happiness. It will take the support of others who do not judge their values or push them to adopt their own, but instead give them the space, as well as the support and inspiration, to sort things out for themselves and to awaken and harness their seeking circuitry to this pursuit. A therapy model that many find helpful is acceptance and commitment therapy, or ACT (Engle & Follette, Chapter 4, this volume; Follette & Pistorello, 2007; Harris, 2009). ACT has a major focus on helping clients sort through their values and goals and then commit to seeking to realize those they believe are most important.

As shown in Figure 12.3, according to this framework the *seeking true goods* healing cycle involves realigning the seeking circuitry with one's deepest needs and longings. A person engaging in this healing cycle is seeking what will be genuinely fulfilling and satisfying, and spending more and more time experiencing that satisfaction and fulfillment. Also, the more people activate their brain's satisfaction circuitry as a result of successful seeking of this kind, and occupy their embodiment circuitry with the sensations of that satisfaction, the less power the circuitries of fear and seeking have over them. That's what it *means* to be satisfied and content: accepting and embracing this moment, without wanting or seeking more from it; accepting whatever may come next, without fear.

As research has shown, when one activates the brain's opioid satisfaction circuitry, activity of the fear and seeking circuitries, including in response to old "triggers" of fear and craving, is actually reduced (e.g., Colasanti, Rabiner, Lingford-Hughes, & Nutt, 2011; Love, Stohler, & Zubieta, 2009; Ribeiro, Kennedy, Smith, Stohler, & Zubieta, 2005; Schreckenberger et al., 2008). When this happens, a person is no longer enslaved to fearing and seeking, nor to the cycles of suffering and addiction. Instead, as shown

---

[2]Buddhist psychology and meditation are also sources of the framework's focus on seeking what is truly good and satisfying. Specifically, in Mahayana Buddhism the greatest motivation, said to be an expression of *bodhicitta* or "mind of enlightenment," is the loving and compassionate motivation to seek enlightenment for the benefit of all beings, so one can help them achieve liberation from suffering and genuine happiness; according to Vajrayana or tantric Buddhism (the Dalai Lama's tradition), as explained in the classic *Introduction to Tantra: The Transformation of Desire* (Yeshe, 2001), "it is only through the skillful use of desirous energy [in biological terms, the seeking circuitry] and by building up the habit of experiencing what we might call true pleasure [biologically based in the satisfaction circuitry] that we can hope to achieve the everlasting bliss and joy of full illumination" (p. 10).

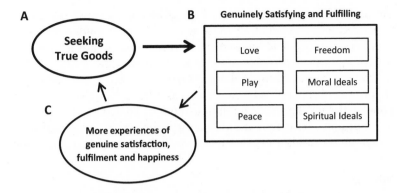

FIGURE 12.3. Healing cycle: Seeking true goods. In this cycle, (A) the seeking circuitry is focused on wanting and pursuing (B) what is genuinely satisfying and fulfilling. This leads to (C) more experiences of genuine satisfaction, fulfillment, and happiness, including the bodily aspects of such experiences as registered by the embodiment circuitry. This in turn increases motivation to seek and enjoy more true goods (rather than quick fixes and other "false goods" that perpetuate suffering), which decreases fear circuitry activation (see text) and suffering in general.

in Figure 12.3, a modulated seeking circuitry can be harnessed to a self-perpetuating seeking true goods cycle: The more one successfully seeks true goods, the more one enjoys the genuine satisfaction, fulfillment, and happiness they bring, and the more one's seeking circuitry becomes focused on seeking true goods that bring healing and happiness.

Contemplative Practices for Seeking to Engage and Transform Suffering

Contemplative practices can be used to carefully attend to and investigate any experience that human beings may have—including those of pain and suffering—and to cultivate capacities for doing so. Employing one's capacities for attention and investigation in this way is central to this framework's *seeking to engage and transform suffering* healing cycle, which involves seeking to know, tolerate, understand, and make positive use of one's pain and suffering.

Preparation

Before directly facing pain and suffering, people need skills for managing painful and unwanted feelings and body sensations, including traumatic memories and addictive cravings. Therapists competent at working with traumatized people, including those with addictions, understand that the *first stage* of recovery is focused on learning and strengthening self-care and self-regulation skills (Herman, 1992; Courtois & Ford, 2009; Fiorillo & Fruzetti, Chapter 5, this volume; Najavits, 2002). For those struggling with the effects of major trauma, there is another prerequisite for safely facing one's pain and suffering: a relationship with someone, often a therapist, who is not only competent at guiding them through the stages of recovery, but truly understands and cares for them (Briere, Chapter 1, this volume).

Mindfulness

A common definition of *mindfulness* is "the awareness that emerges through paying attention on purpose, in the present moment, and nonjudgmentally to the unfolding of experience moment by moment" (Kabat-Zinn, 2003). When someone freely chooses to embark on the *second* stage of recovery from trauma, also known as "remembrance and mourning" (Herman, 1992), mindfulness is an excellent tool for exploring trauma-related memories, feelings, bodily experiences, thought processes, and ways of relating to others. Experiences that had previously felt too unbearable to focus on can be explored and investigated, and seen as passing sensations and thoughts that arise under particular conditions, without resorting to seeking escape. When habitual reactions arise, or suffering cycles begin to unfold, one can mindfully observe and even experientially understand them and not get carried away.[3]

Bodily Awareness as Key

Mindful awareness of bodily sensations—that is, one's *moment-to-moment experiences of embodiment*—is the foundation for attending to and exploring one's emotions, thoughts, behaviors, and relationship patterns (e.g., Chiesa, Serretti, & Jakobsen, 2013; Kerr, Sacchet, Lazar, Moore, & Jones, 2013). Only with that grounding in embodied awareness—of the

---

[3] As meditation masters teach, concentration arising from concentration meditation is a precondition of mindfulness. Without a foundation of concentration, mindfulness is impossible, because attention is swept away by thoughts, emotions, and images that revolve around wants and fears. Also, effective meditative concentration requires both (1) quieting the fear circuitry and (2) adjusting activity of the seeking circuitry to the optimal amount required to sustain meditative focus, as indicated by the Tibetan term for the concentration practice of *shamatha*, which means "calm abiding" (Wallace, 1998). Similarly, in the Buddhist tradition mindfulness itself is a precondition for something more transformative than present-focused awareness, stress reduction, and other benefits for which it is now promoted. That is, mindfulness can be a foundation for liberating insight, or *vipassana*, which includes directly observing how aversion, seeking, and habitual relationships between them—which can otherwise unfold outside of awareness, in just fractions of a second—are causing suffering to oneself and others.

impermanent bodily sensations—can one effectively bring mindful awareness to emotions and thoughts; otherwise, one is repeatedly swept away in
habitual cycles of seeking brief escapes and quick fixes that perpetuate suffering and disconnection from present experience. Researchers have found
that the insula, that key component of the embodiment circuitry which
brings together *all* information coming from the body (see earlier discussion), is larger and has a greater density of "gray matter" in long-term
mindfulness meditators (Lazar et al., 2005; Hölzel et al., 2008). Researchers have also found that mindfulness meditators exhibit brain functioning
in which insula activity dominates the processing of sadness (Farb et al.,
2010) and pain sensations (e.g., Gard et al., 2012; Grant, Courtemanche,
& Rainville, 2011). For people struggling with trauma, this means that
mindfulness can enable direct and safe engagement with the bodily sensations of pain and suffering, which, as several mindfulness researchers have
pointed out (e.g., Farb et al., 2010; Gard et al., 2012), enables one to experience and understand those sensations as "relatively innocuous sensory
information rather than as an affect-laden threat to the self requiring a regulatory response" (Farb et al., 2010, p. 31). Rather than seeking to control
or escape those sensations, which does not bring healing and tends to perpetuate suffering, mindfulness allows tolerance and compassionate understanding of those sensations and other constructive and healing responses
to them. In short, as illustrated by clinical examples in other chapters of
this book (see, e.g., Brach, Chapter 2; Ogden, Chapter 14), mindfulness
enables the transformation of suffering experiences into opportunities for
healing, even spiritual awakening.

Examples of Mindfulness and Successfully Seeking to Engage and Transform Suffering

A female therapy client who was sexually abused as a child learned to
mindfully observe constricted feelings in her chest and visual images of
the abuse, without immediately getting lost in the feelings of disgust and
shame that went with them. She also learned to mindfully observe the disgust and shame, including the transitory bodily sensations that went with
them—again, without getting lost in them or seeking to escape. In time
these memories, feelings, and sensations lost their grip on her, and she discovered peace, strength, and freedom that she had never known were possible. Another client, a male soldier sexually assaulted by his commanding
officer, learned to mindfully observe—without judging himself or being
consumed by fear or shame—memories of the overwhelming helplessness
and betrayal he felt during the assault. Even without (yet) engaging in practices to cultivate self-compassion (see later discussion), new compassionate
understandings of what had happened, and of his reactions to it, spontaneously arose and replaced the guilt and self-hate that he had struggled with
for years.

Special Help for Dissociation and Addiction

Clients who struggle with dissociation will likely need special help to safely and effectively learn and apply mindfulness (Waelde, Chapter 19, this volume). Those who struggle with addictions may need special help to avoid getting addicted to pleasant bodily and mental states that meditation can bring. We are all vulnerable to having our seeking become craving and attachment (i.e., to spoiling and losing true goods by relating to them as quick-fix escapes), but clients with stronger addictive tendencies may need special help avoiding this. And because both dissociative and addictive tendencies can result in mistaking attachment to states of disconnection for "enlightened detachment," careful monitoring and specific methods may be needed to avoid getting stuck in that way (Waelde, Chapter 19, this volume).

For severely traumatized people, attending to body sensations associated with trauma, even unintentionally in the midst of a mindfulness exercise, can be quite triggering (e.g., of traumatic memories and trauma-based emotional reactions) and overwhelming. For them it is safest—and most helpful—if they first experience mindfulness in the context of a relationship with a mindful therapist. Experiencing mindfulness first within a therapy relationship can be healing, especially for those not ready to engage in mindfulness practice on their own, as illustrated by several case vignettes in chapters of this book (see, e.g., Brach, Chapter 2; Emerson & E. K. Hopper, Chapter 11; Fiorillo & Fruzzetti, Chapter 5; Grindler Katonah, Chapter 10; Ogden, Chapter 14; Parker, Chapter 20).

For these reasons and others, mindfulness and other contemplative methods for engaging with and transforming suffering are not quick fixes or panaceas. Even after cultivating the self-care and self-regulation skills needed to engage directly with trauma and suffering, engaging with and transforming suffering can be a long process. We are all creatures of habit, and old habits can be hard to break, especially if they once ensured our physical or psychological survival. But with a foundation of self-regulation skills, regular practice, and relationships that support both, mindfully engaging with one's suffering can facilitate the healing cycle of *seeking to engage and transform suffering*.

Contemplative Practices and Seeking True Goods

Finally, the second healing cycle specified by the framework, *seeking true goods*, includes the use of contemplative practices to *harness the brain's seeking circuitry*—which when wrongly directed causes so much of our suffering—*to the pursuit of true goods that bring genuine happiness*.

Our seeking circuitry is always active. Fortunately, unlike many other aspects of brain function, this one is accessible to us, something we can reflect upon and contemplate. And we can choose: *What shall I seek? What should I seek as my highest priorities? What do I want to seek in this moment?* We can also contemplate and choose our answers to these questions: What *really* makes me happy? What is my *motivation* for doing (or thinking or saying or writing) this? These questions and choices are at the heart of contemplative practices and how we put them into practice in our lives.

What Should We Seek?

Religious and spiritual leaders have long sought (whether wisely or in confusion themselves) to help people seek transcendent "true goods"—obedience to God's law; surrender to God's will; an intimate relationship with God or Jesus; loving others, even our "enemies," as we love ourselves; forever striving to free all beings from suffering. Profit-seeking companies, politicians, and advertisers bombard us with sights, sounds and words designed to harness our seeking circuitry to the (perceived) benefits they seek for themselves.[4] The Declaration of Independence declares it a "self-evident" truth that we are endowed by our creator with unalienable rights, not only to life and liberty, but also to "the pursuit of happiness." In short, the brain's seeking circuitry is central to human life.

The Dalai Lama often says, "We all naturally desire happiness and not to suffer" (e.g., 1999, p. 49). He writes of "genuine happiness"—which has "inner peace" as its principal characteristic, "is rooted in concern for others and involves a high degree of sensitivity and feeling," and provides a basic sense of well-being that cannot be undermined, "no matter what difficulties we encounter in life" (1999, pp. 55–56). He distinguishes this genuine happiness from all those states of mind that, despite being called "happiness" and sought by many, lack those qualities. He is pointing to those central questions at the heart of our lives, about what brings genuine happiness and should be the object of our seeking.

The Seeking Circuitry Has Been Unknown, Unappreciated, and Misunderstood

So far, aside from addiction research, the brain's seeking circuitry has been largely unrecognized and overlooked in psychology and psychiatry. Among

---

[4]This now includes advertising and marketing for "mindfulness-based" techniques that are uncoupled from the ethical and religious contexts in which mindfulness was developed. As Purser and Loy (2013) observe, "While a stripped-down, secularized technique—what some critics are now calling 'McMindfulness'—may make it more palatable to the corporate world, decontextualizing mindfulness from its original liberative and transformative purpose, as well as its foundation in social ethics, amounts to a Faustian bargain. Rather than applying mindfulness as a means to awaken individuals and organizations from the unwholesome roots of greed, ill will and delusion, it is usually being refashioned into a banal, therapeutic, self-help technique that can actually reinforce those roots."

those focused on psychological trauma, attention has been almost entirely on the circuitry of fear (with the exception of Elman and colleagues' work on reward and seeking in PTSD; e.g., Elman et al., 2009; Hopper et al., 2008). Similarly, the focus on mindfulness and other contemplative methods for healing trauma surveyed in this book has involved little consideration of the seeking circuitry.[5]

Discussions of mindfulness often include cautions about the danger of seeking any result, and the concern that doing so is incompatible with mindfulness. Certainly, seeking results can be an obstacle to mindfulness and the unsought and unexpected insights and transformations that it can bring. But as stated in the Buddha's Second Noble Truth, the problem is *craving conditioned by ignorance*—not seeking itself, which need not involve craving and is inseparable from normative brain function, healthy living, and embodied life itself. Furthermore, as Purser and Loy (2013) note, "Buddhists differentiate between Right Mindfulness (*samma sati*) and Wrong Mindfulness (*miccha sati*)," and this distinction addresses "whether the quality of awareness is characterized by wholesome intentions and positive mental qualities that lead to human flourishing and optimal well-being for others as well as oneself." In short, Right Mindfulness entails seeking true goods for oneself and others (beyond nonjudgmental awareness of present experience and any benefits that it automatically engenders whether or not one seeks them).

Tara Brach has movingly written of an experience when, after days of having grasped, resisted, and attempted to control feelings of longing for love, she recognized this reality that seeking is central to life itself:

> Late one evening I sat meditating alone in my room. My attention moved deeper and deeper into longing, until I felt as if I might explode with its heartbreaking urgency. Yet at the same time I knew that was exactly what I wanted—*I wanted to die into longing, into communion, into love itself.* At that moment I could finally let my longing be all that it was. I even invited it. . . . (Brach, 2003, pp. 153–154)

In a recent interview, the widely respected Buddhist teacher, author, and peace activist Thich Nhat Hanh recalled this formative experience when he was 7 or 8 years old:

> One day I saw a picture of the Buddha. . . . [H]e was sitting on the grass very peaceful, smiling, and I was impressed. Around me people were not like that, so I had the desire to be someone like him. And I nourished that kind of desire until the age of 16, when I had the permission from my

---

[5]There are good reasons for this, including lack of knowledge of this critical aspect of brain function; a focus, shared with medicine, on treating illness and reducing suffering rather than promoting health and happiness; and fears of venturing into realms of morality, religion, and spirituality.

parents to go and ordain as a Buddhist monk. . . . We call it the beginner's mind: *the deep intention, the deepest desire that one person may have.* And I can say that since that time, until this day, this beginner's mind is still alive in me. (Nhat Hanh, 2012, emphasis in spoken words)

Similarly, the Dalai Lama is clearly a driven man, as well as an accepting one. Despite many obstacles, he *continually seeks* to be a vehicle of compassion, to serve Tibetans as their spiritual and political leader, and to serve humanity, including by helping to foster integrations of neuroscience with contemplative practices and insights. Yes, seeking can cause problems—when it becomes craving, grasping, clinging, and attachment to passing things that cannot bring genuine happiness. But seeking can be focused on true goods that, when experienced but not clung to, bring genuine happiness and *reduce* craving and attachment.

Seeking Love, Kindness, and Compassion

For Thich Nhat Hanh, it was an image of a happy and loving Buddha; for many Christians, it is an image of Jesus. Every religion and spiritual tradition has its images of wise, loving, and happy beings that can powerfully activate our seeking circuitry and deepest longings. Yet often more effective for cultivating love within oneself—at least initially, for those struggling with trauma—are simpler and more common images easily called to mind or found on the Internet, such as a cute baby, a puppy, or a kitten. The key to successfully utilizing images in this way: bringing the image to mind causes motivations and feelings of love, kindness, and compassion to arise *spontaneously and effortlessly.*

In the *metta* practice of the Theravadin Buddhist tradition, being taught to traumatized people by several authors in this book (e.g., Tara Brach; Christopher Germer and Kristin Neff; David J. Kearney), the focusing of attention on such an image and the bodily sensations of spontaneously arising motivations and feelings are combined with internally repeating phrases like these:

May you be happy.
May you be healthy.
May you be at peace.
May you be free of suffering.

Harnessing the Brain's Seeking Circuitry to Cultivating Embodied and Satisfying Love, Kindness, and Compassion

In this way, according to the framework offered here, during this practice visual imagination and verbal thoughts—typically absorbed in memories, plans, and fantasies of imagined rewards—along with attention to bodily sensations are used to *harness the brain's seeking circuitry to love, kindness, and compassion*. If while doing the practice we *experience in our bodies* feelings of love, kindness, and compassion, we occupy the embodiment circuitry with them. If those good feelings are accompanied by feelings of contentment, peace, and satisfaction, then this practice also involves the satisfaction circuitry. And to the extent that we experience the bodily sensations of contentment, peace, and satisfaction, the embodiment and satisfaction circuitries are not only involved, but are also being transformed.

In this framework, harnessing the seeking, satisfaction, and embodiment circuitries to the cultivation of love, kindness, and compassion is the most basic and powerful form of the *seeking true goods* healing cycle. The benefits of cultivating love, kindness, and compassion toward oneself and others are many—especially for traumatized people who so far have experienced little of these in their lives.[6] As with mindfulness, however, things can be more complex. Given the neglect, losses, abuses, and betrayals that many traumatized people have experienced in their lives, feelings of love, kindness, and compassion can trigger fear (Gilbert et al., 2010). This is normal, and there are many ways clinicians can help their clients to gently and safely explore, understand, and overcome these obstacles to receiving, cultivating, and giving love, kindness, and compassion (Germer, 2009; Germer & Neff, Chapter 3, this volume; Gilbert, 2005, 2010).

Other "True Goods"

There is a good case, made by many for millennia, that *love*—which we can experience and express in many ways—is the greatest good and the greatest source of genuine human happiness. But most of us agree that there are other (if lesser) "true goods" too, other experiences and goals that are most worthy of seeking and most likely to bring genuine happiness. Depending on our personalities, our cultural and religious backgrounds, and several other factors, we may highly value and seek various things along a continuum from false to true goods (e.g., power, money, technology tools and toys, entertainment, sexual stimulation, physical health, beauty, creativity, knowledge, courage, generosity, connection with nature, playfulness, achievement, contributing to others through our work).

---

[6]Germer and Neff (Chapter 3, this volume) discuss several benefits. But one of the greatest benefits—seldom mentioned but worth contemplating, whether we seek healing from trauma or fostering it in others—is this: By focusing one's seeking on love, one harnesses the brain's seeking circuitry to pursuing the greatest good and greatest happiness.

The world's religious and spiritual traditions supremely value wisdom, which includes liberation from ignorance and, to use a central Buddhist conception, "seeing things as they really are"—not as we fear or want them to be. Such wisdom entails accurately perceiving and knowing oneself, per the ancient Delphic maxim. Combining mindfulness with analytical meditations involving self-questioning—and the courage to know oneself—can yield insights into our true motivations for what we do and say (Wallace, 2001). In doing so we find that, for our clients and ourselves, even efforts to pursue true goods are sometimes *largely* motivated by fears of failure, judgment, or rejection; by cravings for lesser goods, such as others' attention or admiration; even by false goods, such as competitive advantage or revenge. Over the course of writing this chapter, I have been motivated by a sincere wish to share something helpful, but also by fears that it won't be good enough, that readers will find it useless, that I won't finish it on time, and by craving for readers' admiration. Seeking the true good of self-knowledge can help us to mindfully and compassionately acknowledge such normal human shortcomings, to gain more freedom from them, and to focus our seeking on true goods and genuine happiness.

In short, there are many contemplative practices—especially but not only those for cultivating love, kindness, and compassion—that can bring healing from trauma and much more, *by harnessing the brain's seeking circuitry to the pursuit of true goods and genuine happiness.*

Conclusion

This chapter offers a framework for understanding key brain and psychological processes involved in trauma, suffering, and healing, particularly healing fostered by contemplative practices for cultivating mindfulness, love, kindness, and compassion. The framework draws on scientific, clinical, and contemplative knowledge to provide an integrative vision. While simplifying things in some ways, the framework also acknowledges the complexity of trauma and healing. Also, appropriate neuroscience reviewers found nothing in this chapter that is inconsistent with current knowledge, although it is important to note that research on interactions between the brain circuitries of fear, seeking, satisfaction, and embodiment is currently limited. Certainly more research is needed. In the meantime those of us seeking to help traumatized people heal and find happiness can better appreciate and explore the power of contemplative practices (used carefully and appropriately) to harness the brain's seeking, satisfaction, and embodiment circuitries to decrease suffering and to cultivate more mindful, loving, and happy human beings.

References

Alcaro, A., & Panksepp, J. (2011). The SEEKING mind: Primal neuro-affective substrates for appetitive incentive states and their pathological dynamics in addictions and depression. *Neuroscience and Biobehavioral Reviews, 35,* 1805–1820.

Akil, H., Owens, C., Gutstein, H., Taylor, L., Curran, E., & Watson, S. (1998). Endogenous opioids: Overview and current issues. *Drug and Alcohol Dependence, 51,* 127–140.

Belova, M. A., Patton, J. J., Morrison, S. E., & Salzman, C. D. (2007). Expectation modulates neural responses to pleasant and aversive stimuli in primate amygdala. *Neuron, 55,* 970–984.

Brach, T. (2003). *Radical acceptance: Embracing your life with the heart of a buddha.* New York: Bantam Books.

Chiesa, A., Serretti, A., & Jakobsen, J. C. (2013). Mindfulness: Top-down or bottom-up emotion regulation strategy? *Clinical Psychology Review, 33,* 82–96.

Colasanti, A., Rabiner E. A., Lingford-Hughes, A., & Nutt, D. J. (2011). Opioids and anxiety. *Journal of Psychopharmacology, 25,* 1415–1433.

Courtois, C. A., & Ford, J. D. (Eds.). (2009). *Treating complex traumatic stress disorders: Scientific foundations and therapeutic models.* New York: Guilford Press.

Craig, A. D. (2002). How do you feel? Interoception: The sense of the physiological condition of the body. *Nature Reviews Neuroscience, 3,* 655–666.

Dalai Lama. (1999). *Ethics for the new millennium.* New York: Riverside Books.

Depue, R. A., & Collins, P. F. (1999). Neurobiology of the structure of personality: Dopamine, facilitation of incentive motivation, and extraversion. *Behavioral and Brain Sciences, 22,* 491–569.

Depue, R. A., & Morrone-Strupinsky, J. V. (2005). A neurobehavioral model of affiliative bonding: Implications for conceptualizing a human trait of affiliation. *Behavioral and Brain Sciences, 28,* 313–395.

Elman, I., Lowen, S., Frederick, B. B., Chi, W., Becerra, L., & Pitman, R. K. (2009). Functional neuroimaging of reward circuitry responsivity to monetary gains and losses in posttraumatic stress disorder. *Biological Psychiatry, 66,* 1083–1090.

Farb, N. A., Anderson, A. K., Mayberg, H., Bean, J., McKeon, D., & Segal, Z. V. (2010). Minding one's emotions: Mindfulness training alters the neural expression of sadness. *Emotion, 10,* 25–33.

Farrin, L., Hull, L., Unwin, C., Wykes, T., & David, A. (2003). Effects of depressed mood on objective and subjective measures of attention. *Journal of Neuropsychiatry and Clinical Neurosciences, 15,* 98–104.

Follette, V. M., & Pistorello, J. (2007). *Finding life beyond trauma: Using acceptance and commitment therapy to heal from post-traumatic stress and trauma-related problems.* Oakland, CA: New Harbinger.

Fransson, P. (2005). Spontaneous low-frequency BOLD signal fluctuations: An fMRI investigation of the resting-state default mode of brain function hypothesis. *Human Brain Mapping, 26,* 15–29.

Gard, T., Hölzel, B. K., Sack, A. T., Hempel, H., Lazar, S. W., Vaitl, D., et al.

(2012). Pain attenuation through mindfulness is associated with decreased cognitive control and increased sensory processing in the brain. *Cerebral Cortex, 22,* 2692–2702.

Germer, C. K. (2009). *The mindful path to self-compassion.* New York: Guilford Press.

Gilbert, D. T., & Wilson, T. D. (2000). Miswanting: Some problems in the forecasting of future affective states. In E. Joseph & P. Forgas (Eds.), *Feeling and thinking: The role of affect in social cognition* (pp. 178–197). New York: Cambridge University Press.

Gilbert, P. (Ed.). (2005). *Compassion: Conceptualizations, research and use in psychotherapy.* London: Routledge.

Gilbert, P. (2010). *Compassion-focused therapy.* London: Routledge.

Gilbert, P., McEwan, K., Matos, M., & Rivis, R. (2010). Fears of compassion: Development of three self-report measures. *Psychology and Psychotherapy: Theory, Research and Practice, 84,* 239–255.

Grabovac, A. D., Lau, M. A., & Willets, B. R. (2011). Mechanisms of mindfulness: A Buddhist psychological model. *Mindfulness, 2,* 154–166.

Grant, J. A., Courtemanche, J., & Rainville, P. (2011). A non-elaborative mental stance and decoupling of executive and pain-related cortices predicts low pain sensitivity in Zen meditators. *Pain, 152,* 150–156.

Greicius, M. D., Krasnow, B., Reiss, A. L., & Menon, V. (2003). Functional connectivity in the resting brain: A network analysis of the default mode hypothesis. *Proceedings of the National Academy of Sciences of the USA, 100,* 253–258.

Gusnard, D. A., & Raichle, M. E. (2001). Searching for a baseline: Functional imaging and the resting human brain. *Nature Reviews Neuroscience, 2,* 685–694.

Harris, R. (2009). *ACT made simple: An easy-to-read primer on acceptance and commitment therapy.* Oakland, CA: New Harbinger.

Herman, J. L. (1992). *Trauma and recovery: The aftermath of violence—from domestic abuse to political terror.* New York: Basic Books.

Hölzel, B. K., Ott, U., Gard, T., Hempel, H., Weygandt, M., Morgen, K., et al. (2008). Investigation of mindfulness meditation practitioners with voxel-based morphometry. *Social Cognitive and Affective Neuroscience, 3,* 55–61.

Hopper, J. W., Frewen, P. A., van der Kolk, B. A., & Lanius, R. A. (2007). Neural correlates of reexperiencing, avoidance, and dissociation in PTSD: Symptom dimensions and emotion dysregulation in responses to script-driven trauma imagery. *Journal of Traumatic Stress, 20,* 713–725.

Hopper, J. W., Pitman, R. K., Su, Z., Heyman, G. M., Lasko, N. B., Macklin, M. L., et al. (2008). Probing reward function in posttraumatic stress disorder: Expectancy and satisfaction with monetary gains and losses. *Journal of Psychiatric Research, 42,* 807–802.

Kabat-Zinn, J. (2003). Mindfulness-based interventions in context: Past, present, and future. *Clinical Psychology: Science and Practice, 10,* 144–156.

Kahneman, D., & Snell, J. (1992). Predicting a changing taste: Do people know what they will like? *Journal of Behavioral Decision Making, 5,* 187–200.

Kerr, C. E., Sacchet, M. D., Lazar, S. W., Moore, C. I., & Jones, S. R. (2013). Mindfulness starts with the body: Somatosensory attention and top-down modulation of cortical alpha rhythms in mindfulness meditation. *Frontiers in Human Neuroscience.* Available at *http://journal.frontiersin.org/Journal/10.3389/fnhum.2013.00012/full.*

Khantzian, E. J. (1999). *Treating addiction as a human process.* Lanham, MD: Aronson.

Khantzian, E. J. (2003). Understanding addictive vulnerability: An evolving psychodynamic perspective. *Neuro-Psychoanalysis, 5,* 5–21.

Klein, D. (1987). Depression and anhedonia. In D. C. Clark & J. Fawcett (Eds.), *Anhedonia and affect deficit states* (pp. 1–14). New York: PMA.

Lanius, R. A., Vermetten, E., Loewenstein, R. J., Brand, B., Schmahl, C., Bremner, J. D., et al. (2010). Emotion modulation in PTSD: Clinical and neurobiological evidence for a dissociative subtype. *American Journal of Psychiatry, 167,* 640–647.

Lazar, S. W., Kerr, C. E., Wasserman, R. H., Gray, J. R., Greve, D. N., Treadway, M. T., et al. (2005). Meditation experience is associated with increased cortical thickness. *Neuroreport, 16,* 1983–1987.

LeDoux, J. E. (2000). Emotion circuits in the brain. *Annual Review of Neuroscience, 23,* 155–184.

LeDoux, J. E. (2012). Evolution of human emotion: A view through fear. *Progress in Brain Research, 195,* 431–442.

Lin, S.-C., & Nicolelis, M. A. (2008). Neuronal ensemble bursting in the basal forebrain encodes salience irrespective of valence. *Neuron, 59,* 138–149.

Love, T. M., Stohler, C. S., & Zubieta, J. K. (2009). Positron emission tomography measures of endogenous opioid neurotransmission and impulsiveness traits in humans. *Archives of General Psychiatry, 66,* 1124–1134.

Machin, A. J., & Dunbar, R. I. M. (2011). The brain opioid theory of social attachment: A review of the evidence. *Behaviour, 148,* 985–1025.

McKiernan, K. A., D'Angelo, B. R., Kaufman, J. N., & Binder, J. R. (2006). Interrupting the "stream of consciousness": An fMRI investigation. *NeuroImage, 29,* 1185–1191.

Najavits, L. M., (2002). *Seeking safety: A treatment manual for PTSD and substance abuse.* New York: Guilford Press.

Naqvi, N. H., & Bechara, A. (2010). The insula and drug addiction: An interoceptive view of pleasure, urges, and decision-making. *Brain Structure and Function, 214,* 435–450.

Naqvi, N. H., Rudrauf, D., Damasio, H., & Bechara, A. (2007). Damage to the insula disrupts addiction to cigarette smoking. *Science, 315,* 531–534.

Nelson, E. E., & Panksepp, J. (1998). Brain substrates of infant–mother attachment: Contributions of opioids, oxytocin, and norepinephrine. *Neuroscience and Biobehavioral Reviews, 22,* 437–452.

Nhat Hanh, T. (2012). *On becoming a monk.* Interview by Oprah Winfrey. Retrieved March 10, 2013, from *www.youtube.com/watch?v=w6CI-jnSo80.*

Olsen, C. M. (2011). Natural rewards, neuroplasticity, and non-drug addictions. *Neuropharmacology, 61,* 1109–1122.

Panksepp, J. (1998). *Affective neuroscience: The foundations of human and animal emotions.* New York: Oxford University Press.

Panksepp, J., & Biven, L. (2012). *The archeology of mind: Neuroevolutionary origins of human emotions.* New York: Norton.

Purser, R., & Loy, D. (2013, July 1). *Beyond McMindfulness*. Retrieved from *www. huffingtonpost.com/ron-purser/beyond-mcmindfulness_b_3519289.html*.

Ribeiro, S. C., Kennedy, S. E., Smith, Y. R., Stohler, C. S., & Zubieta, J. K. (2005). Interface of physical and emotional stress regulation through the endogenous opioid system and mu-opioid receptors. *Progress in Neuropsychopharmacology and Biological Psychiatry, 29*, 1264–1280.

Satpute, A. B., Shu, J., Weber, J., Roy, M., & Ochsner, K. N. (2013). The functional neural architecture of self-reports of affective experience. *Biological Psychiatry, 73*, 631–638.

Schreckenberger, M., Klega, A., Gründer, G., Buchholz, H. G., Scheurich, A., Schirrmacher, R., et al. (2008). Opioid receptor PET reveals the psychobiologic correlates of reward processing. *Journal of Nuclear Medicine, 49*, 1257–1261.

Sherrington, C. S. (1906). *The integrative action of the nervous system*. New York: Scribner.

Shin, L. M., & Handwerger, K. (2009). Is posttraumatic stress disorder a stress-induced fear circuitry disorder? *Journal of Traumatic Stress, 22*, 409–415.

Singer, T., Critchley, H. D., & Preuschoff, K. (2009). A common role of the insula in feelings, empathy and uncertainty. *Trends in Cognitive Sciences, 13*, 335–340.

Smallwood, J., Fitzgerald, A., Miles, L. K., & Phillips, L. H. (2009). Shifting moods, wandering minds: Negative moods lead the mind to wander. *Emotion, 9*, 271–276.

Smallwood, J., O'Connor, R. C., Sudbery, M. V., & Obonsawin, M. C. (2007). Mind wandering and dysphoria. *Cognition and Emotion, 21*, 816–842.

Treadway, M. T., & Zald, D. H. (2011). Reconsidering anhedonia in depression: Lessons from translational neuroscience. *Neuroscience and Biobehavioral Reviews, 35*, 537–555.

Wallace, B. A. (1998). *The bridge of quiescence*. Chicago: Open Court.

Wallace, B. A. (2001). *Buddhism with an attitude*. Ithaca, NY: Snow Lion.

Yeshe, L. T. (2001). *Introduction to tantra: The transformation of desire* (rev. ed.). Boston: Wisdom.

An Interpersonal Neurobiology Approach to Developmental Trauma

The Possible Role of Mindful Awareness in Treatment

Daniel J. Siegel and Moriah Gottman

An Interpersonal Neurobiology View of Developmental Trauma and its Treatment

In this chapter, we provide a brief overview of the field of interpersonal neurobiology (IPNB) and how this interdisciplinary approach can shed light on the developmental aspects of trauma and the potential application of treatment with mindful awareness practices. IPNB uses a consilient (Wilson, 1998) process whereby empirically based findings across a range of scientific disciplines are woven into a unified view of human development and health. Disciplines ranging from anthropology and sociology to psychology and neuroscience are integrated in order to offer a comprehensive definition of the mind and well-being (see Siegel 2012a, 2012b). Naturally, this is only one of many perspectives on the mind and human development, one that hopefully will be able to offer scientifically grounded and useful principles to help alleviate the suffering of individuals who have experienced trauma in their lives.

In IPNB, trauma is viewed as single or multiple experiences an individual, family, or society undergoes that overwhelm the capacity for effective adaptation. For an individual, trauma early in life can induce changes in foundational systems of the growing brain that can have lasting impacts on the developing mind, as well as the synaptic connections and the epigenetic regulation of gene expression in a range of neural circuits. Some of these regions affected by trauma are involved in the modulation of the stress response (Meaney et al., 2007) and the regulation of emotion, attention, memory, and behavior (Choi et al., 2009). Both abuse and neglect have been demonstrated to produce negative impacts on brain function and growth (De Bellis et al., 2002). Developmental trauma is a form of overwhelming experience that occurs early in life and can recursively reinstate the features of the initial abuse or neglect (see van der Kolk, 2006; Sroufe & Siegel, 2011).

One possible mechanism mediating these negative outcomes is the secretion of excessive and prolonged amounts of the stress hormone cortisol, which can have a toxic effect on neurons, negatively affecting their survival, their growth, and their ability to link to other neurons. Work by Choi and colleagues (2009) suggests that parts of the brain that are particularly vulnerable to cortisol damage are those that link widely separated areas to each other, such as the prefrontal region, the hippocampus, and the corpus callosum. This linkage of differentiated parts of a system, which can be called integration, enables the coordination and balance of neural functions distributed throughout the nervous system and body as a whole. Integrative circuits in the brain, such as the middle aspects of the prefrontal cortex that include the medial, orbitofrontal, and ventrolateral prefrontal regions along with the anterior cingulate cortex—vertically and horizontally "middle" areas just behind the forehead—play an important role in coordinating and balancing the whole of the nervous system, as well as in enabling social functions to occur (Siegel, 2007a, 2010a, 2010b).

Within the important attachment relationships that influence the developing brain of the child (Schore, 2003a, 2012; Cozolino, 2011), integration within interpersonal relationships can be viewed as the essential social communication process underlying secure relationships (Siegel, 2012a). A child "feels felt" when he or she is "seen" by the caregiver, giving the child the sense that his or her internal world is experienced authentically and accurately by the caregiver. Being seen, feeling safe, being soothed, and coming to feel secure enable a child to develop optimally. This form of interpersonal communication entails the honoring of differences between parent and child and then the cultivation of compassionate, attuned linkages. In this way, interpersonal integration can be viewed as the basis of secure attachment. In IPNB, healthy relationships are integrative—they honor differences and promote linkages. These integrative forms of communication are viewed as promoting the growth of integrative functioning in the brain—the stimulation and growth of integrative fibers in the brain that link widely differentiated areas to one another. In other words, interpersonal integration fosters neural integration.

Here is the fundamental framework of IPNB: Relationships are seen as the sharing of energy and information between two or more people; the brain is the embodied mechanism of energy and information flow; and a key aspect of the "mind" is viewed as an emergent, self-organizing process, embodied and relational, that regulates the flow of energy and information within our bodies and in our relationships. In this way one aspect of "mind," beyond subjective experience and consciousness, is this self-organizing regulatory embodied and relational process (Siegel, 2012a, 2012b). Energy is the "capacity to do something" from a physics point of view; information is a pattern of energy flow that stands for something other than itself—it has meaning.

Psychological trauma in various degrees of severity can be seen to occur when experiences are nonintegrative—such as when an infant is neglected (excessive differentiation without linkage) or abused (excessive linkage without differentiation). The result of overwhelming experiences that are nonintegrative is the impairment of integrative growth in the brain—as revealed in the deficits in the growth and development of the corpus callosum, prefrontal, and hippocampal integrative regions in the cases of abuse and neglect (Choi et al., 2009). For the corpus callosum, the two halves of the brain are linked; for the hippocampus, widely distributed neural regions involved in memory are integrated; and for the prefrontal cortex, the cortical, limbic, brain stem, bodily, and even social streams of energy and information combine to form complex mental processes (Siegel, 2012a).

From an IPNB perspective, integration is a core mechanism of health. When a system is integrated, it functions in harmony. Elements of the system are coordinated and linked with integration, and the movement of that system is the most flexible, adaptive, coherent, energized, and stable. When linkage and/or differentiation are impaired, however, this nonintegrated state of the system results in chaos, rigidity, or some combination of both within various aspects of physiological, mental, or relational experiences. The developmental consequences of trauma can be seen as characterized by this spectrum of chaos and rigidity (Bluhm et al., 2009; Bremner, Elzinga, Schmahl, & Vermetten, 2008; Choi et al., 2009; De Bellis et al., 2002). For single-event trauma, as well, posttraumatic stress disorder can be seen as comprising chaotic and rigid symptoms. Posttraumatic stress disorder (PTSD) has been defined in the *Diagnostic and Statistical Manual of Mental Disorders* (DSM-5; American Psychiatric Association, 2013) as an anxiety disorder characterized by intrusive symptoms (including distressing memories and recurrent dreams related to the trauma), alterations in arousal, avoidance of trauma-related stimuli, and alterations in cognitions and mood associated with the trauma. Reexperiencing traumatic memories and alterations in arousal are examples of the chaotic end of the spectrum, away from integrative functioning; avoidance and disturbances in mood represent the rigid end. The social and personal dysfunction resulting from trauma, viewed through the lens of IPNB, can thus be seen as the result of blockages to integration.

Treatment from this perspective involves a relationship between therapist and client that fosters experiences that are integrative (Siegel, 2010a). In the therapeutic process, both the attachment aspects of a person being seen, safe, soothed, and secure within the relationship and the offering of specific therapeutic interventions promote the stimulation and growth of integrative fibers in the brain responsible for self-regulation.

Empirical Support for the Notion of Impaired Integration in Trauma

Research by Lanius, Bluhm, and colleagues (Bluhm et al., 2009; Lanius, Bluhm, & Frewen, 2011) helps to elucidate possible neurological roots across PTSD cases. Their work reveals (Bluhm et al., 2009) that the default network in the brain that connects the limbic system, what some consider the emotional core of the brain, to the prefrontal cortex (PFC), the integrative area needed for executive control and conflict processing, exhibits fewer connections to the hippocampus and the amygdala within individuals with PTSD. It is these midline cortical circuits that may be seen as the neural correlates of the self (Northoff et al., 2006). The ways in which these midline structures differentiate and link their functioning is correlated with well-being and the experience of self (Gusnard, Akbudak, Shulman, & Raichle, 2001; Uddin, Kelly, Biswal, Castellanos, & Milham, 2009). Mindfulness training has been shown to increase the integration (functional connectivity) of this same default network in the brain (Brewer et al., 2011)—a finding that may provide a clue as to how mindful awareness might facilitate integrative growth in the brain and the coherence of a sense of self often fragmented after trauma. As mentioned earlier, work by Choi and colleagues further suggests that the three major integrative circuits of the corpus callosum, prefrontal cortex, and hippocampus are those that are negatively affected by developmental trauma, the early, intense, and often chronic experience of abuse and neglect (Choi et al., 2009). Depending on the timing of the trauma, these important regions that coordinate and balance the neural processing of information and the establishment of self-regulation can be differentially affected by these negative experiences. Studies by Eileen Luders and colleagues have also shown that mindfulness training leads to the increased integration of these exact regions (Luders, Clark, Narr, & Toga, 2011).

Disorganized Attachment and Dissociation as Impaired Integration and Regulation

Dissociation has been found to be an outcome of disorganized attachment (Beebee, Jaffe, Markese, Buck, Chen, et al., 2010; Dutra, Ilaria, Siegel, & Lyons-Ruth, 2009) in which interpersonal attunement between infant and caregiver is impaired such that the infant experiences a fear-inducing and a disorganizing set of responses from the primary caregiver. In this situation, two brain circuits within the child are activated simultaneously in such a way as to create a biological paradox. The attachment circuit (about 200 million years old) drives the infant to seek comfort from the attachment figure when terrified; the survival circuit involving the brain stem (about 300 million years old) engages a fight–flight–freeze reaction, causing the child to withdraw from the source of terror. When the attachment figure is the source of the terror, these two circuits are driving the infant *toward* (comfort) and *away* (survival) from the same person. This creates what Mary Main and Erik Hesse (1990) have called "fear without solution." The child is unable to link an organized, adaptive strategy to these experiences. This is a prime example of a developmental trauma as defined as an early set of experiences beyond the capacity to cope effectively.

An IPNB view suggests that the developmental trauma of disorganized attachment creates significant impairments to neural integration in the child that persist into adolescence and adulthood as impediments to self-regulation and as continuing tendencies toward dissociation. This fragmentation of consciousness in turn may make the individual experience more difficulty regulating stress, engaging in supportive relationships, balancing emotions, and maintaining clear thinking under pressure. These behavioral traits may each contribute to the vulnerability to develop PTSD if one is later exposed to overwhelming experiences. With an overwhelming event, the impaired neural integration that existed before the traumatic incident will make the individual less able to recover from the trauma and more likely to develop PTSD in its clinical, formal presentation. It is important to keep in mind that the impact of traumatic experiences in childhood may have significant negative effects on the child's development even if the child does not meet formal diagnostic criteria for PTSD (van der Kolk, 2006).

A number of hypotheses explain how childhood trauma in the form of abuse and/or neglect may lead not only to negative impacts on the regulation of emotion, attention, and behavior but also to a predisposition for PTSD in the event of future stress exposure. In addition to the negative effects on integrative fiber growth discussed previously, another possibility is that maltreatment may alter the ability of the brain to produce cerebrospinal fluid (CSF) and lead to enlargement of the ventricular spaces, similar to what occurs in clients with Alzheimer's disease (De Bellis et al., 2002).

Brain volume decreases with more severe abuse and also appears to be sex-linked, with male brains becoming more affected than those of females. The children in De Bellis's study also had lower levels of white matter when they developed PTSD in comparison with age-matched controls, similar to the results of adult PTSD research.

As distinct from developmental trauma, only 15% of adults who experience an overwhelming, single traumatic event will go on to develop the formal disorder of PTSD (Yehuda, 2003). The exact reasons why some are vulnerable to PTSD and others are not are unclear at this time. One possibility is that a genetically related and/or experientially derived tendency toward dissociation may predispose the individual to develop PTSD following a traumatic event. One study of first responders in the September 11, 2001, attack in New York City suggested that those individuals who dissociated during or immediately following the event were those most prone to developing PTSD (Marmar et al., 2006). Dissociation includes symptoms of depersonalization, derealization, intrusive images and emotions, and other aspects of altered states of consciousness (Neria, DiGrande, & Adams, 2011; Simeon, Greenberg, Nelson, Schmeidler, & Hollander, 2005). There is much to learn to understand these developmental and acute impacts of trauma—but one implication of these findings suggests that prevention of abuse and neglect is vitally important. Because of the neuroplasticity of even the adult brain, ongoing experiences may be able to lead to integrative neural growth that can help overcome these developmental challenges to self-regulation with proper clinical intervention (see Doidge, 2007; Schore, 2003a, 2003b, 2012).

A review by Jovanovic and Ressler (2010) concluded that PTSD stems from the inability of clients to inhibit fear and is, in their view, an amygdala-related difficulty, possibly related in part to genetics, as well as to an experiential diathesis that may be closely related to trauma experienced during childhood. This theory is consistent with the idea that disorganized attachment underlies a propensity to develop PTSD: Impaired integration leads to difficulty in regulating the nervous system and adaptive social interactions. Studies of certain genetic variants affecting neurotransmitter metabolism (Bakermans-Kranenburg & van IJzendoorn, 2007; Bakermans-Kranenburg, van IJzendoorn, Pijlman, Mesman, & Juffer, 2008) suggest that the response to challenging childhood experience may be more intense with certain genetic alleles. Genetic or experientially derived challenges to neural integration may thus predispose an individual to develop impediments to self-regulation and to later develop PTSD. In addition, as reviewed earlier, the regulation of gene expression may be negatively affected by early experience as well. In these ways, epigenetic, genetic, and experiential factors may each contribute to the impact of trauma on the developing mind.

In the face of such experiential, genetic, and epigenetic components that may make a person vulnerable to a range of posttraumatic developmental impacts, how might mindfulness support the movement of an individual toward integration and healing?

How Might Mindfulness Relate to Integration?

Though a formal definition of mindfulness shared by all researchers and clinicians is not yet available (Bishop et al., 2004), for the purposes of this chapter, we use Jon Kabat-Zinn's (2012) description of mindfulness as "paying attention in a particular way; on purpose, in the present moment, and non-judgmentally" (p. 3). The clinical benefits of mindfulness include enhanced pain tolerance, increased flexibility, self-respect, relaxation, fear and arousal inhibition, and emotional clarity (Bishop, Shapiro, Carlson, Anderson, Carmody, et al., 2004; Masicampo & Baumeister, 2007; Fulton, 2005; Young, 1997; Walsh & Shapiro, 2006; Wallace, 2001). In this chapter we suggest that mental training that cultivates mindful awareness is a profoundly integrative intervention, increasing the activity and growth of neural structures that link widely separated brain areas to one another (see Luders et al., 2011; Kilpatrick et al., 2011).

What is it that can be differentiated and then linked within mindful awareness? Here is one possibility. Mindful awareness involves the capacity for an observing stream of energy and information flow to be open and receptive to an experiencing stream of such flow (Siegel, 2007a). Farb and colleagues have identified two neural circuits, a lateralized "experiencing" one and a more medial "observational" or witnessing circuit, that have been shown to become differentiated with mindfulness-based stress reduction (MBSR) training (Farb, Segal, Mayberg, Bean, McKeon, et al., 2007). One can interpret these findings as consistent with the proposal that mindful awareness training promotes the differentiation and then linkage of these fundamental processes in cultivating neural integration (Siegel, 2007b).

Another aspect of mindful awareness is that it involves the capacity to integrate consciousness. Awareness can be seen to entail two distinct components: the sense of "knowing" of consciousness and "that which is known," such as an object of observation—a thought, a feeling, a sensation from the body, or a perception of the outside world. Within mindful awareness, a differentiation is made between the knowing and the known, as well as distinguishing the many forms of the "known," such as enhancing the ability to stably perceive feelings, thoughts, and memories with curiosity, openness, acceptance, and positive regard.

Attention is the process that directs the flow of energy and information—within the brain, within our relationships, and within our mental experience of the subjective awareness. When traumatic experience occurs, especially early in life, it can not only alter the capacity to regulate attention but also can itself draw attention repeatedly to a variety of aspects of the traumatic past. In other words, developmental trauma may affect both the way information is processed in the mind and the content of what is being experienced within awareness.

Awareness is not the same as attention. As stated before, awareness can be defined as the sense of knowing, one that can also involve something that is known—such as a bodily sensation, an image from memory, or an emotion or thought. Mindful awareness can be conceptually understood in broad terms as empowering the mind to sense the impulse and object of attention and to then be able to modulate its path—to choose to focus or not on a memory, feeling, or thought.

In many ways, the layers of experience that become encoded in the brain by way of the pathway from implicit representations (perceptions, emotions, bodily sensations, behavioral impulses, priming, mental models) to the explicit forms of factual and autobiographical memory can be viewed as nonintegrated with trauma. This blockage of the integration of implicit memory into explicit forms and then into a coherent narrative that helps an individual to "make sense of his or her life" by connecting past, present, and future may be a core feature of how trauma continues to have a negative impact on that individual. Rather than being the active author of one's own unfolding story, developmental trauma, and perhaps traumatic experience in its broadest sense, pushes an individual toward being a passive recipient, a recorder of events that simply unfold. The experience of helplessness, hopelessness, shame, despair, and psychological paralysis would emerge in the face of this impaired memory and narrative integration. In the attachment research world, we see such outcomes in the form of unresolved trauma and grief, a form of incoherent narrative outcome that can be identified through the Adult Attachment Interview (see Hesse, 2008). A parent's lack of resolution is associated with his or her child's disorganized attachment and dissociation, and hence the cross-generational passage of impaired integration is perpetuated. A recent study by Amy DiNoble reveals a preliminary finding that an adult's secure attachment status is associated with the mindful traits of that adult (DiNoble, 2009).

Research on mindfulness training reveals what can be considered a neuro-signature of resilience, the "left shift" that supports the idea of a eudemonic state of well-being characterized by a sense of purpose, meaning, connection, and equanimity in the face of stressors (Urry et al., 2006). This movement toward, rather than away from, challenges may be a fundamental way in which mindfulness could be empirically shown to help those with PTSD. The left shift entails the left hemisphere's state of approach, which can be seen as the way the brain enables an individual to move toward challenges rather than withdrawing from them (as with the right-sided frontal activity dominance with withdrawal from stressors, or the "right shift"). Davidson, Kabat-Zinn, and colleagues' study also found a correlation between the left shift and the degree of immune response following a flu vaccine (Davidson et al., 2003).

Amishi Jha and colleagues (Jha, Krompinger, & Baime, 2007, 2009; Baijal, Jha, Kiyonaga, Singh, & Srinivasan, 2011) have also revealed how mindfulness supports improvements in fundamental mental processes that may also be of help in the treatment of trauma. Mindfulness training has been shown to improve the selective attention of working memory, to reduce mind wandering, to decrease ruminating, to produce a disidentification with inner experience, and to reduce self-related preoccupations (Jha et al., 2007; Lutz, Slagter, Dunne, & Davidson, 2008; Lutz et al., 2009; Brefczynski-Lewis, Lutz, Schaefer, Levinson, & Davidson, 2008; Ives-Deliperi, Solms, & Meintjes, 2011). Negative mind wandering has been correlated with unhappiness (Killingsworth & Gilbert, 2010)—and perhaps one way in which mindfulness creates a positive state of living is in cultivating the capacity for being present with life (Parker, Nelson, Epel, & Siegel, in press). In many ways, mindfulness training enables an individual to be present for an experience, to do one thing at a time, to be aware of what is happening as it unfolds, and to approach life's challenges by being present.

Mindfulness, Trauma Treatment, and Integration

Mindfulness training involves the focusing of attention in a mindful way—with curiosity, openness, acceptance, and kind regard—on what is happening as it is happening. With practice, presumably the neural firing that is engaged during that intentionally created state will activate gene expression and protein production in a way that will enhance neural firing and its differentiation and linkage, the outcome of which is the integration of an array of neural regions. Ideally, with regular practice, these intentionally created states will become automatic positive traits. Jha has suggested (2012, personal communication) that in her controlled studies, not yet published, a boundary level of about 12 minutes a day of practice has been revealed.

IPNB's definition of the mind as an embodied and relational process that regulates the flow of energy and information (Siegel, 2012a, 2012b) may help traumatized individuals turn toward mindfulness training for healing. This regulatory aspect of mind suggests that it "resides" within our bodies and within our relationships. Regulation entails both the monitoring and the modification of that which is to be regulated. What is being sensed and shaped? Energy and information flow. From an IPNB viewpoint, mindfulness stabilizes the ability to sense this flow, a flow that occurs both within and between us. Ultimately, mindfulness enables an individual to regulate—monitor and modify—energy and information flow in a way that helps him or her to be present in life in ways that enhance mental, relational, and physiological life (Parker et al., in press). Embedded in this experience of being present for whatever arises is also a way to embrace uncertainty, to be able to thrive in the face of ambiguity.

With developmental trauma, uncertainty has often been coupled with disconnection, terror, and an array of negative interpersonal and internal outcomes. Although these developmental foundations in trauma may make an individual prone to dysregulation of emotion, attention, relationships, and thinking to various degrees, mindfulness may provide an important mental training that directly addresses these forms of impaired regulation and brain integration. Any intervention powerful enough to cultivate significant change has the potential to, perhaps by necessity, disrupt the developmental adaptations to trauma that have been adopted to enable the individual to survive earlier challenges. In this way, mindfulness may evoke awareness of trauma that may flood the individual and create a disabling emotional state of arousal. Teaching self-regulatory tools, such as self-soothing and relaxation, can be an essential aspect of treatment to avoid incapacitating disruptions of function that may emerge from initial forays into mindful awareness training. Caution in the use of such an intervention is naturally advised. Ideally, this powerful form of development of the integrative functioning of the mind may provide important steps in overcoming developmental challenges.

Mindfulness has been shown to increase efficacious self-regulation, effective sleep, and sensitivity to heart rate and breathing and to decrease serum cortisol levels, dissociation and ruminating, and the likelihood of acquiring self-harmful behaviors (Lee, Zaharlick, & Akers, 2011). One perspective suggests that mindfulness may play a role, when taught and then carried forward in a person's life, in altering emotional reactivity and dysfunctional stress responses at the heart of PTSD (Taylor et al., 2011).

By creating a receptive, compassionate stance toward self-experience, by letting go of judgments and learning how to be present for what emerges, IPNB suggests that mindful awareness may enable a form of "internal attunement" to one's own inner subjective reality (Siegel, 2007a). Much like the interpersonal attunement of secure attachment (Siegel, 2012a), the outcomes of mindfulness training also involve the cultivation of many of the self-regulatory capacities that emerge from the integrative circuits of the brain itself. It is these very circuits of secure attachment (Schore, 2012) that have been shown to grow in long-term mindfulness meditators

(Luders et al., 2011; Lazar, Kerr, Wasserman, Gray, Greve, et al., 2005). IPNB views mindfulness as an effective means of cultivating integration in the mind, the brain, and the interpersonal relationships of the individual. This perspective reveals one possible means through which mindfulness may help in the treatment of individuals who have experienced developmental trauma.

A variety of possibly relevant findings related to mindfulness training support this notion. Luders et al. (2011) elucidated some of the positive benefits of daily meditation. Mindfulness meditators have been shown to have (1) thicker cortices; (2) a greater amount of brain tissue overall due to increases in surface area; (3) lower age-linked connective degeneration; and (4) increased gray matter density even after 8 weeks of training in MBSR. Kilpatrick's work has also shown that meditation positively effects brain connectivity and that it can be generalized to newer meditators over an 8-week MBSR workshop (Kilpatrick et al., 2011; Hölzel et al., 2011).

The positive results of such interventions may rest in the basic ways in which mindfulness enhances self-regulation of emotion, attention, and impulse control. This concept has found support in studies suggesting increases in limbic and cortical connectivity and an increase in white matter and volume with mindfulness training (Ivanovski & Malhi, 2007). The focus of mindfulness practice on awareness and acceptance of one's bodily and emotional state, as well as on regulating physiological arousal, makes it a conceptually promising treatment for trauma. Because outcomes of traumatic experiences include dissociation, avoidance, numbing, and flashbacks, an effective treatment may work by calming arousal and helping individuals safely approach the challenges of the emotional horror, interpersonal betrayal, and inner chaos inherent in developmental trauma. As mindfulness makes the left shift of moving toward such challenges a trainable neural propensity and fosters integration within the nervous system and within interpersonal relationships, carefully offering mindfulness training to individuals with developmental trauma is a natural application for this important approach to cultivating well-being.

References

American Psychiatric Association. (2013). *Diagnostic and statistical manual of mental disorders* (5th ed.). Arlington, VA: Author.

Baijal S., Jha, A. P., Kiyonaga, A., Singh, R., & Srinivasan, N. (2011). The influence of concentrative meditation training on the development of attention networks during early adolescence. *Frontiers of Psychology, 2*, 153.

Bakermans-Kranenburg, M. J., & van IJzendoorn, M. H. (2007). Genetic vulnerability or differential susceptibility in child development: The case of attachment. *Journal of Child Psychology and Psychiatry, 48*(12), 1160–1173.

Bakermans-Kranenburg, M. J., van IJzendoorn, M. H., Pijlman, F. T. A., Mesman, J., & Juffer, F. (2008). Experimental evidence for differential susceptibility:

Dopamine D4 receptor polymorphism (DRD4 VNTR) moderates intervention effects on toddlers' externalizing behavior in a randomized controlled trial. *Developmental Psychology*, 44(1), 293–300.

Beebee, B., Jaffe, J., Markese, S., Buck, K., Chen, H., Cohen, P., et al. (2010). The origins of 12-month attachment: A microanalysis of 4-month mother–infant interaction. *Attachment and Human Development*, 12, 3–141.

Bishop, S. R., Shapiro, S., Carlson, L., Anderson, N. D., Carmody, J., Segal, Z. V., et al. (2004). Mindfulness: A proposed operational definition. *Clinical Psychology*, 11, 230–241.

Bluhm, R. L., Williamson, P. C., Osuch, E. A., Frewen, P. A., Stevens, T. K., Boksman, K., et al. (2009). Alterations in default network connectivity in posttraumatic stress disorder related to early-life trauma. *Journal of Psychiatry and Neuroscience*, 34(3), 187–194.

Brefczynski-Lewis, J. A., Lutz, A., Schaefer, H. S., Levinson, D. B., & Davidson, R. J. (2007). Neural correlates of attentional expertise in long-term meditation practitioners. *Proceedings of the National Academy of Sciences of the USA*, 104, 11483–11488.

Bremner, J. D., Elzinga, B., Schmahl, C., & Vermetten, E. (2008). Structural and functional plasticity of the human brain in posttraumatic stress disorder. *Progressive Brain Research*, 167(1), 171–186.

Brewer, J. A., Worhunsky, P. D., Gray, J. R., Tang, Y.-Y., Weber, J., & Kober, H. (2011). Meditation experience is associated with differences in default mode network activity and connectivity. *Proceedings of the National Academy of Sciences of the USA*, 108(20), 20254–20259.

Choi, J., Joeng, B., Rohan, M. L., Polcari, A. M., & Teicher, M. H. (2009). Preliminary evidence for white matter tract abnormalities in young adults exposed to parental verbal abuse. *Biological Psychiatry*, 65(3), 227–234.

Cozolino, L. (2011). *The neuroscience of relationships*. New York: Norton.

Davidson, R. J., Kabat-Zinn, J., Schumacher, J., Rosenkranz, M., Muller, D., & Santorelli, S. F. (2003). Alterations in brain and immune function produced by mindfulness meditation, *Psychosomatic Medicine*, 65(4), 564–570.

Davis, D. M., & Hayes, J. A. (2011). What are the benefits of mindfulness?: A practice review of psychotherapy-related research. *Psychotherapy*, 48(2), 198–208.

De Bellis, M. D., Keshevan, M. S., Shifflett, H., Iyengar, S., Beers, S. R., Hall, J., et al. (2002). Brain structures in pediatric maltreatment-related posttraumatic stress disorder: A sociodemographically matched study. *Biological Psychiatry*, 52(11), 1066–1078.

DiNoble, A. (2009). *Examining the relationship between adult attachment style and mindfulness traits*. Unpublished doctoral dissertation, California Graduate Institute of the Chicago School of Professional Psychology, Chicago.

Doidge, N. (2007). *The brain that changes itself* (2nd ed.). Denver, CO: Penguin.

Dutra, L., Ilaria, B., Siegel, D. J., & Lyons-Ruth, K. (2009). The relational context of dissociative phenomena. In P. F. Dell & J. A. O'Neil (Eds.), *Dissociation and the dissociative disorders, DSM-V and beyond* (pp. 83–92). New York: Routledge.

Epel, E. S., Lin, J., Dhabhar, F. S., Wolkowitz, O. M., Puterman, E., Karan, L., et al. (2010). Dynamics of telomerase activity in response to acute psychological stress. *Brain, Behavior, and Immunity*, 24(4), 531–539.

Farb, N. A. S., Segal, Z. V., Mayberg, H., Bean, J., McKeon, D., Fatima, Z., et al. (2007). Attending to the present: Mindfulness meditation reveals distinct neural modes of self-reference. *Social, Cognitive, and Affective Neuroscience, 2*(4), 313–322.

Fulton, P. R. (2005). Mindfulness as clinical training. In C. K. Germer, R. D. Siegel, & P. R. Fulton (Eds.), *Mindfulness and psychotherapy* (pp. 55–72). New York: Guilford Press.

Galea, S., Resnick, H., Ahern, J., Gold, J., Kilpatrick, D., Stuber, J., et al. (2002). Posttraumatic stress disorder in Manhattan, New York City, after the September 11th terrorist attacks. *Journal of Urban Health, 79*(3), 340–353.

Gusnard, D. A., Akbudak, E., Shulman, G. L., & Raichle, M. E. (2001). Medial prefrontal cortex and self-referential mental activity: Relation to a default mode of brain function. *Proceedings of the National Academy of Sciences of the USA, 98,* 4259–4264.

Hesse, E. (2008). The Adult Attachment Interview: Protocol, method of analysis, and empirical studies. In J. Cassidy & P. R. Shaver (Eds.), *Handbook of attachment: Theory, research, and clinical applications* (2nd ed., pp. 552–598). New York: Guilford Press.

Hölzel, B. K., Carmody, J., Vangel, M., Congleton, C., Yerramsetti, S. M., Gard, T., et al. (2011). Mindfulness practice leads to increases in regional brain gray matter density. *Psychiatry Research: Neuroimaging, 191*(1), 36–43.

Ivanovski, B., & Malhi, G. S. (2007). The psychological and neurophysiological concomitants of mindfulness forms of meditation. *Acta Neuropsychiatrica, 19*(2), 76–91.

Ives-Deliperi, V. L., Solms, M., & Meintjes, E. M. (2011). The neural substrates of mindfulness: An fMRI investigation. *Social Neuroscience, 6*(3), 231–242.

Jha, A. P., Krompinger, J., & Baime, M. J. (2007). Mindfulness training modifies subsystems of attention. *Cognitive, Affective, and Behavioral Neuroscience, 7*(2), 109–119.

Jovanovic, T., & Ressler, K. J. (2010). How the neurocircuitry and genetics of fear inhibition may inform our understanding of PTSD. *American Journal of Psychiatry, 167*(6), 648–662.

Kabat-Zinn, J. (2012). *Mindfulness for beginners: Reclaiming the present moment—and your life.* Boulder, CO: Sounds True.

Killingsworth, M. A., & Gilbert, D. T. (2010). A wandering mind is an unhappy mind. *Science, 330,* 932.

Kilpatrick, L. A., Suyenobu, B. Y., Smith, S. R., Bueller, J. A., Goodman, T., Creswell, J. D., et al. (2011). Impact of mindfulness-based stress reduction training on intrinsic brain connectivity. *NeuroImage, 56*(1), 290–298.

Kohls, N., Sauer, S., Offenbächer, M., & Giordano, J. (2011). Spirituality: An overlooked predictor of placebo effects? *Philosophical Transactions of the Royal Society of Biological Sciences, 366*(1572), 1838–1848.

Kroes, M. C., Rugg, M. D., Whalley, M. G., & Brewin, C. R. (2011). Structural brain abnormalities common to posttraumatic stress disorder and depression. *Journal of Psychiatry and Neuroscience, 36*(4), 256–265.

Kroes, M. C., Whalley, M. G., Rugg, M. D., & Brewin, C. R. (2011). Association between flashbacks and structural brain abnormalities in posttraumatic stress disorder. *Journal of the Association of European Psychiatrists, 26*(8), 525–531.

Krystal, J. H., & Neumeister, A. (2009). Noradrenergic and serotonergic mechanisms in the neurobiology of posttraumatic stress disorder and resilience. *Brain Research, 1293*(1), 13–23.

Lanius, R. A., Bluhm, R. L., & Frewen, P. A. (2011). How understanding the neurobiology of complex post-traumatic stress disorder can inform clinical practice: A social cognitive and affective neuroscience approach. *Acta Psychiatrica Scandinavica, 124*(5), 331–348.

Lazar, S. W., Kerr, C. E., Wasserman, R. H., Gray, J. R., Greve, D. N., & Treadway, M. T. (2005). Meditation experience is associated with increased cortical thickness. *NeuroReport, 16*, 1893–1897.

Lee, M., Zaharlick, A., & Akers, D. (2011). Meditation and treatment of female trauma survivors of interpersonal abuses: Utilizing clients' strengths. *Families in Society, 92*(1), 41–49.

Liberzon, I., Taylor, S. F., Amdur, R., Jung, T. D., Chamberlain, K. R., Minoshima, S., et al. (1999). Brain activation in PTSD in response to trauma-related stimuli. *Biological Psychiatry, 45*(7), 817–826.

Luders, E., Clark, K., Narr, K. L., & Toga, A. W. (2011). Enhanced brain connectivity in long-term meditation practitioners. *NeuroImage, 57*(4), 1308–1316.

Luders, E., Toga, A. W., Lepore, N., & Gaser, C. (2009). The underlying anatomical correlates of long-term meditation: Larger hippocampal and frontal volumes of gray matter. *NeuroImage, 45*, 672–678.

Lutz, A., Slagter, H. A., Dunne, J. D., & Davidson, R. J. (2008). Attention regulation and monitoring in meditation. *Trends in Cognitive Sciences, 12*(4), 163–169.

Lutz, A., Slagter, H. A., Rawlings, N. B., Francis, A. D., Greischar, L. L., & Davidson, R. J. (2009). Mental training enhances attentional stability: Neural and behavioral evidence. *Journal of Neuroscience, 29*, 13418–13427.

Lyons-Ruth, K. (2004). *The relational context of trauma: Fear, dissociation, and the early caregiving environment.* Paper presented at the Conference on Attachment, University of California at Los Angeles.

Main, M., & Hesse, E. D. (1990). Parents' unresolved traumatic experiences are related to infant disorganized attachment status: Is frightened and/or frightening parental behavior the linking mechanism? In M. Greenberg, D. Cicchetti, & M. Cummings (Eds.), *Attachment in the preschool years* (pp. 161–184). Chicago: University of Chicago Press.

Marmar, C. R., McCaslin, S. E., Metzler, T. J., Best, S., Weiss, D. S., Fagan, F., et al. (2006). Predictors of posttraumatic stress in police and other first responders *Annals of the New York Academy of Sciences, 1071*, 1–18.

Masicampo, E. J., & Baumeister, R. F. (2007). Relating mindfulness and self-regulatory processes. *Psychological Inquiry, 18*, 255–258.

McGowan, P. O., Sasaki, A., D'Alessio, A. C., Dymov, S., Labonté, B., Szyf, M., et al. (2009). Epigenetic regulation of hippocampal glucocorticoid receptor gene expression associates with childhood abuse in human suicide victims. *Nature Neuroscience, 12*(3), 342–348.

Meaney, M. J., Szyf, M., & Seckl, J. R. (2007). Epigenetic mechanisms of perinatal programming of hypothalamic–pituitary–adrenal function and health. *Trends in Molecular Medicine, 13*(7), 269–277.

Moore, A., & Malinowski, P. (2009). Meditation, mindfulness and cognitive flexibility. *Consciousness and Cognition, 18*(1), 176–186.

Neria, Y., DiGrande, L., & Adams, B. G. (2011). Posttraumatic stress disorder following the September 11, 2001, terrorist attacks: A review of the literature among highly exposed populations. *American Psychologist, 66*(6), 429–446.

Northoff, G., Heinzel, A., de Greck, M., Bermopohl, F., Dobrowolny, H., & Panksepp, J. (2006) Self-referential processing in our brain: A meta-analysis of imaging studies on the self. *NeuroImage, 31*, 440–457.

Osuch, E., & Engel, C. C., Jr. (2004). Research on the treatment of trauma spectrum responses: The role of the optimal healing environment and neurobiology. *Journal of Alternative and Complementary Medicine, 10*(Suppl. 1), S211–S221.

Parker, S. C., Nelson, B. W., Epel, E., & Siegel, D. J. (in press). The science of presence: A central mediator in the interpersonal benefits of mindfulness. In K. W. Brown, J. D. Creswell, & R. M. Ryan (Eds.), *Handbook of mindfulness: Theory and research*. New York: Springer.

Price, C. J., McBride, B., Hyerle, L., & Kivlahan, D. R. (2007). Mindful awareness in body-oriented therapy for female veterans with post-traumatic stress disorder taking prescription analgesics for chronic pain: A feasibility study. *Alternative Therapies in Health and Medicine, 13*(6), 32–40.

Ravindran, L. N., & Stein, M. B. (2009). Pharmacotherapy of PTSD: Premises, principles, and priorities. *Brain Research, 1293*(1), 24–39.

Schore, A. N. (2001). Effects of a secure attachment relationship on right brain development, affect regulation, and infant mental health. *Infant Mental Health Journal, 22*, 7–66.

Schore, A. N. (2003). *Affect regulation and the disruption of the self*. New York: Norton.

Schore, A. N. (2012). *The science of the art of psychotherapy*. New York: Norton.

Siegel, D. J. (2007a). *The mindful brain: Reflection and attunement in the cultivation of well-being*. New York: Norton.

Siegel, D. J. (2007b). Mindfulness training and neural integration: Differentiation of distinct streams of awareness and the cultivation of well-being. *Journal of Social, Cognitive, and Affective Neuroscience, 2*(4), 259–263.

Siegel, D. J. (2010a). *Mindsight: The new science of personal transformation*. New York: Bantam.

Siegel, D. J. (2010b). *The mindful therapist: A clinician's guide to mindsight and neural integration*. New York: Norton.

Siegel, D. J. (2012a). *The developing mind: How relationships and the brain interact to shape who we are* (2nd ed.). New York: Guilford Press.

Siegel, D. J. (2012b). *Pocket guide to interpersonal neurobiology: An integrative handbook of the mind*. New York: Norton.

Simeon, D., Greenberg, J., Nelson, D., Schmeidler, J., & Hollander, E. (2005). Dissociation and posttraumatic stress 1 year after the World Trade Center disaster: Follow-up of a longitudinal survey. *Journal of Clinical Psychiatry, 66*(2), 231–237.

Sobolewski, A., Holt, E., Kublik, E., & Wróbel, A. (2011). Impact of meditation on emotional processing: A visual ERP study. *Neuroscience Research, 71*(1), 44–48.

Sroufe, L. A., Egeland, B., Carlson, E. A., & Collins, W. A. (2005). *The development of the person: The Minnesota Study of Risk and Adaptation from Birth to Adulthood.* New York: Guilford Press.

Sroufe, L. A., & Siegel, D. J. (2011, March–April). The verdict is in: The case for attachment theory. *Psychotherapy Networker.* Available at *www.psychother-apynetworker.org/magazine/recentissues/1271-the-verdict-is-in.*

Tang, Y.-Y., Lu, Q., Xiujuan, G., Stein, E. A., Yang, Y., & Posner, M. I. (2010). Short-term meditation induces white matter changes in the anterior cingulate. *Proceedings of the National Academy of Sciences of the USA, 107,* 15649–15652.

Taylor, V. A., Grant, J., Daneault, V., Scavone, G., Breton, E., Roffe-Vidal, S., et al. (2011). Impact of mindfulness on the neural responses to emotional pictures in experienced and beginner meditators. *NeuroImage, 57*(5), 1524–1533.

Tronick, E. (2004). Why is connection with others so critical?: Dyadic meaning making, messiness and complexity governed selective processes which co-create and expand individuals' states of consciousness. In J. Nadel & D. Muir (Eds.), *Emotional development* (pp. 86–111). New York: Norton.

Uddin, L. Q., Kelly, A. M., Biswal, B. B., Castellanos, F. X., & Milham, M. P. (2009) Functional connectivity of default mode network components: Correlation, anticorrelation, and causality. *Human Brain Mapping, 30,* 625–637.

Urry, H. L., van Reekum, C. M., Johnstone, T., Kalin, N. H., Thurow, M. E., Schaefer, H. S., et al. (2006). Amygdala and ventromedial prefrontal cortex are inversely coupled during regulation of negative affect and predict the diurnal pattern of cortisol secretion among older adults. *Journal of Neuroscience, 26*(16), 4415–4425.

van den Hout, M. A., Engelhard, I. M., Beetsma, D., Slofstra, C., Hornsveld, H., Voutveen, J., et al. (2011). EMDR and mindfulness: Eye movements and attentional breathing tax working memory and reduce vividness and emotionality of aversive ideation. *Journal of Behavior Therapy and Experimental Psychiatry, 42*(4), 423–431.

van der Kolk, B. A. (2006). Clinical implications of neuroscience research in PTSD. *Annals of the New York Academy of Sciences, 1071,* 277–293.

Vasile, D., & Vasiliu, O.(2010). *Matching psychotropics to neurobiological mechanisms in the aftermath of a traumatic event: A literature review.* Proceedings of the World Medical Conference.

Vermetten, E., & Bremner, J. D. (2002). Circuits and systems in stress: II. Applications to neurobiology and treatment in posttraumatic stress disorder. *Depression and Anxiety, 16*(1), 14–38.

Vujanovic, A. A., Niles, B., Pietresfesa, A., Schmertz, S. K., & Potter, C. M. (2011). Mindfulness in the treatment of posttraumatic stress disorder among military veterans. *Professional Psychology: Research and Practice, 42*(1), 24–31.

Waelde, L. C., Uddo, M., Marquett, R., Ropelato, M., Freightman, S., Pardo, A., et al. (2009). A pilot study of meditation for mental health workers following Hurricane Katrina. *Journal of Traumatic Stress, 21*(5), 497–500.

Wang, F., Kalmar, J. H., Edmiston, E., Chepenick, L. G., Bhagwagar, Z., Spencer, L., et al. (2008). Abnormal corpus callosum integrity in bipolar disorder: A diffusion tensor imaging study. *Biological Psychiatry, 64*(8), 730–733.

Wilson, E. O. (1998). *Consilience: The unity of knowledge.* New York: Vintage Press

Yehuda, R. (2003). Clinical relevance of biologic findings in PTSD. *Psychiatric Quarterly, 73*(2), 123–133.

Zylowska, L., Ackerman, D. L., Yang, M. H., Futrell, J. L., Horton, N. L., Hale, T. S., et al. (2008). Mindfulness meditation training in adults and adolescents with ADHD: A feasibility study. *Journal of Attention Disorders, 11,* 737–746.

Embedded Relational Mindfulness

A Sensorimotor Psychotherapy Perspective on the Treatment of Trauma

Pat Ogden

Trauma, particularly early attachment trauma, strongly influences unconscious processes that underlie explicit content in the therapy hour. Trauma-related implicit processes—visibly reflected in nonverbal behaviors of gesture, posture, prosody, facial expressions, eye gaze, and affect—persist in spite of attempts to regulate them with top-down executive control. Clients often feel at the mercy of an overwhelming cascade of dysregulated emotions, upsetting physical sensations, intrusive images, pain, smells, constriction, and numbing. These in turn influence cognitive distortions such as "I am damaged," "I am a bad person," or "I cannot protect myself."

These trauma-related unconscious processes speak to the dominance of what Schore (2009) calls the nonverbal, affective, and bodily-based "implicit self" over the verbal, linguistic "explicit self." A therapist's exclusive reliance on the "talking cure" to resolve symptoms of trauma and address implicit processing dynamics can limit clinical efficacy, because forming a coherent verbal narrative of past trauma is typically problematic. Traumatic memories are often not explicitly encoded. Instead, the past is "remembered as a series of *unconscious expectations*" (Cortina & Liotti, 2007, p. 205, emphasis added), which are all the more potent precisely because memories of the events that shaped them are not available for reflection and revision. Memories may be dissociated—split off from conscious awareness—and many survivors "remember" only isolated affective, sensory, or motor aspects of traumatic experience. During trauma, functioning of the prefrontal cortex or "executive brain," responsible for clear thinking and decision making, and of the hippocampus, involved in the consolidation of emotional and verbal memory, is selectively impaired and enhanced in ways that increase emotional processes and their encoding while decreasing conceptual processes and their encoding (Arnsten 2009; Schwabe, Joels, Roozendaal, Wolf, & Oitzl, 2012). Attempting to describe the processes that precipitate implicit "remembering" only leads to failure and frustration, or, worse, to reliving.

The primary raw ingredients of therapeutic change lie not in what is explicitly spoken but in the constantly changing experiential context that remains generally unsymbolized in ordinary verbal exchange (Bromberg, 2010). A paradigm shift is indicated that privileges mindful awareness of the moment-by-moment *experience* of implicit patterns over formulating a cohesive narrative, engaging in conversation, or "talking about" (Kurtz, 1990; Ogden & Minton, 2000; Ogden, Minton, & Pain, 2006). This chapter offers a practical overview of a clinical map for using mindfulness embedded within what transpires between therapist and client and delineates interventions from sensorimotor psychotherapy (Ogden et al., 2006) that directly address the in-the-moment experience of implicit processes.

What Is "Mindfulness"?

Definitions of mindfulness vary. Williams and colleagues (Williams, Teasdale, Segal, & Kabat-Zinn, 2007) describe it as "the awareness that emerges through paying attention on purpose, in the present moment, and non-judgmentally to things as they are," a perspective that takes into account internal experience, as well as "those aspects of life that we most take for granted or ignore" (p. 47). Included in most descriptions is an attitude of openness and receptivity to whatever arises, as a "quality of attention which notices without choosing, without preference" (Goldstein & Kornfield, 1987, p. 19). Many mindfulness practices encourage such unrestricted receptivity, whereas others, described as "concentration practices," promote focusing attention upon particular elements of either internal experience (such as the breath, body sensation, or mantra) or the external environment (such as a candle flame). Several psychotherapeutic methods have been developed that teach mindfulness through structured exercises, practices, and sets of skills. In Linehan's (1993) model, for example, clients are taught mindfulness "what" skills of observing, describing, and participating, as well as "how" skills of focusing on one thing at a time and being effective.

Kurtz (2004), building on Buddhist perspectives, describes the essence of mindfulness:

to be fully present to our [internal] experience, whatever it is: our thoughts, images, memories, breath, body sensations, the sounds and smells and tastes, moods and feelings and the quality of our whole experience as well as of the various parts. Mindfulness is not our notions about our experience, but even noticing the notions. (p. 39)

Sensorimotor Psychotherapy, influenced by Kurtz, employs a specific clinical "map" and a set of therapeutic skills for the purpose of inquiring into the direct moment-by-moment internal experience of the effects of trauma. Mindfulness is not taught through structured exercises or practices but is integrated with and embedded within what transpires moment-to-moment between therapist and client.

A Map for the Use of Mindfulness in Clinical Practice

In Sensorimotor Psychotherapy, the clinician maintains a dual focus: One is following the client's narrative or "story." The other, more important focus is tracking the five "building blocks" of present-moment internal experience—emotions, thoughts, five-sense perception, movements, and body sensations—that emerge spontaneously in the therapy hour and become the focal points of mindful exploration and transformation (cf. Ogden et al., 2006). These building blocks are elaborated in Figure 14.1. Reflecting implicit processes, these five elements comprise the present-moment internal experience of every waking moment—at least potential internal experience, as they often occur outside of awareness. They change in response to themselves, with internal thoughts affecting emotions, which in turn associatively evoke internal perceptions, and so on. They also change in response to external stimuli. The building blocks are dramatically affected by both internal and external traumatic reminders that bring the past abruptly into the experiential present. When triggered by such reminders, clients report disturbing body sensations, movements, intrusive images, smells or sounds, fear, shame, panic or rage, and thoughts—all of which can spin out of control—even while realizing cognitively that these reactions do not match current reality. As one client put it, "I know I'm safe, but my body is running amok. I shake, I panic, I see my father's face, and I feel like I will die."

Rather than conversation, the focus of therapy becomes *the spontaneous fluctuations of these five elements.* The therapist is on the lookout for specific building blocks that point to implicit processes that reflect unresolved trauma, as well as those that reflect self-regulatory resources, positive affect, competency, and mastery. Together, therapist and client interrupt the automaticity of these building blocks by becoming mindful of them. In this way, the client can identify and observe, rather than identify

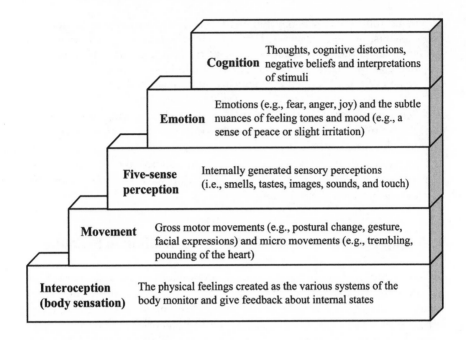

FIGURE 14.1. Five "building blocks" of moment-by-moment here-and-now internal experience. Illustration by Anne Westcott.

with, the effects of the past trauma, and discover more adaptive actions (cf., Ogden et al., 2006).

Mindfulness is "motivated by curiosity" (Kurtz, 1990, p. 111), and thus "allow[s]' difficult thoughts and feelings [and images, body sensations and movements] simply to be there . . . to adopt toward them a more 'welcome' than a 'need to solve' stance" (Segal, Teasdale, & Williams, 2002, p. 55). The therapist, by example and encouragement, helps the client cultivate an attitude of curiosity, neutrality, and receptivity toward internal experience. However, unrestricted mindfulness toward any and all of the five building blocks can be disturbing and overwhelming to people with posttraumatic stress disorder (PTSD) and thus is often met with dismay, judgment, self-criticism, and further dysregulation. To help prevent this, a sensorimotor psychotherapy approach employs mindfulness in very specific way, termed "directed mindfulness," which entails carefully and firmly directing the client's mindful attention toward one or more of the five building blocks considered important to therapeutic goals (Ogden, 2007, 2009). For example, if an internal image of past trauma or an external traumatic reminder, such as the sound of a siren, causes hyperarousal, a therapist might direct a client to become mindful of the sensation in his or her legs to promote grounding, rather than to the internally generated image, because grounding supports the goal of stabilization.

Safety, Danger, and Mindfulness in the Therapeutic Relationship

Critically, mindfulness in sensorimotor psychotherapy is not a solitary activity but is firmly embedded in what occurs within the therapeutic dyad. It is imperative that mindfulness is employed in a way that increases clients' experience of relational safety and fosters their ability to connect to and engage with the therapist. However, maintaining the moment-by-moment therapeutic alliance is precarious, because both external reminders of the trauma and recurring internal images, thoughts, emotions, and sensations are implicitly triggering, which elicits primitive defenses and dysregulated arousal. If danger is (implicitly or explicitly) detected, this produces either mobilization behaviors (fight–flight), accompanied by hyperarousal and tense muscles that prepare for defensive fight-or-flight behaviors, or immobilization behaviors accompanied by hypoarousal, shut down or "feigned death," and a loss of muscular tension. Social behaviors can continue only if these defenses can be inhibited sufficiently so that clients can experience some degree of relational safety.

Porges (2004, 2011) introduced the term *neuroception,* to be distinguished from *perception,* in order to emphasize the brain's automatic detection of environmental features that are safe, dangerous, and life threatening. This detection is usually implicit and strongly affects physiological state to produce social, active defensive, or shutdown behaviors. When safety is neurocepted, levels of autonomic arousal fluctuate within a "window of tolerance" (Siegel, 1999) in which behaviors typical of engagement with others can take place. In therapy, clients must automatically detect or neurocept some degree of safety in order to remain engaged with the therapist; otherwise, therapy cannot take place. However, as stated, clients with trauma are often unable, based on prior conditioning, to detect accurately whether the environment is safe or another person is trustworthy. This difficulty is exacerbated in therapy when traumatic material is deliberately stimulated, which it must be in order to resolve the past. The therapist intends to bring clients' experience of the past into the therapy hour, but this can cause the client to implicitly neurocept danger, which activates the brain's fear circuitry, stimulates the sympathetic nervous system, and mobilizes fight–flight–shutdown defenses.

It is important to note that the client's neuroception of the environment as safe or dangerous occurs implicitly, triggering defensive or social behaviors usually without any conscious awareness. As Porges (2011, p. 11) states, "Even though we may not be aware of danger on a cognitive level, on a neurophysiological level, our body has already started a sequence of neural processes that would facilitate adaptive defense behaviors such as fight, flight, or [shut down]." Clients and therapists alike are often baffled by the client's unexpected change from social to defensive behaviors. The stimulus that provoked the change is typically not conscious for either party.

Therapists must pay exquisite attention to the nonverbal signals that suggest state changes from regulated arousal (the client's neuroception of safety) to dysregulated arousal and defensive responses (the client's neuroception of danger and life threat) and take steps to help clients inhibit defensive systems enough so that their social engagement can continue or return. Taking place within an attuned dyad, mindfulness must be used not only to activate clients' experience of trauma and dysregulated arousal but also to *ensure that their social engagement is intact.* In other words, the client must detect safety and danger simultaneously. Detecting only safety would preclude addressing past trauma, and detecting only danger would lead to reliving the trauma. The simultaneous evocation of both implicit trauma-related dysregulating processes and safe social engagement can result in a depth of intersubjectivity and connectedness that exceeds that which ensues from conversation alone. However, for this to occur, a specific set of relational mindfulness interventions must be privileged over ordinary conversation, discussion, or "talking about" (Kurtz, 1990; Ogden et al., 2006) and over solitary mindfulness exercises or practices.

Directed Mindfulness Therapeutic Skills and Embedded Relational Mindfulness

In sensorimotor psychotherapy, therapists closely and unobtrusively "track" the client's unfolding experience of body sensations, movements, five-sense perceptions, emotions, and thoughts in response to particular stimuli, such as a description of past trauma or current difficulty. The therapist is on the lookout for changes in sensation (such as flushing or blanching), shifts in movement (posture or gesture), internally generated perceptions (reports of images, smells, tastes, sounds), emerging emotions (moist eyes, facial expression, or prosody), or beliefs and cognitive distortions that emerge from the client's narrative. In addition, connections among the building blocks are noted; for example, the thought "It's my fault," expressed as the client reports the image of her mother's unwelcoming face when she turned to her for comfort, emerges as her posture slumps, her face blanches, and her expression reflects sadness.

These tracked elements of present-moment experience typically remain unnoticed by the client until the therapist brings attention to them, through a "contact statement" that describes what has been noticed, such as, "As you see your mother's face, your posture slumps," or "You seem to feel hopeless right now." Therapists of all persuasions are skillful at reflective statements that convey their understanding of the narrative ("That must have been so painful for you"; "You were devastated by that experience"). Although it is important for the client to know that the therapist is following the narrative details, it is essential to contact present-moment experience in order to facilitate mindfulness. If therapists only verbalize their understanding of the narrative, clients will assume that the narrative, rather than present-moment experience, is of the greatest import, influencing them to continue the conversation. Contacting present experience repeatedly shifts the client's attention "to the various things going on outside of the flow of conversation, to experiences" (Kurtz, 2004, p. 40) that can then be further explored through mindful awareness.

Contact statements should convey empathic understanding of the client's present experience (Kurtz, 1990; Ogden et al., 2006). Thus it is not only the words therapists say but also their nonverbal body language, affect, and prosody that modulate clients' fear circuitry and stimulate the systems underlying experiences of safety and social engagement. These contact statements emerge from the clinician's own implicit processing as "the therapist resonates with the patient's internal state of arousal dysregulation, modulates it, communicates it back prosodically in a more regulated form, and then verbally labels his/her states experiences" (Schore, 2003, p. 30). Such resonance followed by "labeling" or naming allows clients to contact here-and-now experience and paves the way for mindful exploration of that experience.

The therapist and client collaborate to determine what to explore through mindful attention. This decision constitutes a commitment to a certain direction for the session in general—whether to start by exploring the present-moment effects of trauma, such as an intrusive image, cognitive distortion, or physical constriction, or instead something that points to resources, such as relaxation, a sense of joy, a "positive" cognition, or a peaceful image. The therapist may have tracked and contacted shifts in experience as the client talks about a memory ("It seems your shoulders and arms start to tighten when you talk about this memory") and may suggest, "Let's find out more about the tightening that emerges when you think about the memory." If the client agrees, the tension becomes the stimulus for mindful study.

Only after tracking, contacting, and deciding to explore an element of present experience does the therapist ask directed mindfulness questions that require awareness of present-moment experience. If the tension in the shoulders and arms is chosen, the induction to mindfulness might be, "As you sense that tension, what can you learn about it—how is it pulling? Is it the same in both shoulders and arms?" If the thought "I know I'm OK" is chosen, the induction to mindfulness might be a questions such as, "Stay with that thought, 'I know I'm OK.' Repeat the words in your mind, and notice what happens. What images, body sensations, or emotions come up by themselves?" Note that mindfulness is directed so that clients become aware of the spontaneous emergence of the building blocks in response to a particular stimulus (the tension or the thought).

Case Example

Sensorimotor Psychotherapy is conducted within a phase-oriented treatment approach, identified by Janet (1898) as comprising three phases: symptom reduction and stabilization; treatment of traumatic memory; and personality integration and rehabilitation. Excerpts from Suzi's treatment will illustrate how the clinical map and therapeutic skills for mindfulness are utilized at each phase of treatment. Suzi, sexually abused as a child and currently 27 years old, began treatment reporting that she lived in fear, with frequent escalation in heart rate and a constant sense of impending danger.

Early in treatment, as Suzi discussed her history, I tracked her shallow breathing, the fear in her widened eyes, the vivid image of her father's contorted face, and the thread of a cognitive distortion heard in the words she chose and her prosody ("I never should have been born," said in a self-deprecating, hopeless manner). Naming specific elements of Suzi's present experience ("You don't seem to be breathing fully") was followed by Suzi's report that she felt numb, especially in her legs. I collaborated with her in deciding to focus on the numb sensation in the hope that she could "ground" herself and bring her arousal into a window of tolerance. Thus numbness became the stimulus for directed mindful exploration: "What happens when you sense that numb feeling? Can you describe that sensation of numbness? Do you feel it equally in both legs?" Note the difference between these questions and nondirective general mindfulness question, such as "What do you notice right now?" In sensorimotor psychotherapy, mindfulness includes the client's labeling of internal experience using language, which engages the prefrontal cortex (Siegel, 2007).

As Suzi described the numbness, she noticed an achy pressure—a feeling that changed to "energized" as she experimented, at my suggestion, with pressing her feet into the floor, an action intended to facilitate grounding (Ogden et al., 2006). This action became the second stimulus for mindful study, as I asked Suzi to notice what occurred as she did it. She took a deep breath, then said she felt less fearful and that she could "be here." Her arousal returned to within a window of tolerance, in accord with the "stabilization" goal of Phase 1 of trauma treatment. Outside of therapy, to help her regulate her arousal, Suzi practiced pushing her feet into the floor over and over.

In Phase 2 of treatment, Suzi discovered her forgotten, dormant defensive impulse to protect herself. As she remembered how she became frozen and did not resist her father's sexual advances, the building block I contacted was the tension of her arms, saying, "It looks like your arms are tensing up as you talk of your father." I selected the tension because I hypothesized that the tension was a preparatory movement of pushing away—an instinctual defensive response that Suzi had unconsciously refrained from executing at the time of the trauma when active resistance would have only made her father angry. Suzi was not aware of the tension until I named it. Together, we decided that it would be the stimulus to study in mindfulness. To illustrate the use of mindfulness of a stimulus, Kurtz (2004) used the metaphor of tossing a pebble in a pond and watching the ripples. The quieter the pond is, the more the ripples are visible. I asked Suzi to take her time to gently become aware of the tension and asked, "What happens when you sense this tension? Is the tension in both arms equally? How is it pulling?" This was a turning point in the session, because the focus shifted from conversation about her abuse to mindful study of a specific here-and-now manifestation of her body's response to the abuse while talking about it—the tension. This "telling" elicits implicit processing, reflected in present-moment alterations in the internal experience of the five building blocks, as illustrated in Figure 14.2.

As Suzi became mindful, she first reported feeling "frozen," but her fingers lifted slightly, which I tracked and named. Suzi was surprised and curious that her fingers lifted, and I asked, "As you sense the lifting of your fingers, what does your body want to do?," directing Suzi to take her time to sense the impulse from her body itself, not her "idea" of the impulse. She reported, "My arms want to push away but I feel scared to do it. I

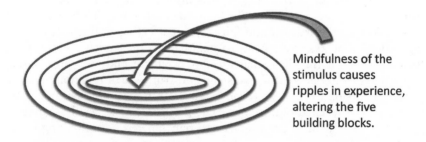

Mindfulness of the stimulus causes ripples in experience, altering the five building blocks.

Implicit processing is made explicit as the patient mindfully studies and reports how the building blocks change in response to the stimulus.

FIGURE 14.2. Directed mindfulness: Eliciting and discovering implicit processing. Copyright 2012 by Pat Ogden.

keep seeing my father's face." I firmly directed her mindful attention exclusively to her body: "Let's just sense your body. Put the fear and the image of your father aside for now. Let's just follow what your body wants to do." This exclusive focus on physical sensation and impulses enabled Suzi to execute an "act of triumph" (Janet, 1925) by pushing against a pillow that I held. The execution of this empowering defensive response elicited a feeling of satisfaction and pleasure, and Suzi reported, "I feel strong! This is a new feeling, and it feels good!" Through directing mindful attention to her body rather than to the image of her father's face, the instinctive impulses to push away—which Suzi could not act upon at the time of the abuse—developed into an action that led to the discovery of her lost ability to defend herself. The connection between the two of us deepened as this long-dormant, empowering action emerged spontaneously, was executed and deeply experienced by her, and was accepted by me.

Over many sessions, after the stabilizing skills gained in Phase 1 treatment and the working through of traumatic memory in Phase 2, Suzi was ready to address Phase 3 treatment goals of increasing her capacity for intimacy and challenging her "implicit relational knowing" (Lyons-Ruth, 1998). Although Suzi desperately longed for a mate, her habits of implicit processing reflected in frozen tension and fear had prevented her from seeking an intimate relationship. These habits became our focus in Phase 3 treatment.

Proximity-seeking actions are abandoned or distorted when they are persistently ineffective in producing the desired outcome from attachment figures. These can become the targets of mindful exploration in Phase 3 treatment. I asked Suzi if she would be interested in noticing what happened if she reached out with her arm or arms toward me. She agreed, and this movement of reaching, a proximity-seeking action, became the stimulus to explore. As Suzi reached out, the part of her that had inhibited that action came forward, and Suzi reported feeling frightened. Exploring actions that are alternatives to habitual action tendencies can bring forward parts of the client that are "inhospitable and even adversarial, sequestered from one another as islands of 'truth,' each functioning as an insulated version of reality" (Bromberg, 2010, p. 21). Suzi became more fearful as she reached out, saying "The thought comes up, 'I'm going to get hurt.'" She avoided eye contact and remembered how climbing up on her father's lap would lead to abuse. Eventually, Suzi discovered a new action: Raising one arm, palm outward in front of her body in a protective motion, Suzi reached toward me with the other arm. She reported that with this dual action she felt calm and strong. Her spine straightened, and she was able to maintain eye contact with me. I wondered if these gestures could be translated into words, and Suzi replied, "I can both defend and connect." Remembering the words and the action helped Suzi feel safe enough to begin to venture out into new social situations that she had previously avoided.

Conclusions

Mindfulness develops "the skill of seeing [the] internal world, and . . . shapes it toward integrative functioning" (Siegel, 2010, p. 223). It focuses attention on interrupting old implicit processing and creating new experiences: "the brain changes physically in response to experience, and new mental skills can be acquired with intentional effort with focused awareness and concentration" (Siegel, 2010, p. 84). In sensorimotor psychotherapy, mindfulness—specifically mindfulness embedded in the moment-to-moment interaction between therapist and client—is privileged over conversation. The therapist repeats directed mindfulness skills throughout the clinical hour, as illustrated in Figure 14.3.

The verbal narrative, although indispensable in clinical practice, cannot provide the same in-the-moment revelations about the client's implicit processing that mindfulness can, nor can it facilitate new physical actions within the relationship. Even when the content that implicit processing represents remains unarticulated, or even unremembered, mindful attention toward the here-and-now effects of past trauma can bring about therapeutic change. Sensorimotor Psychotherapy (Ogden et al., 2006), with its

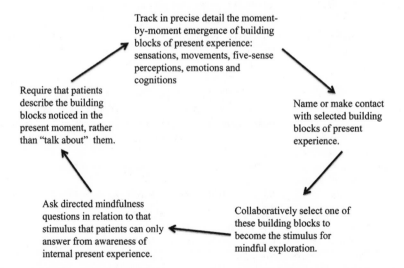

FIGURE 14.3. Clinical map for using directed mindfulness in psychotherapy practice.

embedded relational mindfulness and directed mindfulness techniques, provides a map and tools for healing trauma in this way.

Acknowledgment

I wish to thank Dr. Kekuni Minton for his contribution to this chapter.

References

Arnsten, A. F. T. (2009). Stress signaling pathways that impair prefrontal cortex structure and function. *Nature Reviews Neuroscience, 10,* 410–422.

Bromberg, P. M. (2010). Minding the dissociative gap. *Contemporary Psychoanalysis, 46*(1), 19–31.

Cortina, M., & Liotti, G. (2007). New approaches to understanding unconscious processes: Implicit and explicit memory systems. *International Forum of Psychoanalysis, 16,* 204–212.

Goldstein, J., & Kornfield, J. (1987). *Seeking the heart of wisdom: The path of insight meditation.* Boston: Shambhala.

Janet, P. (1898). *Neuroses et idées fixe.* Paris: Felix Alcan.

Janet, P. (1925). *Principles of psychotherapy.* London: George Allen.

Kurtz, R. (1990). *Body-centered psychotherapy: The Hakomi method.* Mendocino, CA: LifeRhythm.

Kurtz, R. (2004). *Level 1 handbook for the refined Hakomi method.* Retrieved January 4, 2012, from *http://hakomi.com.*

Linehan, M. M. (1993). *Skills training manual for treating borderline personality disorder.* New York: Guilford Press.

Lyons-Ruth, K. (1998). Implicit relational knowing: Its role in development and psychoanalytic treatment. *Infant Mental Health Journal, 19,* 282–289.

Ogden, P. (2007, October). *Beyond words: A clinical map for using mindfulness of the body and the organization of experience in trauma treatment.* Paper presented at Mindfulness and Psychotherapy Conference, Los Angeles, CA.

Ogden, P. (2009). Emotion, mindfulness and movement: Expanding the regulatory boundaries of the window of tolerance. In D. Fosha, D. Siegel, & M. Solomon (Eds.), *The healing power of emotion: Perspectives from affective neuroscience and clinical practice* (pp. 204–231). New York: Norton.

Ogden, P., & Minton, K. (2000). Sensorimotor psychotherapy: One method for processing traumatic memory. *Traumatology, 6,* 1–20.

Ogden, P., Minton, K., & Pain, C. (2006). *Trauma and the body: A sensorimotor approach to psychotherapy.* New York: Norton.

Porges, S. W. (2004). Neuroception: A subconscious system for detecting threats and safety. *Zero to Three.* Retrieved August 8, 2005, from *http://bbc.psych.uic.edu/pdf/Neuroception.pdf.*

Porges, S. W. (2011). *The polyvagal theory: Neurophysiological foundations of emotions, attachment, communication, and self-regulation.* New York: Norton.

Schore, A. (2003). *Affect regulation and the repair of the self.* New York: Norton.

Schore, A. N. (2009). Right-brain affect regulation: An essential mechanism of development, trauma, dissociation, and psychotherapy. In D. Fosha, D. Siegel, & M. Solomon (Eds.), *The healing power of emotion: Affective neuroscience, development and clinical practice* (pp. 112–144). New York: Norton.

Schwabe, L., Joels, M., Roozendaal, B., Wolf, O. T., & Oitzl, M. S. (2012). Stress effects on memory: An update and integration. *Neuroscience and Biobehavioral Reviews, 36,* 1740–1749.

Segal, Z., Teasdale, J., & Williams, M. (2002). *Mindfulness-based cognitive therapy for depression.* New York: Guilford Press.

Siegel, D. (1999). *The developing mind.* New York: Guilford Press.

Siegel, D. (2007). *The mindful brain: Reflection and attunement in the cultivation of well-being.* New York: Norton.

Siegel, D. (2010). *The mindful therapist: A clinician's guide to mindsight and neural integration.* New York: Norton.

Williams, M., Teasdale, J., Segal, Z., & Kabat-Zinn, J. (2007). *The mindful way through depression: Freeing yourself from chronic unhappiness.* New York: Guilford Press.

Part IV

SPECIAL APPLICATIONS AND POPULATIONS

Mindfulness-Based Stress Reduction for Underserved Trauma Populations

Mary Ann Dutton

Trauma exposure, including physical and sexual abuse, is all too common in the United States and it can often lead to adverse health and mental health consequences. According to the National Intimate Partner and Sexual Violence Survey, nearly 1 in 5 women and 1 in 71 men have been raped in their lifetime. Almost half of women experienced the first rape before age 18 years, and 28% of male victims of rape were first raped when they were 10 years old or younger. One in 4 women and 1 in 7 men have been the victims of intimate partner violence in their lifetimes (Black et al., 2011). Given this high prevalence of trauma exposure, attention is needed to its aftermath.

Exposure to traumatic stressors can lead to a wide range of emotional reactions and psychological problems, including depression, posttraumatic stress disorder (PTSD) and other anxiety-related problems, sleep difficulties, somatic symptoms, and an increased risk of substance abuse (Dutton et al., 2006; Mellman & Hipolito, 2006; Schnurr & Green, 2004; Zayfert, Dums, Ferguson, & Hegel, 2002). Cumulative trauma exposure further increases the risk for adverse outcomes (Anda et al., 2006). Moreover, chronic trauma exposure can often result in a wide range of impairments beyond PTSD. The notion of "complex trauma" encompasses these reactions, which involve a broader range of functioning. Complex trauma has been described as affecting three domains of function: dysregulation of emotion (e.g., psychic numbing, impairment in emotional expression), the self (e.g., self-loathing or perception of damage), and interpersonal relations (e.g., expectancy of betrayal, boundary diffusion; Courtois & Ford, 2013).

Many evidence-based trauma treatments focus on specific outcomes, such as PTSD or depression (Lang et al., 2012), even though "recovery" from the effects of trauma exposure may require a great deal more than reducing these symptoms. It is as yet unclear whether a reduction in hallmark trauma symptoms such as PTSD and depression conveys a significant therapeutic impact to the broad range of other trauma-related outcomes that are often experienced, for example, somatic symptoms, interference with self-capacities (relationship to oneself), and disruption in interpersonal relations. Although the reduction of hallmark symptoms of PTSD may greatly increase quality of life for the survivor of chronic trauma, there is much room for improvement if one is left with an internal sense of failure, an inability to self-soothe, and difficulty maintaining satisfying relationships.

Trauma exposure places a greater burden on high-risk groups. A combination of risk factors affecting primarily low-income ethnic and racial minority groups begins with a high prevalence of trauma exposure, often inadequate legal response, and poor access to and substandard quality of health care (Woods-Giscombe & Black, 2010), as well as social injustice, prejudice, and discrimination (Gary, 2005; Walters & Simoni, 2002). Only a handful of survivors of trauma ever receive mental health treatment, and this is especially true for those who face formidable barriers to care, such as the stigma of mental health treatment and limited access to health insurance, transportation, and culturally sensitive treatment (U.S. Department of Health and Human Services, 2001). Approaches that effectively overcome these barriers are needed to adequately address the high burden of suffering that chronic trauma exposure exacts on underserved populations in particular.

Rationale for Mindfulness-Based Stress Reduction for Underserved Trauma Populations

Decades of research have produced a collection of evidence-based mental health treatments that are effective for reducing hallmark trauma symptoms of PTSD and depression. However, evidence-based mental health treatments are not effective for everyone (Schottenbauer, Glass, Arnkoff, Tendick, & Gray, 2008). Two evidence-based treatments for PTSD, prolonged exposure (PE), and cognitive processing therapy (CPT), although effective, are also limited (Orsillo & Batten, 2005). First, cognitive-behavioral therapies (CBTs), like PE and CPT, require users to focus primarily on negative experiences, such as fear and flashbacks, and less on other emotional responses (e.g., anger, sadness, shame, guilt) that often accompany trauma. Further, "problems in living" (e.g., functioning, quality of life, concentration) that often accompany PTSD are not primary outcomes that are addressed by most traditional CBTs for PTSD. Importantly, a significant number of CBT clients also do not show clinical improvements in PTSD after treatment (Belleville, Guay, & Marchand, 2011). Although these current evidence-based gold standard treatments are effective for reducing PTSD and depression, the development of further alternative or complementary options that can lead to even greater benefit is needed.

Mindfulness practices are indigenous to daily life in many parts of the world, and mindfulness-based instruction is increasingly accessible in the United States (*http://nccam.nih.gov/health/meditation/overview.htm*). The research that examines mindfulness practices, such as MBSR, for improving emotional and physical well-being is burgeoning (Dakwar & Levin, 2009; Ludwig & Kabat-Zinn, 2008; Toneatto & Nguyen, 2007). There is a clear theoretical "fit" between the focus on awareness and nonjudgmental acceptance characteristic of mindfulness meditation and the often broad impact of trauma exposure, such as problems with affect regulation, relationships with oneself and others, and sleep disturbance. Mindfulness practice is well suited for adoption by individuals within underserved populations who have been exposed to traumatic stressors and who are experiencing a wide range of physical and emotional reactions that are distressing and that interfere with living a fulfilling life. Following is a discussion of several of these specific factors.

What Is MBSR?

A well-accepted and readily available approach to teaching mindfulness skills is MBSR (Biegel, Brown, Shapiro, & Schubert, 2009; Carlson & Garland, 2005; Goldin & Gross, 2010; Grossman, Tiefenthaler-Gilmer, Raysz, & Kesper, 2007; Lengacher et al., 2009; Reibel, Greeson, Brainard, & Rosenzweig, 2001), developed by Jon Kabat-Zinn in the early 1970s. MBSR professional education and training is available through several MBSR training centers[1], and MBSR courses are available through many local communities. Using a holistic approach, MBSR encourages individuals to develop a new orientation to their experience of life (Bishop et al., 2004) by teaching how to focus attention in a nonjudgmental or

---

[1]Oasis Institute, Center for Mindfulness at the University of Massachusetts Medical School (*http://www.umassmed.edu/cfm/oasis/index.aspx*); Center for Mindfulness, University of California San Diego (*http://health.ucsd.edu/specialties/mindfulness/Pages/default.aspx*).

accepting way on what is happening in the present moment (Kabat-Zinn, 2003) rather than concentrating on the past or future. Participants cultivate awareness and attention to events and experiences as they occur in real time, learning an ever-changing and unfolding landscape of moment-to-moment cognitive, emotional, kinesthetic, and sensory experiences (Biegel et al., 2009). In addition, participants are taught how to allow negative or intrusive thoughts to pass quickly, rather than to be consumed or restrained by them (Biegel, et al., 2009; Brown & Ryan, 2003). Mindful inquiry (curiosity about present-moment experience) and nonjudgmental acceptance of one's own experience are central tenets of MBSR (Carmody & Baer, 2008; Kabat-Zinn, 1990).

The standard MBSR training curriculum (Kabat-Zinn, 1990) includes eight weekly 2½-hour group sessions and a day-long "silent retreat." Formal MBSR practices involve meditation during sitting, walking, and lying down postures, as well as gentle stretching. A key feature of MBSR is the "body scan," which is the practice of systematically bringing one's nonjudgmental and accepting awareness to each part of the body in sequence. MBSR also teaches informal techniques, such as "mindful listening" (giving full attention to another person while he or she is talking), "mindful eating" (giving full attention to the experience of eating every bite), and a "three breaths break" (pausing and paying attention to three subsequent breaths). These techniques encourage participants to more fully appreciate the value of routine, day-to-day activities such as eating, conversation, washing dishes, or taking a shower. MBSR encourages people to practice mindfulness on a daily basis, including both formal and informal practice (Shapiro, Carlson, Astin, & Freedman, 2006).

MBSR Avoids the Stigma Associated with Mental Health Treatment

Seeking mental health treatment is often associated with considerable stigma, especially among low-income and minority individuals (U.S. Department of Health and Human Services, 2001), and this prevents people from obtaining help even when it is available. Being labeled with a psychiatric diagnosis such as often occurs in traditional mental health settings, although useful for professional communication and insurance reimbursement, can lead to further stigma and shame. Although this is a concern for everyone seeking traditional mental health services, it is of special concern for low-income, minority individuals for whom echoes of (even unintended) discrimination are historically associated with overdiagnosis, overmedication, and culturally insensitive or incompetent treatment. Psychiatric diagnoses can have tangible detrimental consequences for individuals embroiled in the legal and social services systems struggling to maintain custody of their children, for example. Nevertheless, there is a need to ameliorate the adverse effects of chronic trauma for those individuals experiencing these effects. Mindfulness practice may avoid many of these pitfalls associated with mental health treatment, either as an alternative or complement to traditional mental health treatment.

MBSR Assumes a Nonjudgmental Stance Regarding One's Own Internal Experience

MBSR assumes a nonjudgmental stance toward one's own experience (Kabat-Zinn, 2003). Our inner experience is not our "fault"; it just is our experience in the moment. Nonjudgment is often confused with "condoning" or "approval," but it is not at all the same thing. The mindfulness practitioner is taught to welcome present-moment reality, that is, sensations or thoughts or feelings—including painful or difficult experiences—without judgment as plainly "what is in this moment." The next moment's experience is equally welcomed, and so on, without "holding on" to the moment that has just passed. This awareness of moment-to-moment experience allows one to discover shifts in and out of different and varied experiences, without holding on to them as if they are "truth" about oneself. It is possible to fine-tune awareness of one's experience enough to discover moments of delight, happiness, lightness, or curiosity, for example, even with someone who has been chronically distressed. Nonjudgmental awareness of sensation, thoughts, and feelings can serve to counter negative experience (e.g., negative self-concept, low self-esteem, shame) that is common among survivors of trauma.

MBSR Enhances Empowerment

Empowerment stems from a sense of self-acceptance, self-mastery, or self-efficacy. Mindfulness practice teaches students to validate their own experience instead of labeling it as right or wrong. Mindfulness practice does not try to change what is, but to honor it. It is worth restating that accepting one's experience is not the same as approval or resignation. Owning one's experience is empowering because no one else can define what it is. From a place of acceptance, one can often more easily take action toward self-care. In fact, increased mindfulness skills have been linked to greater health-related self-management (Gregg, Callaghan, Hayes, & Glenn-Lawson, 2007). In one example, a woman explained, "I am finally able to break up with him [an abusive partner]," and another stated, "I can put my mind to anything."

MBSR Facilitates a Sense of Community

Mindfulness practice taught in a group can create a sense of belonging and social support that has long been associated with a wide range of health and mental health outcomes (Goodman, Bennett, & Dutton, 1999; Kocot & Goodman, 2003). Learning mindfulness in the context of a group creates an immediate community of group members who meet together weekly for a period of time. Meditation communities within local communities can also support one's meditation practices. Importantly, many online meditation communities and forums are available that can offer a sense of belonging to a worldwide community of meditators and in which access to (often free) online meditation sessions and related resources is abundant.

MBSR Embraces the Whole Self

Trauma exposure challenges every aspect of the self: emotions, thoughts, sensations, meaning. Mindfulness practice deliberately embraces the whole self, not privileging one over the other, by valuing and exploring subjective experience at all levels. In this way, mindfulness practice honors rather than compartmentalizes all aspects of the individual with trauma, enhancing a sense of integrity or wholeness. Mental health treatments often maintain a more narrow focus on thoughts and feelings without integration with the whole self, especially existential or spiritual aspects.

MBSR Increases Mindfulness Skills: A Pathway to Reducing PTSD Symptoms

Mindfulness practice is uniquely suited to addressing many symptoms associated with PTSD. PTSD is characterized by a prototypic pattern of avoidance (emotional numbing and behavioral avoidance), hyperarousal (e.g., sleep disturbance, difficulty concentrating, anger, irritability), and intrusive (e.g., intrusive reminders, flashbacks) symptoms and is often accompanied by other associated problems (e.g., cognitive dysregulation related to self and others, affect dysregulation, interpersonal difficulties; American Psychiatric Association, 2000). Present-moment awareness of one's experience is antithetical to experiencing avoidance or numbing, one of the leading hallmark symptoms of PTSD. Learning to allow one's thoughts and feelings to arise in the moment can promote emotion regulation, reducing emotional reactivity (Goldin, Ziv, Jazaieri, Hahn, & Gross, 2013). Mindfulness practice has been shown to reduce markers of physiological stress and sleep disturbance, a pervasive problem associated with PTSD (Brand, Holsboer-Trachsler, Naranjo, & Schmidt, 2012; Carlson, Speca, Faris, & Patel, 2007). Mindfulness practice has been shown to increase mindfulness skills, as well as trauma-related mental health outcomes, including symptoms associated with PTSD and depression (Baer, Carmody, & Hunsinger, 2012; Kearney, McDermott, Malte, Martinez, & Simpson, 2012b; Kimbrough, Magyari, Langenberg, Chesney, & Berman, 2010). Further, those with higher trait mindfulness skills have been associated with better baseline mental health and greater improvement following mindfulness practice (Shapiro, Brown, Thoresen, & Plante, 2011), suggesting that increases in mindfulness skills precede and mediate improvements in mental health outcomes (Baer et al., 2012).

MBSR Does Not Require Processing the Trauma Narrative

A hallmark characteristic of most empirically based trauma treatments includes explicit emotional processing of one's trauma memory or narrative or changing the meaning of traumatic events (Resick et al., 2008). The nature of this processing varies with the particular treatment. For example, PE (Foa & Rauch, 2004) gradually exposes the individual to greater and greater intensity of trauma-related stimuli, with the idea of extinguishing the associated fear response. Similarly, exposure to the specific traumatic narrative occurs through writing in CPT (Resick, Nishith, Weaver, Astin, & Feuer, 2002; Resick & Schnicke, 1992) and in Pennebaker's expressive writing intervention (Hughes, Uhlmann, & Pennebaker, 1994; Pennebaker & Susman, 1988). In contrast, mindfulness practice does not require the person to revisit the trauma narrative; rather, mindfulness practice involves directly encountering whatever experience arises, which, for survivors of trauma, will likely include the effects of trauma exposure on the mind and body. Thus one might understand mindfulness practice to involve the mechanisms of exposure to the direct experience resulting from trauma, but not through the narrative of the story.

Adaptations of MBSR for Trauma

Although MBSR teaches mindfulness skills that have been associated with reduced posttraumatic stress symptoms (Chopko & Schwartz, 2013; Kearney, McDermott, Malte, Martinez, & Simpson, 2012a; Owens, Walter, Chard, & Davis, 2012; Smith et al., 2011; Tyler Boden et al., 2012), there are a number of adaptations to the process of delivery that are suggested to make the practice of mindfulness safer for survivors of trauma, as well as more accessible. We identified these based on a recent study of MBSR, funded by the National Institute of Mental Health, with low-income, predominately African American women with chronic trauma exposure (Bermudez et al., 2013; Dutton, Bermudez, Mátas, & Meyers, 2011). (Study results indicating efficacy for PTSD and depression are forthcoming.) The following adaptations were made based on focus groups, interviews with case managers and the shelter director, and feedback from MBSR participants.

Facilitating Safe Attachment to the MBSR Instructor

Individual orientation sessions are designed to facilitate a positive attachment to the instructor and to the MBSR group itself, in part through the collection of relevant information, including reason for participating. Much like a clinical intake session, individual orientation sessions are also helpful for discerning specific challenges that might be relevant to individual participants in order to better facilitate their active participation in the MBSR group process, including with at-home practice. In addition to the usual information, such as personal goals and current concerns, other information might include the nature, recency, and extent of trauma exposure; participants' adaptive coping skills for dealing with possible emotional distress; and history of high-risk coping strategies (e.g., substance abuse, self-harm).

Attending to Perception of Threat

As practiced by Magyari (Kimbrough et al., 2010), it is important to arrange and secure the room to enhance a sense of safety. Survivors of trauma may have difficulty relaxing, closing their eyes, or lying on the floor related to perceived threat.

Providing a Rationale for the Mechanism of Action Early in the Process

The standard MBSR curriculum includes a module pertaining to physiological stress response and how stress affects mind and body. Moving this module to the first or second session provides a solid rationale for participating in a process, especially for individuals who are less familiar with mindfulness or meditation, including those who have been referred to an MBSR group rather than seeking it out independently.

Increasing the Sense of Self-Efficacy

To increase a sense of mastery, we found several structural adaptations to be useful. For example, providing a standard transition into each MBSR session with music helps participants to transition from a busy day. In addition, we reduced the session length (e.g., from 2½ to 1½ hours) to increase the likelihood that participants could better tolerate sessions. Finally, creating a "no fail" perspective for home practice is important; for example, reducing the expectation for formal practice by emphasizing informal practice or "real life" application can be very important to build a sense of success and self-efficacy with the new skill of mindfulness practice.

Providing Tools for Self-Regulation

Beginning mindfulness practice can increase emotional distress when people initially become more aware of distressing emotions that may previously have been numbed or avoided. We included the "3-minute breathing space" from mindfulness-based cognitive therapy (MBCT; Segal, Teasdale, & Williams, 2004) to provide participants with a concrete and simple tool to help them cope with increased arousal or simply restlessness as they gain more gradual additional benefits of mindful awareness and acceptance.

Enhancing the Nurturing Quality of the MBSR Experience

Loving-kindness meditation (Salzberg, 1995) was incorporated into the MBSR sessions to directly help counter negative trauma-related affect and cognitions (e.g., shame, guilt, low self-esteem). Loving-kindness is a meditation practice, a way of paying full attention to and taking an interest in the "good within us" (Salzberg, 2011) without pretending that we have no problems.

Encouraging Self-Empowerment

Meditation participants were encouraged to make decisions that take charge of their own meditation practice—and their lives. Regardless of the instruction, participants were always encouraged to "take care of themselves." That may mean choosing to open one's eyes, sitting in a chair rather than on the floor, or leaving the room to ground oneself rather than to continue with the practice. Although participants were not encouraged to avoid negative feelings or discomfort, they were given permission to regulate the experience at their own pace. Although within any meditation training this is always implicitly the case, here we made this message explicit.

Reducing the Risk of Emotional Flooding

Gradually increasing the formal practice time from 5 or 10 minutes to more than 40 minutes at a time, we helped participants to "learn" to tolerate their experience. This approach allowed participants to experiment with the experience of immersing themselves in the flow of new awareness, while minimizing the possibility of emotional flooding.

Conclusions

Based on our experience working with low-income, minority women with chronic trauma exposure, we believe that mindfulness practice is feasible and acceptable as an approach to relieving the trauma-related suffering that too often has become a way of life. Importantly, women in our study were not seeking mental health treatment for distress related to their trauma exposure prior to joining our study. We have learned that many trauma survivors have no expectation that mental health treatment will promote a life of greater ease or less distress. Instead, they "live with" their trauma symptoms, without necessarily understanding the link to their trauma exposure, with negative self-judgment and sometimes with maladaptive ways of coping with the traumatic effects Through mindfulness training using MBSR, women in our study reported a reduction of symptoms (study results are forthcoming), but they gained more than symptom reduction, including envisioning hope, increased self-compassion, and improved interpersonal relationships (Bermudez et al., 2013; Dutton, Bermudez, Mátas, Majid, & Myers, 2013). Much more work is needed to consider the ways in which mindfulness practice can best be offered to survivors of trauma in ways that promote healing in the most beneficial fashion.

References

American Psychiatric Association. (2013). *Diagnostic and statistical manual of mental disorders* (5th ed.). Arlington, VA: Author.

Anda, R. F., Felitti, V. J., Bremner, J. D., Walker, J. D., Whitfield, C., Perry, B. D., et al. (2006). The enduring effects of abuse and related adverse experiences in childhood: A convergence of evidence from neurobiology and epidemiology. *European Archives of Psychiatry and Clinical Neuroscience, 256*(3), 174–186.

Baer, R. A., Carmody, J., & Hunsinger, M. (2012). Weekly change in mindfulness and perceived stress in a mindfulness-based stress reduction program. *Journal of Clinical Psychology, 68*(7), 755–765.

Belleville, G., Guay, S., & Marchand, A. (2011). Persistence of sleep disturbances following cognitive-behavior therapy for posttraumatic stress disorder. *Journal of Psychosomatic Research, 70*(4), 318–327.

Bermudez, D., Benjamin, M. T., Porter, S. E., Saunders, P., Myers, N. A. L., & Dutton, M. A. (2013). A qualitative analysis of beginning mindfulness experiences for women with post-traumatic stress disorder and a history of intimate partner violence. *Complementary Therapies in Clinical Practice, 19*(2). Retrieved from *http://dx.doi.org/10.1016/j.ctcp.2013.02.004.*

Biegel, G. M., Brown, K. W., Shapiro, S. L., & Schubert, C. M. (2009). Mindfulness-based stress reduction for the treatment of adolescent psychiatric outpatients: A randomized clinical trial. *Journal of Consulting and Clinical Psychology, 77*(5), 855–866.

Bishop, S. R., Lau, M., Shapiro, S., Carlson, L., Anderson, N. D., Carmody, J., et al. (2004). Mindfulness: A proposed operational definition. *Clinical Psychology: Science and Practice, 11*(3), 230–241.

Black, M. C., Basile, K. C., Breiding, M. J., Smith, S. G., Walters, M. L., Merrick,

M. T., et al. (2011). *The National Intimate Partner and Sexual Violence Survey (NISVS): 2010 summary report.* Atlanta, GA: Centers for Disease Control and Prevention, National Center for Injury Prevention and Control.

Brand, S., Holsboer-Trachsler, E., Naranjo, J. R., & Schmidt, S. (2012). Influence of mindfulness practice on cortisol and sleep in long-term and short-term meditators. *Neuropsychobiology, 65*(3), 109–118.

Brown, K. W., & Ryan, R. M. (2003). The benefits of being present: Mindfulness and its role in psychological well-being. *Journal of Personality and Social Psychology, 84*(4), 822–848.

Carlson, L. E., & Garland, S. N. (2005). Impact of mindfulness-based stress reduction (MBSR) on sleep, mood, stress and fatigue symptoms in cancer outpatients. *International Journal of Behavioral Medicine, 12*(4), 278–285.

Carlson, L. E., Speca, M., Faris, P., & Patel, K. D. (2007). One year pre–post intervention follow-up of psychological, immune, endocrine and blood pressure outcomes of mindfulness-based stress reduction (MBSR) in breast and prostate cancer outpatients. *Brain, Behavior, and Immunity, 21*(8), 1038–1049.

Carmody, J., & Baer, R. A. (2008). Relationships between mindfulness practice and levels of mindfulness, medical and psychological symptoms and well-being in a mindfulness-based stress reduction program. *Journal of Behavioral Medicine, 31*(1), 23–33.

Chopko, B. A., & Schwartz, R. C. (2013). The relation between mindfulness and posttraumatic stress symptoms among police officers. *Journal of Loss and Trauma, 18*(1), 1–9.

Courtois, C. A., & Ford, J. D. (2013). *Treatment of complex trauma: A sequenced, relationship-based approach.* New York: Guilford Press.

Dakwar, E., & Levin, F. R. (2009). The emerging role of meditation in addressing psychiatric illness, with a focus on substance use disorders. *Harvard Review of Psychiatry, 17*(4), 254–267.

Dutton, M. A., Bermudez, D., Mátas, A., Majid, H., & Myers, N. (2013). Mindfulness-based stress reduction for PTSD with low-income women with a history of intimate partner violence. *Cognitive and Behavioral Practice, 20*, 23–32.

Dutton, M. A., Bermudez, D., Mátas, A., & Meyers, N. L. (2011, October). *MBSR for PTSD among low-income women with chronic trauma.* Paper presented at the International Scientific Conference for Clinicians, Researchers and Educators: Investigating and Integrating Mindfulness in Medicine, Health Care, and Society, Norwood, MA.

Dutton, M. A., Green, B. L., Kaltman, S. I., Roesch, D. M., Zeffiro, T. A., & Krause, E. D. (2006). Intimate partner violence, PTSD, and adverse health outcomes. *Journal of Interpersonal Violence, 21*(7), 955–968.

Foa, E. B., & Rauch, S. A. M. (2004). Cognitive changes during prolonged exposure versus prolonged exposure plus cognitive restructuring in female assault survivors with posttraumatic stress disorder. *Journal of Consulting and Clinical Psychology, 72*(5), 879–884.

Gary, F. A. (2005). Stigma: Barrier to mental health care among ethnic minorities. *Issues in Mental Health Nursing, 26*(10), 979–999.

Goldin, P., Ziv, M., Jazaieri, H., Hahn, K., & Gross, J. J. (2013). MBSR vs. aerobic exercise in social anxiety: fMRI of emotion regulation of negative self-beliefs. *Social Cognitive and Affective Neuroscience, 8*(1), 65–72.

Goldin, P. R., & Gross, J. J. (2010). Effects of mindfulness-based stress reduction (MBSR) on emotion regulation in social anxiety disorder. *Emotion, 10*(1), 83–91.

Goodman, L., Bennett, L., & Dutton, M. A. (1999). Obstacles to victims' cooperation with the criminal prosecution of their abusers: The role of social support. *Violence and Victims, 14*(4), 427–444.

Gregg, J. A., Callaghan, G. M., Hayes, S. C., & Glenn-Lawson, J. L. (2007). Improving diabetes self-management through acceptance, mindfulness, and values: A randomized controlled trial. *Journal of Consulting and Clinical Psychology, 75*(2), 336–343.

Grossman, P., Tiefenthaler-Gilmer, U., Raysz, A., & Kesper, U. (2007). Mindfulness training as an intervention for fibromyalgia: Evidence of postintervention and 3-year follow-up benefits in well-being. *Psychotherapy and Psychosomatics, 76*(4), 226–233.

Hughes, C. F., Uhlmann, C., & Pennebaker, J. W. (1994). The body's response to processing emotional trauma: Linking verbal text with autonomic activity. *Journal of Personality, 62*(4), 565–585.

Kabat-Zinn, J. (1990). *Full catastrophe living: Using the wisdom of your body and mind to face stress, pain, and illness.* New York: Delacorte Press.

Kabat-Zinn, J. (2003). Mindfulness-based interventions in context: Past, present, and future. *Clinical Psychology: Science and Practice, 10*(2), 144–156.

Kearney, D. J., McDermott, K., Malte, C., Martinez, M., & Simpson, T. L. (2012a). Association of participation in a mindfulness program with measures of PTSD, depression and quality of life in a veteran sample. *Journal of Clinical Psychology, 68*(1), 101–116.

Kearney, D. J., McDermott, K., Malte, C., Martinez, M., & Simpson, T. L. (2012b). Effects of participation in a mindfulness program for veterans with posttraumatic stress disorder: A randomized controlled pilot study. *Journal of Clinical Psychology, 69*(1), 14–27.

Kimbrough, E., Magyari, T., Langenberg, P., Chesney, M., & Berman, B. (2010). Mindfulness intervention for child abuse survivors. *Journal of Clinical Psychology, 66*(1), 17–33.

Kocot, T., & Goodman, L. (2003). The roles of coping and social support in battered women's mental health. *Violence against Women, 9*, 323–346.

Lang, A. J., Schnurr, P. P., Jain, S., Raman, R., Walser, R., Bolton, E., et al. (2012). Evaluating transdiagnostic treatment for distress and impairment in veterans: A multi-site randomized controlled trial of acceptance and commitment therapy. *Contemporary Clinical Trials, 33*(1), 116–123.

Lengacher, C. A., Johnson-Mallard, V., Post-White, J., Moscoso, M. S., Jacobsen, P. B., Klein, T. W., et al. (2009). Randomized controlled trial of mindfulness-based stress reduction (MBSR) for survivors of breast cancer. *Psychooncology, 18*(12), 1261–1272.

Ludwig, D. S., & Kabat-Zinn, J. (2008). Mindfulness in medicine. *Journal of the American Medical Association, 300*(11), 1350–1352.

Mellman, T. A., & Hipolito, M. M. (2006). Sleep disturbances in the aftermath of trauma and posttraumatic stress disorder. *CNS Spectrums, 11*(8), 611–615.

Orsillo, S. M., & Batten, S. V. (2005). Acceptance and commitment therapy in the treatment of posttraumatic stress disorder. *Behavior Modification, 29*(1), 95–129.

Owens, G. P., Walter, K. H., Chard, K. M., & Davis, P. A. (2012). Changes in mindfulness skills and treatment response among veterans in residential PTSD treatment. *Psychological Trauma: Theory, Research, Practice, and Policy, 4*(2), 221–228.

Pennebaker, J. W., & Susman, J. R. (1988). Disclosure of traumas and psychosomatic processes. *Social Science and Medicine, 26*(3), 327–332.

Reibel, D. K., Greeson, J. M., Brainard, G. C., & Rosenzweig, S. (2001). Mindfulness-based stress reduction and health-related quality of life in a heterogeneous patient population. *General Hospital Psychiatry, 23*(4), 183–192.

Resick, P. A., Galovski, T. E., O'Brien Uhlmansiek, M., Scher, C. D., Clum, G. A., & Young-Xu, Y. (2008). A randomized clinical trial to dismantle components of cognitive processing therapy for posttraumatic stress disorder in female victims of interpersonal violence. *Journal of Consulting and Clinical Psychology, 76*(2), 243–258.

Resick, P. A., Nishith, P., Weaver, T. L., Astin, M. C., & Feuer, C. A. (2002). A comparison of cognitive-processing therapy with prolonged exposure and a waiting condition for the treatment of chronic posttraumatic stress disorder in female rape victims. *Journal of Consulting and Clinical Psychology, 70*(4), 867–879.

Resick, P. A., & Schnicke, M. K. (1992). Cognitive processing therapy for sexual assault victims. *Journal of Consulting and Clinical Psychology, 60*(5), 748–756.

Salzberg, S. (1995). *Lovingkindness: The revolutionary art of happiness.* Boston: Shambhala.

Salzberg, S. (2011). *Real happiness: The power of meditation: A 28-day program.* New York: Workman.

Schnurr, P. P., & Green, B. L. (2004). *Trauma and health: Physical health consequences of exposure to extreme stress.* Washington, DC: American Psychological Association.

Schottenbauer, M. A., Glass, C. R., Arnkoff, D. B., Tendick, V., & Gray, S. H. (2008). Nonresponse and dropout rates in outcome studies on PTSD: Review and methodological considerations. *Psychiatry, 71*(2), 134–168.

Segal, Z. V., Teasdale, J. D., & Williams, J. M. G. (2004). Mindfulness-based cognitive therapy: Theoretical rationale and empirical status. In S. C. Hayes, V. M. Follette, & M. M. Linehan (Eds.), *Mindfulness and acceptance: Expanding the cognitive-behavioral tradition* (pp. 45–65). New York: Guilford Press.

Shapiro, S. L., Brown, K. W., Thoresen, C., & Plante, T. G. (2011). The moderation of mindfulness-based stress reduction effects by trait mindfulness: Results from a randomized controlled trial. *Journal of Clinical Psychology, 67*(3), 267–277.

Shapiro, S. L., Carlson, L. E., Astin, J. A., & Freedman, B. (2006). Mechanisms of mindfulness. *Journal of Clinical Psychology, 62*(3), 373–386.

Smith, B. W., Ortiz, J. A., Steffen, L. E., Tooley, E. M., Wiggins, K. T., Yeater, E. A., et al. (2011). Mindfulness is associated with fewer PTSD symptoms, depressive symptoms, physical symptoms, and alcohol problems in urban firefighters. *Journal of Consulting and Clinical Psychology, 79*(5), 613–617.

Toneatto, T., & Nguyen, L. (2007). Does mindfulness meditation improve anxiety and mood symptoms?: A review of the controlled research. *Canadian Journal of Psychiatry*, 52(4), 260–266.

Tyler Boden, M., Bernstein, A., Walser, R. D., Bui, L., Alvarez, J., & Bonn-Miller, M. O. (2012). Changes in facets of mindfulness and posttraumatic stress disorder treatment outcome. *Psychiatry Research*, 200(2–3), 609–613.

U.S. Department of Health and Human Services. (2001). *Mental health, culture, race, and ethnicity—A supplement to mental health: A report of the Surgeon General*. Washington, DC: U.S. Department of Health and Human Services, Substance Abuse and Mental Health Services Administration, Center for Mental Health Services.

Walters, K. L., & Simoni, J. M. (2002). Reconceptualizing Native women's health: An "indigenist" stress-coping model. *American Journal of Public Health*, 92(4), 520–524.

Woods-Giscombe, C. L., & Black, A. R. (2010). Mind–body interventions to reduce risk for health disparities related to stress and strength among African American women: The potential of mindfulness-based stress reduction, loving-kindness, and the NTU therapeutic framework. *Complementary Health Practice Review*, 15(3), 115–131.

Zayfert, C., Dums, A. R., Ferguson, R. J., & Hegel, M. T. (2002). Health functioning impairments associated with posttraumatic stress disorder, anxiety disorders, and depression. *Journal of Nervous And Mental Disease*, 190(4), 233–240.

16

Mindfulness in the Treatment of Trauma-Related Chronic Pain

Ronald D. Siegel

When we experience bodily pain, we naturally assume that it is due to an injury, illness, or structural abnormality. And although most acute pain indeed does signal such conditions, countless clients suffer from chronic pain that has little or no relationship to tissue damage. The origin of this pain often lies in psychological trauma.

A steadily growing body of research demonstrates that psychological trauma is a risk factor for developing chronic physical pain. Studies show this association for a remarkably wide variety of syndromes, including chronic regional and widespread pain (Ablin et al., 2010; Kendall-Tackett, Marshall, & Ness, 2003), chronic low back pain (Schofferman, Anderson, Hines, Smith, & Keane, 1993), chronic pelvic pain (Roelofs & Spinhoven, 2007), self-reported arthritis (Kopec & Sayre, 2004), chronic orofacial pain (Burris, Cyders, de Leeuw, Smith, & Carlson, 2009), fibromyalgia (Naring, van Lankveld, & Geenen, 2007; Amital et al., 2006), and chronic headaches (Tietjen et al., 2009a, 2009b, 2009c; Peterlin et al., 2009).

How Might Psychological Trauma Cause Physical Pain?

At first glance, the mechanisms by which psychological trauma predisposes someone to chronic physical pain seem mysterious. In fact, many medical practitioners, and most clients, are reluctant to consider psychological trauma as a likely source. The reason is partly that we all learn early in life to associate physical pain with tissue damage. After all, when we cut a finger, the relationship between seeing blood and feeling pain is unmistakable. It is also partly due to the remarkable progress medicine has made in developing imaging techniques that reveal structural abnormalities, which physicians naturally assume are the cause of clients' distress. Yet without understanding the role of psychological trauma in chronic pain, the likelihood of successful treatment for many people is seriously diminished.

There are several ways in which psychological trauma predisposes clients to developing chronic pain and by which that pain in turn becomes psychologically traumatizing, further perpetuating the disorder. Fortunately, mindfulness practices can be enormously useful in interrupting these processes.

Autonomic Reactivity

People with trauma histories often experience ambiguous stimuli as dangerous and hence are prone to autonomic arousal (Tucker et al., 2010; Pole et al., 2007). When we walk in a dangerous neighborhood at night and hear a rustling in the bushes, we are likely to react with fear. The same rustling in a safe neighborhood may escape our attention entirely. People who have experienced psychological trauma rarely feel themselves to be in a safe neighborhood.

This assumption of danger becomes a risk factor for chronic pain. All mammals share an ancient, sophisticated emergency "fight–freeze–flight" response system. When a mammal is threatened, its sympathetic nervous system and hypothalamic–pituitary–adrenal (HPA) axis are activated, resulting in increased epinephrine (adrenaline) in the bloodstream and many other physiological changes (Sapolsky, 2004). Respiration, heart rate, body temperature, and muscle tension all increase—the better to fight an enemy or flee from danger.

Imagine, for example, that a rabbit grazing in a field notices a fox. The rabbit freezes, hoping not to be noticed, while becoming more vigilant and physiologically aroused in preparation to flee (rabbits aren't big fighters). In this state of high arousal and preparation for action, both sympathetic and parasympathetic branches of the autonomic nervous are highly activated, with the faster acting parasympathetic vagus nerve applying a "brake" that can be rapidly withdrawn to release the full force of the sympathetic activation it holds in check. If the fox wanders off, soon the rabbit's sympathetic activity will decrease, while the parasympathetic nervous system helps the animal calm down until its physiology returns to baseline. This system works wonderfully for rabbits and undoubtedly has contributed to their survival.

But what if the rabbit were to possess a highly evolved cerebral cortex, allowing for language and complex symbolic, anticipatory thought? Once the fox left, the rabbit might think: "Will he return?" "Will he find my family?" (not to mention whether it can save up enough carrots for retirement). Such thoughts would continue to activate its fight–or–flight system, which would remain stuck "on," eventually causing what has been called an *allostatic load*—stress-induced strain on organ systems that can lead to a host of physical ailments (McEwen, 2000).

Consider further what might happen to such a rabbit that had experienced a trauma, such as actually being captured by a fox before narrowly escaping. It would regularly imagine foxes in the bushes, so that virtually any ambiguous situation would throw its body into a state of high arousal. This is, of course, what happens for many human trauma survivors. They are repeatedly "triggered" by ordinary life events that others see as non-threatening.

Illness Anxiety: It's Probably Something Serious

Of all the stimuli that can trigger a fight–freeze–flight response, the most problematic in chronic pain syndromes is often the pain itself. We see in mindfulness practice that the body produces an endless stream of sensations— aches, itches, tingles, numbness. If we are young, have lived relatively safe lives, and come from ethnic groups that do not overly attend to bodily sensations, we tend to interpret them as "probably nothing." If, however, we are older, have encountered serious medical problems, or have had other reasons to see the universe as threatening, we tend to interpret the same sensations as indications of injury or illness. A critical factor in developing a chronic pain syndrome is the belief that the body is damaged. It is only by realizing that pain is not actually due to illness or structural damage, and therefore need not be feared, that clients can resume normal activity and, by so doing, resolve their pain syndromes. In my clinical work, I find that many survivors of trauma find it difficult to believe that their pain might be harmless, and they tend toward hypervigilance, scanning the body for signs of injury or illness, reacting to the sensations they notice with fear.

Often, believing that pain indicates a serious problem leads to kinesiophobia (fear of movement), which causes the body to lose strength, flexibility, and endurance, predisposing it to injury. Then the pain itself, if interpreted as dangerous, becomes another trigger for autonomic arousal.

There are other survivors of trauma, however, who become dissociated from their bodies, hypoaroused, or depressed and may encounter an opposite problem—they may fail to notice pain signals that require attention. Although these individuals may not have difficulty with hypervigilance, they are often unaware of emotional reactions, which, as will be discussed shortly, can also predispose them to chronic pain.

From Fear to Pain

There are two major ways that fear can create or exacerbate bodily pain. The first involves muscle tension. Take a moment to act terrified. You will probably notice that your skeletal muscles contract. Tight muscles can be painful—whether it's the aching tightness in our neck and shoulders after a stressful day or the intense pain of a charley horse when a calf muscle goes into spasm. If we then become frightened of the pain, our muscles tighten further, creating a vicious cycle. A wide variety of chronic neck, back, jaw, foot, pelvic, and chest pain is caused this way.

Fear also amplifies the subjective experience of pain. We have known for decades that the experience of pain is not simply proportionate to the degree of disturbance to tissues (Melzack & Wall, 1965). People experience a given stimulus as far more painful if they are frightened than if they feel safe (Beecher, 1946; Burgmer et al., 2011). In a classic experiment, participants' hands are placed in ice water. If they are told that the experiment will only last a minute, their pain ratings at 30 seconds are relatively low. If told, however, that they will need to keep their hands in the ice water for 10 minutes (a more frightening prospect), pain ratings at 30 seconds are much higher.

Difficulty Self-Soothing

A critical variable in whether emotional distress passes or persists involves our capacity to self-soothe. We all regularly become upset, but some of us are much better at self-soothing than others. Survivors of childhood trauma often have particular difficulty self-soothing, because many of them were not supported in learning self-regulation skills or lacked caregivers who could modulate their arousal through caring presence. Without effective strategies to manage discomfort or memories of "it's OK, sweetheart" in which to take refuge, people with early trauma histories typically become quite distressed about pain, which in turn makes it persist.

Fear of Unwanted Mental Contents

All animals have an instinctual aversion to pain. Humans have particularly sophisticated ways of trying to avoid it, especially when that pain is emotional or psychological. We employ a wide variety of strategies to distract ourselves or actively push out of awareness painful thoughts, feelings, images, instinctual urges, and memories. But these efforts are usually only partially effective: *When we bury feelings, we bury them alive.* Disavowed mental contents are easily reawakened, and when they get close to our awareness, we feel fear. Freud (1926/1959) called this fear "signal anxiety." We respond to tigers within ourselves with a system designed for tigers in the outside world.

Not surprisingly, there is evidence that (1) people who have difficulty acknowledging affect suffer disproportionately from stress-related disorders (Schwartz, 1990), (2) being unaware of feelings can interfere with successful rehabilitation from chronic pain syndromes (Burns et al., 2012), and (3) learning to identify and safely express emotion can reduce the frequency of symptoms (Pennebaker, Keicolt-Glaser, & Glaser, 1988).

Our propensity to feel anxiety when unwanted mental contents are aroused is proportional to how much of our experience we have split off or disavowed. Survivors of trauma usually have many memories, thoughts, and feelings that their minds work to keep out of awareness. This is another factor predisposing them to fear and, hence, to chronic pain syndromes that are caused, maintained, or exacerbated by such fear.

As mentioned earlier, some survivors of trauma do not experience much overt fear; instead, they experience deadening, numbing, and hypoarousal. Yet many of these clients also suffer with chronic pain. Here the mechanism of action is less clear—it is as though the acute emotional pain one might expect to accompany the memory of trauma manifests instead as physical symptoms. One explanation is that in trauma, the body can become stuck in a freeze response, causing it to shut down, which over time leads to chronic pain or other organ system dysfunction. Treatments such as somatic experiencing (Levine, 2008; Scaer, 2007), which attempt to release such freeze responses by helping people reconnect with disavowed memories and associated feelings, have received considerable anecdotal support.

Mindfulness Practices

For any given client, one or more of the mechanisms just described may be most salient to his or her pain condition. Mindfulness practices, in conjunction with other interventions, can be used to address any or all of them in the context of a comprehensive approach that includes (1) a *medical evaluation* to rule out treatable injuries or illnesses and give the client authoritative permission to move freely; (2) *cognitive restructuring* to understand the role of tension, fear, and behavioral avoidance in the condition; (3) *resuming normal activities* to treat kinesiophobia and to regain muscle strength, endurance, and flexibility; and (4) *working with negative emotions* to understand and deal with the role in the disorder of psychological factors, including thoughts, feelings, and memories associated with trauma. One program utilizing this approach, called *Back Sense,* integrates cognitive, psychodynamic, behavioral, and systemic interventions along with explicit teaching of mindfulness practice to treat chronic back and neck pain (Siegel, Urdang, & Johnson, 2001). Clients can participate in the program following the self-treatment guide[1] or by working with a mental health or rehabilitation professional.

---

[1] *Back Sense: A Revolutionary Approach to Halting the Cycle of Chronic Back Pain* (Siegel et al., 2001).

Mindfulness for Autonomic Reactivity

Several controlled studies and countless anecdotal reports suggest that mindfulness practices can help us to be less physiologically reactive to perceived threats (e.g., Brewer et al., 2009; Goldin & Gross, 2010). How does this work? First, by practicing *being with* unpleasant thoughts, feelings, and sensations when they arise, allowing them to come and go, we are less inclined to generate strong aversion responses and therefore less likely to become aroused by a desperate desire to escape discomfort. Second, by gradually learning to see all phenomena, pleasant and unpleasant, as changing impersonal events, we are more likely to allow events to take their course without resistance. Finally, by seeing ourselves as part of the larger world and noticing how our sense of a separate self is constructed moment by moment, we become less preoccupied with self-preservation and have fewer defensive arousal reactions.

Mindfulness for Illness Anxiety

As long as a client believes that his or her chronic pain is due to a serious illness or injury rather than to the effects of anxiety and muscle tension or a persistent freeze and shutdown response, he or she is unlikely to become free of a trauma-related chronic pain syndrome. Such beliefs increase fear, disrupting normal body functioning by further tensing muscles, disturbing other organ systems, amplifying subjective pain signals, and prompting avoidance of the normal life activities that are necessary for health.

A competent medical evaluation, ideally by a physician who understands the role of psychological factors in chronic pain, is required. I usually ask clients to inquire whether the doctor has "evidence that were I to engage in normal life activities I'd irreparably damage my body." Because there are now considerable data, particularly in the case of the neck and back, that it is safe to exercise vigorously in the presence of chronic pain (e.g., Chou et al., 2007; Rainville, Sobel, Hartigan, Monlux, & Bean, 1997), most physicians will respond to this question with permission to move normally.

Once such permission is granted, for hypervigilant clients, psychoeducation about the stress–response system and the role of fear in tensing muscles, disrupting normal body functioning, and amplifying pain sensations is usually needed. Mindfulness practices can provide enormous support for this by illustrating how often worried pain-related thoughts arise (usually every few seconds) and how much tension is held in the body (usually a lot). They can foster and support the ability to observe the interplay among pain, fear, and behavior, illuminating the role that thoughts and emotions play in the pain.

Although the effect is gradual, mindfulness practice can also increase cognitive flexibility. By observing the arising and passing of thoughts without following or judging them, clients become less identified with their content. They see how thought is socially influenced—how their minds are full of ideas picked up from doctors, friends, and others. Developing such metacognitive awareness helps chronic pain clients consider that their assumptions about structural damage or disease are changeable constructs, not objective conclusions about reality.

Mindfulness for the Experience of Pain

There is a well-known sutra, called the story of the two arrows or two darts, in which the Buddha describes our typical response to pain:

> When touched with a feeling of pain, the uninstructed run-of-the-mill person sorrows, grieves, & laments, beats his breast, becomes distraught. So he feels two pains, physical & mental. Just as if they were to shoot a man with an arrow and, right afterward, were to shoot him with another one, so that he would feel the pains of two arrows. (Thanissaro, 2012, p. 1)

This ancient realization—that the sensation of pain is followed immediately by a response of aversion and suffering—is easily observed in mindfulness practice. When I introduced this idea to a client who works at the Massachusetts Institute of Technology (MIT), he said (as people from MIT often do) "there's a mathematical formula for that." He went on to present it: *pain × resistance = suffering*. So when pain is very intense—one has literally been shot by an arrow—suffering will likely be great unless one is extraordinarily skilled at acceptance. But when pain is not too severe, by lowering our resistance, we can alleviate suffering. The reason is that fear and resistance cause painful muscle tension and amplify the subjective experience of pain. Mindfulness practices, by training the mind to *be with* and *accept* discomfort, reduce tension and the amplification of pain sensations created by fear.

Mindfulness for Self-Soothing

Of the three core aspects of mindfulness practice, (1) concentration (or focused attention), (2) mindfulness per se (or open monitoring), and (3) acceptance (Siegel, 2010; Germer, 2013; Pollak, Pedulla, & Siegel, 2014), the last is most helpful for self-soothing in the face of chronic pain. Practices of loving-kindness or *metta* (Pollak, Pedulla, & Siegel, 2014; Siegel, 2010) and self-compassion (Germer, 2009) can help traumatized clients develop a sense of safety in the midst of physical discomfort. The very structure of meditation, in which we adopt a dignified physical posture and sit with the intention to be open to experience, can provide a form of the emotional "holding" famously described by D. W. Winnicott (1960).

Mindfulness of Unwanted Mental Contents

For many clients, learning that their pain is not due to serious disease or tissue damage, seeing for themselves the roles of fear and behavioral avoidance in their problem, and resuming full normal life activity are sufficient to free them from their pain. For others, especially those with a trauma history, a return to normal functioning is not enough. Here emotional difficulties beyond concerns about pain often contribute to persistent fear and hypervigilance, which in turn are perpetuating the disorder. Exploration of unwelcome emotions is usually needed, and mindfulness practice can provide support.

If you lie on a psychoanalyst's couch long enough and say whatever comes to mind, sooner or later everything you have ever wanted *not* to think, feel, or remember will come into awareness. Similarly, if you spend enough time mindfully following the breath or other object of awareness, sooner or later disavowed thoughts, feelings, and memories will surface.

Mindfulness practice not only brings previously unnoticed or rejected mental contents into consciousness, but it also helps clients to tolerate them. As we sit with difficult material and see that it arises, is experienced, and eventually passes, it becomes easier to bear. Anxiety about what might arise drops away as we become increasingly comfortable with the contents of our minds.

Do No Harm

For survivors of trauma who habitually block out painful memories or emotions, the power of mindfulness practices to reintegrate split-off contents can also pose serious risks. In 1976, I worked at a psychiatric treatment facility near the Insight Meditation Society in Barre, Massachusetts. We saw several clients who had had psychotic breaks or were seriously destabilized during silent meditation retreats. Even outside of a retreat setting, some people will become overwhelmed after only a few minutes of following their breath. For these people, the ratio between the "holding" effects of the practice and its power to bring into awareness disavowed experience is tilted too far toward opening the door to unwanted contents.

Clients most at risk for being destabilized by mindfulness meditation include those with unresolved trauma histories, rigid personality organizations, fears of fragmentation or loss of sense of self, or who are suffering from psychosis. With all of these populations, clinicians need to be particularly careful about which practices they introduce when.

A good rule of thumb is to be sure to establish safety before engaging in practices that work to reintegrate split-off contents (Herman, 1997; Cloitre, Cohen, & Koenen, 2006). A wide variety of approaches, including establishing a supportive therapeutic alliance; creating stable, safe living arrangements; cultivating a social support network; and teaching cognitive-behavioral therapy techniques that foster emotion regulation and rational thought can all contribute to such safety.

Another way to help traumatized chronic pain clients establish safety and not be overwhelmed is to introduce mindfulness exercises that turn the attention toward the outer, rather than the inner, world. Relatively safe options include walking meditation, nature meditation (attending to the sights and sounds of trees, clouds, birds), eating or listening meditation, and mindful yoga. These practices are not only unlikely to destabilize a client, but they can also be used in difficult situations to provide stabilization, as illustrated in the following clinical encounter.

Andy, a long-term client with a terrible trauma history, came to my office looking particularly distressed. Our early work had focused on his chronic back and bladder pain, which he had successfully resolved by understanding these to be psychophysiological disorders; by resuming normal activity; by learning to accept, rather than fight, the pain sensations; and by turning his attention to other thoughts and feelings that he might be having difficulty acknowledging.

Andy had grown up in a very abusive household and readily became overwhelmed when people spoke harshly to him. He had recently had an encounter with someone who bullied him and was now consumed with anxiety, struggling against persistent, intrusive images, and was becoming concerned about a new bout of back pain and gastrointestinal distress. After discussing what had brought him to this state, I invited him to try a practice to help him better tolerate his experience. I asked him to stand with me at the window and look at a tree—to start at the top and describe everything he saw in detail—the leaves, branches, colors, and textures. Then we moved on to another tree and eventually to everything else we could see. I told him we were not trying to make his anxiety go away, to wipe out feelings about the hostile encounter, to get rid of the intrusive images, nor to eliminate his physical symptoms; rather, we were trying to bring some of his attention to the reality of the external world here and now so that he could notice his thoughts, feelings, and sensations arising against a backdrop of relatively safe and stable present reality. After focusing on nature in this way for a little while, he began to feel more confident. Because our session was ending, I suggested he spend the next hour walking around the neighborhood continuing to notice the trees and plants, bringing his attention to them as we had done at the window. He did this, and when I saw him at my next break between clients he felt able to drive home and continue with his day. The practice had helped him establish a sense of safety.

Mindfulness-Based Programs for Chronic Pain

One of the first medical treatment programs explicitly to teach mindfulness to clients, mindfulness-based stress reduction (MBSR), was designed for the management of chronic pain (Kabat-Zinn, 1982). Since then, mindfulness-based programs have been used to treat a wide variety of pain syndromes. In the early years, encouraging outcomes were frequently reported, but studies often lacked control groups or randomized designs (see Baer, 2003, and Grossman, Niemann, Schmidt, & Walach, 2004, for reviews). More recent studies are often better controlled (see Veehof, Oskam, Schreurs, & Bohlmeijer, 2011, and Siegel, 2013, for reviews). Overall, they demonstrate that mindfulness practice yields modest benefits in reducing pain intensity and more significant benefits in improving other quality-of-life measures. It is likely that the limited benefits of mindfulness meditation in reducing pain intensity are due to the fact that most studies involved teaching mindfulness alone, rather than integrating it into a more comprehensive rehabilitation program that addresses clients' beliefs about their pain, fear of movement, and the effects of anxiety related to disavowed thoughts, feelings, and memories. Anecdotal evidence indicates that such a more comprehensive approach can be quite effective (Siegel et al., 2001).

Programs such as MBSR are usually conducted in groups and include considerable meditation practice involving internal objects of awareness, such as the sensations of the breath. These programs can therefore readily flood traumatized individuals with unwanted thoughts, feelings, and images. Individual treatments, in which the type of mindfulness practice can be tailored to the changing safety needs of the client, are probably better alternatives for traumatized populations.

Psychological and Neurobiological Mechanisms of Action

As mindfulness practices are being increasingly used for chronic pain and evidence is mounting for their efficacy, researchers have begun investigating their mechanisms of action. One set of studies measures the level of mindfulness of clients with chronic pain to see how it relates to their physical, social, cognitive, and emotional functioning. Data suggest that higher levels of mindfulness correspond to better functioning, primarily by lessening pain-related anxiety and patterns of avoidance and disability (Cho, Heiby, McCracken, Lee, & Moon, 2010; Schutze, Rees, Preece, & Schutze, 2010).

Another area of investigation has looked at how experienced meditators react to experimentally induced pain. The evidence suggests that (1) experienced meditators perceive painful stimuli as less unpleasant than do inexperienced controls (Brown & Jones, 2010); (2) experienced meditators report stronger tendencies to observe pain sensations nonreactively (Grant & Rainville, 2009); (3) open monitoring (mindfulness per se) results in a significant reduction of pain unpleasantness among experienced meditators, but not novices (Perlman, Salomons, Davidson, & Lutz, 2010); and (4) experienced meditators, but not inexperienced controls, have significant decreases in anticipatory pain anxiety when in a mindful state (Gard et al., 2011). Interestingly, one study found that whereas concentration increased pain intensity for inexperienced controls, it did not do so for more experienced meditators—suggesting that the latter group was able to *be with* painful stimuli without having a strong aversive reaction to it (Grant & Rainville, 2009).

The central mechanism suggested by all of these studies parallels the Buddha's story of the two arrows. By accepting pain sensations, rather than fighting, fearing, or trying to avoid them, we are able to tolerate more pain with less distress, whether the pain is caused by a medical condition or induced in the laboratory (Thompson & McCracken, 2011).

Another exciting line of research examines the brain regions that are activated when participants adopt different meditative attitudes toward experimentally induced pain. Two of these attitudes are (1) concentration or focused attention, in which we repeatedly return attention to a single object, and (2) mindfulness per se or open monitoring, in which we attend to whatever arises in awareness (Lutz, Slagter, Dunne, & Davidson, 2008). Investigators have found that experienced meditators who were exposed to painful stimuli while practicing open monitoring had decreased activity in the lateral prefrontal cortex (lPFC), an area associated with executive control and cognitive evaluation (Grant, Courtemanche, & Rainville, 2011; Gard et al., 2011). The meditators simultaneously showed increased activation in the posterior insula (Grant et al., 2011; Gard et al., 2011), which is understood to be involved in interoceptive and sensory processing (Craig, 2009). These findings suggest that mindfulness practice decreases the experience of pain and pain-related anxiety through increased processing of the pain sensations themselves, coupled with letting go of resistance. Researchers seem to be observing on a neurobiological level how experienced meditators experience less distress by opening to pain sensations with acceptance.

Mindfulness Practices for Chronic Pain

The following practices can be offered to clients within the context of comprehensive treatment for chronic pain, as outlined earlier. The first exercise is designed to open to the experience of pain while letting go of habitual fear and other aversion reactions. Because it involves an inward focus, it should be used cautiously with trauma survivors who struggle with split-off, disavowed thoughts, feelings, and memories (further suggestions for the use of this meditation can be found in Siegel, 2010).

Separating the Two Arrows[2]

Begin by settling into your meditation seat and finding your breath. First simply attend to the breath, wherever it's most clearly felt in the body. Every time your mind wanders away from the sensations of breathing, gently bring it back. Try to observe the breath with as much precision as possible. Notice the texture of each breath and examine its complex and varied qualities. See if you can develop an attitude of interest or curiosity toward all of these sensations. (Continue for 10–15 minutes.)

Now that the mind has settled a bit, begin to shift your focus to wherever you feel discomfort, whether mild or strong. Allow the breath to settle into the background and bring your attention to the painful or uncomfortable sensations. Begin by attending to the general area of the pain. Relax and settle into the physical sensations. Try to carefully observe their nature—whether burning, tight, piercing, dull, sharp, and so forth.

Next, narrow your attention to zero in on the particular spot in your body that hurts the most. Try to bring the same attitude of precision, interest, curiosity, and acceptance to the discomfort that you brought to the breath. You're not trying to change it, but rather to just experience it clearly. Notice how the sensations vary subtly from moment to moment. Perhaps one second they throb, while the next they burn or ache. See if you can observe that "pain" is actually a series of momentary sensations strung together like frames in a movie, creating an illusion of continuity.

If the pain is very intense, and the mind recoils from the pain sensations, experiment with bringing your attention back to the general area of the pain or even back to the breath for a while, before returning your attention to the pain's precise source. Shifting your focus in this way will help you stay with the experience longer. As you stay with the pain sensations, notice any thoughts that arise in the mind. You might experiment with labeling them: for example, fearing, hating, worrying. The idea is to notice that the thoughts come and go independent of the pain sensations. (Continue for the next 10 minutes or so.)

Urge Surfing for Pain[2]

This practice is designed to help clients overcome kinesiophobia and engage in normal physical activity. It is presented here to help deal with pain that comes on when sitting, though it can be adapted to most situations in which pain interferes with an activity

---

[2]Adapted with permission from Siegel (2010). Copyright 2010 by Ronald D. Siegel. Available free of charge in audio at *www.mindfulness-solution.com*.

Close your eyes and first bring your attention to your breath for a few minutes. Next allow yourself to be with the pain sensations, attending to them with curiosity and interest, as in the previous exercise. See how they change from moment to moment.

If the urge to get up or stop your activity arises, notice exactly where in your body you feel the urge. Bring your full attention to it, noticing its intensity and texture. See how the urge to get up or stop is distinct from the pain sensations themselves.

Now return your attention partially to your breath. Using your breath as a surfboard, ride each wave of urgency from its beginning as a small wavelet to the point where it crests. Allow each wave to rise up as high as it wants, trusting that it will reach a crescendo and then subside again.

Conclusion

Although many instances of pain are indeed due to the effects of illness, injury, or structural abnormality, others are caused or maintained by psychological processes. For individuals with significant unresolved trauma who struggle to keep painful thoughts, feelings, and memories out of awareness or who generally experience the world as threatening, the likelihood of getting stuck in psychogenic pain syndromes is increased. Luckily, mindfulness practices introduced by a skilled clinician, in the context of a comprehensive rehabilitation program, can help many people to break free of these disorders.

References

Ablin, J. N., Cohen, H., Clauw, D. J., Shalev, R., Ablin, E., Neumann, L., et al. (2010). A tale of two cities: The effect of low intensity conflict on prevalence and characteristics of musculoskeletal pain and somatic symptoms associated with chronic stress. *Clinical and Experimental Rheumatology, 28*(6, Suppl. 63), S15–S21.

Amital, D., Fostick, L., Polliack, M. L., Segev, S., Zohar, J., Rubinow, A., et al. (2006). Posttraumatic stress disorder, tenderness, and fibromyalgia syndrome: Are they different entities? *Journal of Psychosomatic Research, 61*(5), 663–669.

Baer, R. (2003). Mindfulness training as a clinical intervention: A conceptual and empirical review. *Clinical Psychology: Science and Practice, 10*(2), 125–142.

Beecher, H. K. (1946). Pain in men wounded in battle. *Annals of Surgery, 123*(1), 96–105.

Brewer, J. A., Sinha, R., Chen, J. A., Michalsen, R. N., Babuscio, T. A., Nich, C., et al. (2009). Mindfulness training and stress reactivity in substance abuse: Results from a randomized, controlled stage I pilot study. *Substance Abuse, 30*(4), 306–317.

Brown, C. A., & Jones, A. K. (2010). Meditation experience predicts less negative appraisal of pain: Electrophysiological evidence for the involvement of anticipatory neural responses. *Pain, 150*(3), 428–438.

Burgmer, M., Petzke, F., Giesecke, T., Gaubitz, M., Heuft, G., & Pfleiderer, B. (2011). Cerebral activation and catastrophizing during pain anticipation in patients with fibromyalgia. *Psychosomatic Medicine, 73*(9), 751–759.

Burns, J. W., Quartana, P. J., Gilliam, W., Matsuura, J., Nappi, C., & Wolfe, B. (2012). Suppression of anger and subsequent pain intensity and behavior among chronic low back pain patients: The role of symptom-specific physiological reactivity. *Journal of Behavioral Medicine, 35*(1), 103–114.

Burris, J. L., Cyders, M. A., de Leeuw, R., Smith, G. T., & Carlson, C. R. (2009). Posttraumatic stress disorder symptoms and chronic orofacial pain: An empirical examination of the mutual maintenance model. *Journal of Orofacial Pain, 23*(3), 243–252.

Cho, S., Heiby, E. M., McCracken, L. M., Lee, S. M., & Moon, D. E. (2010). Pain-related anxiety as a mediator of the effects of mindfulness on physical and psychosocial functioning in chronic pain patients in Korea. *Journal of Pain, 11*(8), 789–797.

Chou, R., Qaseem, A., Snow, V., Casey, D., Cross, J. T., Shekelle, P., et al. (2007). Diagnosis and treatment of low back pain: A joint clinical practice guideline from the American College of Physicians and the American Pain Society. *Annals of Internal Medicine, 147*(7), 478–491.

Cloitre, M., Cohen, L. R., & Koenen, K. C. (2006). *Treating survivors of childhood abuse: Psychotherapy for the interrupted life.* New York: Guilford Press.

Craig, A. D. (2009). How do you feel—now?: The anterior insula and human awareness. *Nature Reviews Neuroscience, 10*(1), 59–70.

Freud, S. (1959). Inhibitions, symptoms and anxiety. In J. Strachey (Ed. & Trans.), *The standard edition of the complete psychological works of Sigmund Freud* (Vol. 20, pp. 87–157). London: Hogarth Press. (Original work published 1926)

Gard, T., Holzel, B. K., Sack, A. T., Hempel, H., Lazar, S. W., Vaitl, D., et al. (2011). Pain attenuation through mindfulness is associated with decreased cognitive control and increased sensory processing in the brain. *Cerebral Cortex, 22,* 2692–2702. Available at *http://cercor.oxfordjournals.org/content/early/2011/12/14/cercor.bhr352.abstract.*

Germer, C. K. (2009). *The mindful path to self-compassion: Freeing yourself from destructive thoughts and emotions.* New York: Guilford Press.

Germer, C. K. (2013). Mindfulness: What is it? What does it matter? In C. K. Germer, R. D. Siegel, & P. R. Fulton (Eds.), *Mindfulness and psychotherapy* (2nd ed., pp. 3–35) New York: Guilford Press.

Goldin, P. R., & Gross, J. J. (2010). Effects of mindfulness-based stress reduction (MBSR) on emotion regulation in social anxiety disorder. *Emotion, 10*(1), 83–91.

Grant, J. A., Courtemanche, J., & Rainville, P. (2011). A non-elaborative mental stance and decoupling of executive and pain-related cortices predicts low pain sensitivity in Zen meditators. *Pain, 152*(1), 150–156.

Grant, J. A., & Rainville, P. (2009). Pain sensitivity and analgesic effects of mindful states in Zen meditators: A cross-sectional study. *Psychosomatic Medicine*, 71(1), 106–114.

Grossman, P., Niemann, L., Schmidt, S., & Walach, H. (2004). Mindfulness-based stress reduction and health benefits: A meta-analysis. *Journal of Psychosomatic Research*, 57(1), 35–43.

Herman, J. (1997). *Trauma and recovery: The aftermath of violence—from domestic abuse to political terror.* New York: Basic Books.

Kabat-Zinn, J. (1982). An outpatient program in behavioral medicine for chronic pain patients based on the practice of mindfulness meditation: Theoretical considerations and preliminary results. *General Hospital Psychiatry, 4,* 33–47.

Kendall-Tackett, K. A., Marshall, R., & Ness, K. E. (2003). Chronic pain syndromes and violence against women. *Women and Therapy, 26,* 45–56.

Kopec, J. A., & Sayre, E. C. (2004). Work-related psychosocial factors and chronic pain: A prospective cohort study in Canadian workers. *Journal of Occupational and Environmental Medicine, 46*(12), 1263–1271.

Levine, P. A. (2008). *Healing trauma: A pioneering program for restoring the wisdom of your body.* Louisville, CO: Sounds True.

Lutz, A., Slagter, H. A., Dunne, J. D., & Davidson, R. J. (2008). Attention regulation and monitoring in meditation. *Trends in Cognitive Sciences, 12*(4), 163–169.

McEwen, B. S. (2000). Allostasis and allostatic load: Implications for neuropsychopharmacology. *Neuropsychopharmacology, 22*(2), 108–124.

Melzack, R., & Wall, P. D. (1965). Pain mechanisms: A new theory. *Science, 150*(699), 971–979.

Naring, G. W., van Lankveld, W., & Geenen, R. (2007). Somatoform dissociation and traumatic experiences in patients with rheumatoid arthritis and fibromyalgia. *Clinical and Experimental Rheumatology, 25*(6), 872–877.

Pennebaker, J. W., Keicolt-Glaser, J. K., & Glaser, R. (1988). Disclosure of traumas and immune function: Health implications for psychotherapy. *Journal of Consulting and Clinical Psychology, 56*(2), 239–245.

Perlman, D. M., Salomons, T. V., Davidson, R. J., & Lutz, A. (2010). Differential effects on pain intensity and unpleasantness of two meditation practices. *Emotion, 10*(1), 65–71.

Peterlin, B. L., Tietjen, G. E., Brandes, J. L., Rubin, S. M., Drexler, E., Lidicker, J. R., et al. (2009). Posttraumatic stress disorder in migraine. *Headache, 49*(4), 541–551.

Pole, N., Neylan, T. C., Otte, C., Metzler, T. J., Best, S. R., Henn-Haase, C., et al. (2007). Associations between childhood trauma and emotion-modulated psychophysiological responses to startling sounds: A study of police cadets. *Journal of Abnormal Psychology, 116*(2), 352–361.

Pollak, S. M., Pedulla, T., & Siegel, R. D. (2014). *Sitting together: Essential skills for mindfulness-based psychotherapy.* New York: Guilford Press.

Rainville, J., Sobel, J., Hartigan, C., Monlux, G., & Bean, J. (1997) Decreasing disability in chronic back pain through aggressive spine rehabilitation. *Journal of Rehabilitation Research and Development, 34*(4), 383–393.

Roelofs, K., & Spinhoven, P. (2007). Trauma and medically unexplained symptoms:

Towards an integration of cognitive and neuro-biological accounts. *Clinical Psychology Review, 27*(7), 798–820.

Sapolsky, R. M. (2004). *Why zebras don't get ulcers* (3rd ed.). New York: Holt.

Scaer, R. C. (2007). *The body bears the burden: Trauma, dissociation, and disease* (2nd ed.). New York: Routledge.

Schofferman, J., Anderson, D., Hines, R., Smith, G., & Keane, G. (1993). Childhood psychological trauma and chronic refractory low-back pain. *Clinical Journal of Pain, 9*(4), 260–265.

Schutze, R., Rees, C., Preece, M., & Schutze, M. (2010). Low mindfulness predicts pain catastrophizing in a fear-avoidance model of chronic pain. *Pain, 148*(1), 120–127.

Schwartz. G. E. (1990). Psychobiology of repression and health: A systems approach. In J. L. Singer (Ed.), *Repression and dissociation: Defense mechanisms and personality styles: Current theory and research* (pp. 405–434). Chicago: University of Chicago Press.

Siegel, R. D. (2010). *The mindfulness solution: Everyday practices for everyday problems.* New York: Guilford Press.

Siegel, R. D. (2013). Psychophysiological disorders: Embracing pain. In C. K. Germer, R. D. Siegel, & P. R. Fulton (Eds.), *Mindfulness and psychotherapy* (2nd ed., pp. 184–207). New York: Guilford Press.

Siegel, R. D., Urdang, M. H., & Johnson, D. R. (2001). *Back sense: A revolutionary approach to halting the cycle of back pain.* New York: Broadway Books.

Thanissaro, B. (Trans.). (2012). *Sallatha Sutta [The Arrow].* Retrieved January 18, 2012, from *www.accesstoinsight.org/canon/sutta/samyutta/sn36-006.html#shot.*

Thompson, M., & McCracken, L. M. (2011). Acceptance and related processes in adjustment to chronic pain. *Current Pain and Headache Reports, 15*(2), 144–151.

Tietjen, G. E., Brandes, J. L., Peterlin, B. L., Eloff, A., Dafer, R. M., Stein, M. R., et al. (2010a). Childhood maltreatment and migraine: Part I. Prevalence and adult revictimization: A multicenter headache clinic survey. *Headache, 50*(1), 20–31.

Tietjen, G. E., Brandes, J. L., Peterlin, B. L., Eloff, A., Dafer, R. M., Stein, M. R., et al. (2010b). Childhood maltreatment and migraine: Part II. Emotional abuse as a risk factor for headache chronification. *Headache, 50*(1), 32–41.

Tietjen, G. E., Brandes, J. L., Peterlin, B. L., Eloff, A., Dafer, R. M., Stein, M. R., et al. (2010c). Childhood maltreatment and migraine: Part III. Association with comorbid pain conditions. *Headache, 50*(1), 42–51.

Tucker, P., Pfefferbaum, B., North, C. S., Kent, A., Jeon-Slaughter, H., & Parker, D. E. (2010). Biological correlates of direct exposure to terrorism several years postdisaster. *Annals of Clinical Psychiatry, 22*(3), 186–195.

Veehof, M. M., Oskam, M. J., Schreurs, K. M., & Bohlmeijer, E. T. (2011). Acceptance-based interventions for the treatment of chronic pain: A systematic review and meta-analysis. *Pain, 152*(3), 533–542.

Winnicott, D. (1960). The theory of the parent–child relationship. *International Journal of Psychoanalysis, 41,* 585–595.

17

Mindfulness-Based Stress Reduction and Loving-Kindness Meditation for Traumatized Veterans

David J. Kearney

Veterans are in need of programs to help them live meaningful, productive lives in the face of significant challenges and difficulties. A significant proportion of returning war veterans meet criteria for at least one mental health condition. For example, a study of approximately 104,000 veterans of Operations Enduring Freedom and Iraqi Freedom (OEF/OIF) who accessed care at a Veterans Administration (VA) health care facility found that 25% promptly received a mental health diagnosis and that among those receiving a mental health diagnosis, more than half were diagnosed with two or more distinct mental health conditions (Seal, Bertenthal, Miner, Sen, & Marmar, 2007). The most common mental health diagnosis code was posttraumatic stress disorder (PTSD), which affected 13% of OEF/OIF veterans who accessed VA health care. Other studies have found prevalence rates of PTSD (assessed conservatively, years after the conflict) of 10% for veterans of the first Gulf War (Kang, Mahan, Lee, Magee, & Murphy, 2000) and of 8.5% for female and 15.2% for male Vietnam veterans (Schlenger et al., 1992). Without help, for those veterans with trauma and posttraumatic stress disorder (PTSD), the toll across the lifespan for both the veteran and his or her family is likely to be large. It is estimated that a person with PTSD will experience active symptoms for at least 20 years across the lifespan (Kessler, 2000). PTSD often disrupts interpersonal relationships, reduces the ability to work, impairs quality of life, and increases the risk of affective disorders (Davidson, 2001; Kessler, Sonnega, Bromet, Hughes, & Nelson, 1995), alcohol/substance abuse disorders (Kessler et al., 1995), and suicidality (Kessler, Borges, & Walters, 1999). It is important to note that a significant proportion of PTSD among veterans is not combat-related; many who serve in the military have experienced other forms of trauma, including sexual trauma, which occurs at alarming rates (Murdoch, Polusny, Hodges, & O'Brien, 2004; Williams & Bernstein, 2011). In a recent study of veterans with PTSD in a large urban VA hospital, the average number of *different categories* of trauma reported by veterans over the course of their lives was *10* (Kearney, McDermott, Malte, Martinez, & Simpson, 2012a).

Chronic physical pain conditions commonly co-occur with PTSD and can present additional difficulties for a person with a history of trauma who is seeking to regain a sense of functionality and well-being. For example, in an analysis of 92 veterans with a high prevalence of PTSD who participated in a mindfulness program at our facility, 67% had a chronic pain condition and 45% had *two or more* conditions associated with chronic pain (Kearney, McDermott, Malte, Martinez, & Simpson, 2012b). Other research has shown that people with PTSD are at increased risk for physical illnesses, including hypertension, cardiovascular disease, asthma, fibromyalgia, and digestive disorders and overall mortality (Boscarino, 2004), after adjusting for other risk factors. The co-occurrence of multiple physical and mental health conditions with PTSD often leads to lower ratings of general health (Hoge, Terhakopian, Castro, Messer, & Engel, 2007). Thus programs designed to enhance functionality and quality of life across multiple domains of health are greatly needed. One type of program that appears promising in this regard is teaching mindfulness.

Mindfulness Programs for Veterans with PTSD

At our facility, we have begun to offer mindfulness teaching as an adjunct to the care of veterans with a wide range of problems, including PTSD. The format we use to teach mindfulness is a standardized 8-week class series called mindfulness-based stress reduction (MBSR; Kabat-Zinn, 1990), which is widely available. A pragmatic goal of MBSR is to provide a format that results in sufficient understanding and familiarity with mindfulness practices so that participants can continue these self-care practices on their own after leaving the program. In this setting, participation in a mindfulness program is not considered a primary treatment package for PTSD. Rather, participation in a structured mindfulness program is offered as a method of working with persistent suffering and pain, to enhance self-compassion, promote healing, enhance well-being, and improve quality of life. Although multiple studies indicate a large decrement in health-related quality of life for people with PTSD (Olatunji, Cisler, & Tolin,

2007), interventions with quality-of-life improvement as a primary goal (not necessarily symptom reduction) have received little attention (Mogotsi, Kaminer, & Stein, 2000). Although there are psychological processes influenced by mindfulness practice that might plausibly lead to reductions in PTSD symptoms (discussed later), another possibility is that development of compassion can bring enhanced freedom and functionality even in the face of persistent symptoms.

In our setting, we have found that programs based on teaching meditation appear acceptable to—even popular among—veterans. This finding is consistent with the larger literature on complementary and alternative medicine (CAM) use by veterans, who use various CAM interventions at high rates (Baldwin, Long, Kroesen, Brooks, & Bell, 2002; Micek et al., 2007). High daily stress, chronic medical illness, and a perceived negative impact of military service on mental or physical health are predictors of CAM use among veterans (Baldwin et al., 2002). Qualitative research among veterans indicates that dissatisfaction with reliance on prescription medications and neglect of social and spiritual aspects of health serve as motivating factors for CAM use (Kroesen, Baldwin, Brooks, & Bell, 2002).

Theoretical Rationale for Mindfulness Programs in PTSD Treatment

Although at this time scientific data are limited, psychological processes influenced by mindfulness practice can be hypothesized to have favorable impact on the lives of people with PTSD. The following comments remain speculative and are provided as possible avenues for future research.

Mindfulness has been operationally defined as "the awareness that emerges by way of paying attention on purpose, in the present moment, and nonjudgmentally to the unfolding of experience moment by moment" (Kabat-Zinn, 2002). Although there is some debate as to whether this definition of mindfulness agrees precisely with the definition provided in the Buddhist historical record (Gethin, 2011), I have found this definition to be helpful in teaching and understanding mindfulness practice. Enhanced mindfulness has been hypothesized to foster acceptance, constructive cognitive change, and constructive behavioral changes and to represent a form of exposure therapy (Baer, 2003). Creation of an attuned and responsive internal environment through mindfulness practice has also been described as mimicking the "holding environment" of an attuned and attentive parent (Epstein, 2013). Mindfulness practices encourage an approach-oriented attitude toward, rather than avoidance of, distressing thoughts, feelings, and physical sensations. Thus consistent engagement in mindfulness practice might result in decreased avoidance behaviors for people with PTSD over time (Kimbrough, Magyari, Langenberg, Chesney, & Berman, 2010; Vujanovic, Niles, Pietrefesa, Schmertz, & Potter, 2011). The attitudinal qualities taught in MBSR run counter to deeply ingrained tendencies to avoid potentially distressing situations or suppress pervasive feelings of shame and guilt, which are hallmarks of PTSD. In MBSR, when habitual patterns of shame, guilt, self-criticism, or judgment arise in meditation practice, participants are encouraged to notice these patterns with an attitude of kindness and self-compassion, to disengage from judgments, and to regard these phenomena in a broader field of awareness.

An additional mechanism by which mindfulness practice might favorably influence PTSD symptoms is through reduced reactivity to intrusive thoughts. In mindfulness meditation practice, thoughts are regarded as passing events and temporary objects of attention, not phenomena to be identified with, avoided, or suppressed. For people with PTSD, thought suppression paradoxically increases reexperiencing (Shipherd & Beck, 2005), and enhanced mindfulness is associated with reduced thought suppression (Bowen, Witkiewitz, Dillworth, & Marlatt, 2007). For people with depression who participate in a mindfulness program, enhanced self-compassion has been shown to play a key role in improved outcomes by changing the relationship to dysfunctional thoughts; improvements in depressive symptoms occur despite the continued presence of dysfunctional attitudes, beliefs, and rules (Kuyken et al., 2010). Enhanced self-compassion could be hypothesized to play a similar role in PTSD.

Enhanced mindfulness also results in reduced rumination (Williams, 2008), and reduced rumination is another potential mechanism by which mindfulness interventions could lessen PTSD symptoms; prior research indicates that rumination plays a role in worsening PTSD symptoms (Bennett & Wells, 2010). There is a tendency for people to adopt an evaluative, ruminative stance regarding trauma, and mindfulness courses teach people to see these ruminative patterns more clearly and to learn the skill of "letting go" and disengaging from these patterns (Grabovac, Lau, & Willett, 2011). Also, what is commonly shared in class discussions are beliefs about oneself, others, and the world at large, which have been deeply influenced by prior trauma. For example, there may be beliefs that others are ungenerous or uncaring, that personal growth or intimacy is no longer possible, or simply that they cannot sit for 30 minutes and follow their breath. When these types of thoughts and beliefs are shared, the participants are encouraged to see them clearly as ideas and beliefs, which may or may not represent reality. These ideas are greeted with curiosity, openness, and kindness by the teacher.

Preliminary Studies of MBSR for PTSD

Preliminary studies of outcomes associated with participation in mindfulness programs for traumatized people are reviewed in this section. Large-scale randomized controlled trials are needed and are currently under way.

A common clinical method of teaching mindfulness is a standardized class series of MBSR, which has previously been described in detail (Kabat-Zinn, 1990). Two before-and-after studies have assessed the efficacy of MBSR for PTSD, with evidence of improved PTSD symptoms and depression (Kearney et al., 2012b; Kimbrough et al., 2010). The first of these studies assessed the efficacy of an 8-week MBSR program (modified slightly for adult survivors of childhood sexual abuse) in 27 participants (15 of whom met criteria for PTSD). Findings included reductions in symptoms of depression and PTSD and a significant increase in mindfulness, with large effect sizes at a 4-month follow-up assessment (Kimbrough et al., 2010). The second outcome study was our own, of 92 veterans who took part in an 8-week MBSR program as an adjunct to usual care, with assessments at baseline, immediately post-MBSR, and 4 months later (Kearney et al., 2012b). MBSR was delivered in heterogeneous groups of 20–30 veterans, of whom nearly three-quarters met symptom criteria for PTSD. The MBSR courses followed closely the format originally developed at the University of Massachusetts Medical School (Kabat-Zinn, 1982), and similar to Kimbrough et al. (2010), we included instructions that encouraged participants to trust their intrinsic wisdom regarding whether to continue forward or pull back during any meditation practice. We found significant improvements in measures of mental health (including PTSD, depression, experiential avoidance, and behavioral activation) and mental and physical health-related quality of life over 4-month follow-up, with medium to large standardized effect sizes. At the immediate post-MBSR and 4-month follow-up time points, 31% and 34%, respectively, of those who screened positive for PTSD at baseline no longer met criteria for PTSD. Mindfulness skills increased significantly, and in a mediation model, mindfulness skills mediated the relationship between MBSR participation and improvement in key clinical outcomes (Kearney et al., 2012b).

In a follow-up pilot study, 47 veterans with PTSD were randomized to MBSR plus usual care, or usual care only, and assessed immediately post-MBSR and 4 months later. Those randomized to MBSR in addition to usual care showed significant improvements in mindfulness skills and improved functional status, but not in PTSD symptoms, in this small study (Kearney et al., 2012a). In a post hoc analysis in which reliable change in *both* functional status *and* PTSD symptoms was defined as treatment "success," 27% of veterans randomized to MBSR met this criterion for treatment success, as compared with 0% of those randomized to usual care; this was highly significant. In "completer" analyses, in which veterans randomized to MBSR who attended at least four MBSR classes (84%) were compared with those randomized to usual care, the MBSR arm also showed improvement in depressive symptoms and enhanced behavioral activation. Overall, the results showed that veterans with PTSD are able to learn mindfulness skills and that MBSR may hold promise as a resource for enhancing functionality and reducing depressive symptoms for veterans with PTSD.

Based on our overall experience teaching MBSR to a large number of veterans, MBSR appears safe for veterans with PTSD. We have not had veterans report flashbacks during the meditation practices taught in MBSR classes. The overall safety may in part be due to client self-selection, as well as to the client setting (most participants are actively engaged in additional mental health care). Of note, the meditation instructions in published studies of MBSR for PTSD also suggest a balance between wise effort and safety; participants are encouraged to trust their intrinsic wisdom and sometimes pause, stop meditation practice, or pull back in their effort if it feels wise and to do so without judgment (Kearney et al., 2012a, 2012b; Kimbrough et al., 2010). The apparent safety of these practices in the setting of trauma may also be due to the intrinsically gentle and gradual nature of the practices themselves.

Exclusion Criteria for Clinical Participation in MBSR

In our setting, we offer MBSR as a hospital-wide course. Veterans may either self-refer or be referred by a provider. We accept all veterans who have a desire to participate in MBSR after attending an orientation session and who do not have one of the following exclusion criteria noted in the medical record: psychotic disorder, poorly controlled bipolar disorder with mania, borderline or antisocial personality disorder, substance use disorder or alcohol use that poses a safety concern or is associated with an inability to keep appointments, suicide attempt or suicidal ideation with intent or plan, or self-harm within the past month. These exclusion criteria were adopted because of concerns that some conditions could disrupt the group process or would require closer monitoring than is possible in a large group setting.

Future Directions

The published literature regarding MBSR for PTSD has reported outcomes associated with participation in MBSR in its widely available form, that is, without significant modification of course content or structure for PTSD. However, it is possible that people with PTSD might experience greater benefit from MBSR if the program included PTSD-specific teaching aimed at bringing mindful awareness and understanding to subtle clinical manifestations of PTSD, such as emotional numbing and avoidance patterns in daily life. Thus one direction for future clinical applications could be to evaluate whether a modified MBSR course is more effective at influencing the core symptoms of PTSD. A small randomized controlled trial suggests that a telehealth mindfulness intervention (based on MBSR) may be a feasible mode of PTSD delivery for veterans (Niles et al., 2012). Other precedents for tailoring mindfulness interventions for specific clinical populations include mindfulness-based cognitive therapy (MBCT) for depression (Teasdale et al., 2000) and a modified version of MBSR that addresses prominent issues among teens (Biegel, Brown, Shapiro, & Schubert, 2009).

An additional challenge will be to assess whether MBSR is acceptable and efficacious to the younger generation of veterans returning from the wars in Iraq and Afghanistan (OIF/OEF/Operation New Dawn [OND] veterans) and how it might be modified to enhance acceptability and efficacy. The age of veterans involved in our programs has averaged in the fifth decade of life, although there have also been OIF/OEF veterans who have participated and benefited. Whether the current form of MBSR is the optimal format for returning OIF/OEF/OND veterans is an unanswered and important question.

Another possible future role for mindfulness training would be to offer participation in a mindfulness program to people before they participate in trauma-focused therapies for PTSD, such as prolonged exposure (PE) therapy or cognitive processing therapy. The ability to "stay with" difficult experience, as developed in mindfulness practice, with an attitude of self-compassion might hold the potential to decrease dropout rates from PE (shown to be 38% among a randomized controlled trial of female veterans; Schnurr et al., 2007) and thus improve the effectiveness of the intervention. For cognitive processing therapy, learning mindfulness skills could also be hypothesized to facilitate the ability to bring attention to fixed, limiting beliefs that can develop in the aftermath of trauma. In these ways, mindfulness training might be synergistic with existing, empirically supported treatments for PTSD.

An additional future direction is to explore meditation practices specifically intended to enhance compassion for oneself and others in people with a history of trauma. There is growing evidence that self-compassion is positively associated with healthy psychological functioning (Neff, Rude, & Kirkpatrick, 2007) and negatively associated with self-criticism, rumination, thought suppression, anxiety, and depression—all of which commonly occur in the setting of PTSD (Bennett & Wells, 2010). One study found that a measure of self-compassion accounted for as much as 10 times more unique variance in anxiety, depression, worry, and quality of life than a measure of mindfulness (Van Dam, Sheppard, Forsyth, & Earleywine, 2011). Another study, of a yoga-based intervention for young adults, found that although both mindfulness and self-compassion mediated effects of the group on quality of life, only self-compassion mediated the effect on perceived stress (Gard et al., 2012). Loving-kindness meditation (LKM) is a meditation practice that cultivates kindness and compassion for oneself and others. Practices that foster self-compassion and the ability to self-soothe may hold the potential to be particularly helpful for people with a history of trauma, given that many people with PTSD have long histories of traumatic experiences and have rarely felt safe or reassured. In MBSR, LKM is typically introduced during the day-long mindfulness retreat between weeks 6 and 7 of the 8-week course. We have begun to offer a 12-week LKM course for veterans with PTSD, with encouraging preliminary results (Kearney et al., 2013). In LKM, participants silently repeat phrases of positive intention. Example phrases include: "May I (you) be free from suffering. May I (you) be happy. May I (you) be safe." The participant is asked to first direct the phrases of positive intention to someone the participant holds in positive regard, followed by oneself, then a neutral person, and then for a person with whom they have experienced difficulty, and eventually to all beings (Salzberg, 1995). Many people with a history of severe trauma find this form of practice to be very helpful. The cultivation of positive emotions through LKM can be hypothesized to benefit the constrictive symptoms characteristic of chronic PTSD, which can present as feelings of chronic alienation, emotional numbness, and deadness. Further study is needed.

Conclusion

PTSD is a common consequence of trauma and is a worldwide problem. Despite the availability of medications and psychotherapy, many people with PTSD experience persistent symptoms and reduced quality of life. Given the large number of people with PTSD, not all of whom will benefit sufficiently or elect to participate in existing treatments, additional treatments suitable for broad implementation are needed. Recently, interventions that facilitate development of enhanced mindfulness, kindness, and self-compassion have been proposed as viable alternatives or complements to the standard trauma-focused interventions for PTSD. Our clinical experience and research, along with that of others, suggests that these interventions hold promise for traumatized veterans.

Acknowledgment

This material is based upon work supported by the U. S. Department of Veterans Affairs, Office of Research and Development, Clinical R&D Program.

References

Baer, R. A. (2003). Mindfulness training as a clinical intervention: A conceptual and empirical review. *Clinical Psychology: Science and Practice, 10*(2), 125–143.

Baldwin, C. M., Long, K., Kroesen, K., Brooks, A. J., & Bell, I. R. (2002). A profile of military veterans in the southwestern United States who use complementary and alternative medicine: Implications for integrated care. *Archives of Internal Medicine, 162*(15), 1697–1704.

Bennett, H., & Wells, A. (2010). Metacognition, memory disorganization and rumination in posttraumatic stress symptoms. *Journal of Anxiety Disorders*, 24(3), 318–325.

Biegel, G. M., Brown, K. W., Shapiro, S. L., & Schubert, C. M. (2009). Mindfulness-based stress reduction for the treatment of adolescent psychiatric outpatients: A randomized clinical trial. *Journal of Consulting and Clinical Psychology*, 77(5), 855–866.

Boscarino, J. A. (2004). Posttraumatic stress disorder and physical illness: Results from clinical and epidemiologic studies. In R. Yehuda & B. McEwen (Eds.), *Annals of the New York Academy of Sciences: Vol. 1032. Biobehavioral stress response: Protective and damaging effects* (pp. 141–153). New York: New York Academy of Sciences.

Bowen, S., Witkiewitz, K., Dillworth, T. M., & Marlatt, G. A. (2007). The role of thought suppression in the relationship between mindfulness meditation and alcohol use. *Addictive Behaviors*, 32(10), 2324–2328.

Davidson, J. R. T. (2001). Recognition and treatment of posttraumatic stress disorder. *Journal of the American Medical Association*, 286(5), 584–588.

Epstein, M. (2013). *The trauma of everyday life: A guide to inner peace*. New York: Penguin.

Gard, T., Brach, N., Holzel, B. K., Noggle, J. J., Conboy, L. A., & Lazar, S. W. (2012). Effects of a yoga-based intervention for young adults on quality of life and perceived stress: The potential mediating roles of mindfulness and self-compassion. *Journal of Positive Psychology*, 7(3), 165–175.

Gethin, R. (2011). On some definitions of mindfulness. *Contemporary Buddhism*, 12(1), 263–279.

Grabovac, A., Lau, M., & Willett, B. (2011). Mechanisms of mindfulness: A Buddhist psychological model. *Mindfulness*, 2(3), 154–166.

Hoge, C. W., Terhakopian, A., Castro, C. A., Messer, S. C., & Engel, C. C. (2007). Association of posttraumatic stress disorder with somatic symptoms, health care visits, and absenteeism among Iraq war veterans. *American Journal of Psychiatry*, 164(1), 150–153.

Kabat-Zinn, J. (1982). An outpatient program in behavioral medicine for chronic pain patients based on the practice of mindfulness meditation: Theoretical considerations and preliminary results. *General Hospital Psychiatry*, 4(1), 33–47.

Kabat-Zinn, J. (1990). *Full catastrophe living: Using the wisdom of your body and mind to face stress, pain and illness*. New York: Bantam Doubleday Dell.

Kabat-Zinn, J. (2002). Commentary on Majumdar et al.: Mindfulness meditation and health. *Journal of Alternative and Complementary Medicine*, 8(6), 731–735.

Kang, H. K., Mahan, C. M., Lee, K. Y., Magee, C. A., & Murphy, F. M. (2000). Illnesses among United States veterans of the Gulf War: A population-based survey of 30,000 veterans. *Journal of Occupational and Environmental Medicine*, 42(5), 491–501.

Kearney, D. J., Malte, C. A., McManus, C., Martinez, M., Felleman, B., & Simpson, T. L. (2013). Loving-kindness meditation for posttraumatic stress disorder: A pilot study. *Journal of Traumatic Stress*, 26(4), 426–434.

Kearney, D. J., McDermott, K., Malte, C., Martinez, M., & Simpson, T. L. (2012a).

Effects of participation in a mindfulness program for veterans with posttraumatic stress disorder (PTSD): A randomized controlled pilot study. *Journal of Clinical Psychology, 69*(1), 14–27.

Kearney, D. J., McDermott, K., Malte, C. A., Martinez, M., & Simpson, T. L. (2012b). Association of participation in a mindfulness program with measures of PTSD, depression and quality of life in a veteran sample. *Journal of Clinical Psychology, 68*(1), 101–116.

Kessler, R. C. (2000). Posttraumatic stress disorder: The burden to the individual and to society. *Journal of Clinical Psychiatry, 61*(Suppl. 15), 4–12.

Kessler, R. C., Borges, G., & Walters, E. E. (1999). Prevalence of and risk factors for lifetime suicide attempts in the National Comorbidity Survey. *Archives of General Psychiatry, 56*(7), 617–626.

Kessler, R. C., Sonnega, A., Bromet, E., Hughes, M., & Nelson, C. B. (1995). Posttraumatic stress disorder in the National Comorbidity Survey. *Archives of General Psychiatry, 52*(12), 1048–1060.

Kimbrough, E., Magyari, T., Langenberg, P., Chesney, M., & Berman, B. (2010). Mindfulness intervention for child abuse survivors. *Journal of Clinical Psychology, 66*(1), 17–33.

Kroesen, K., Baldwin, C. M., Brooks, A. J., & Bell, I. R. (2002). U.S. military veterans' perceptions of the conventional medical care system and their use of complementary and alternative medicine. *Family Practice, 19*(1), 57–64.

Kuyken, W., Watkins, E., Holden, E., White, K., Taylor, R. S., Byford, S., et al. (2010). How does mindfulness-based cognitive therapy work? *Behaviour Research and Therapy, 48*(11), 1105–1112.

Micek, M. A., Bradley, K. A., Braddock, C. H., Maynard, C., McDonell, M., & Fihn, S. D. (2007). Complementary and alternative medicine use among Veterans Affairs outpatients. *Journal of Alternative and Complementary Medicine, 13*(2), 190–193.

Mogotsi, M., Kaminer, D., & Stein, D. J. (2000). Quality of life in the anxiety disorders. *Harvard Review of Psychiatry, 8*(6), 273–282.

Murdoch, M., Polusny, M. A., Hodges, J., & O'Brien, N. (2004). Prevalence of in-service and post-service sexual assault among combat and noncombat veterans applying for Department of Veterans Affairs posttraumatic stress disorder disability benefits. *Military Medicine, 169*(5), 392–395.

Neff, K. D., Rude, S. S., & Kirkpatrick, K. L. (2007). An examination of self-compassion in relation to positive psychological functioning and personality traits. *Journal of Research in Personality, 41*(4), 908–916.

Niles, B. L., Klunk-Gillis, J., Ryngala, D. J., Silberbogen, A. K., Paysnick, A., & Wolf, E. J. (2012). Comparing mindfulness and psychoeducation treatments for combat-related PTSD using a telehealth approach. *Psychological Trauma: Theory, Research, Practice, and Policy, 4*(5), 538–547.

Olatunji, B. O., Cisler, J. M., & Tolin, D. F. (2007). Quality of life in the anxiety disorders: A meta-analytic review. *Clinical Psychology Review, 27*(5), 572–581.

Salzberg, S. (1995). *Lovingkindness: The revolutionary art of happiness.* Boston: Shambhala.

Schlenger, W. E., Kulka, R. A., Fairbank, J. A., Hough, R. L., Jordan, B. K., Marmar, C. R., et al. (1992). The prevalence of posttraumatic stress disorder in the Vietnam generation: A multimethod, multisource assessment of psychiatric disorder. *Journal of Traumatic Stress, 5*(3), 333–363.

Schnurr, P. P., Friedman, M. J., Engel, C. C., Foa, E. B., Shea, M. T., Chow, B. K., et al. (2007). Cognitive-behavioral therapy for posttraumatic stress disorder in women: A randomized controlled trial. *Journal of the American Medical Association, 297*(8), 820–830.

Seal, K. H., Bertenthal, D., Miner, C. R., Sen, S., & Marmar, C. (2007). Bringing the war back home: Mental health disorders among 103,788 U.S. veterans returning from Iraq and Afghanistan seen at Department of Veterans Affairs facilities. *Archives of Internal Medicine, 167*(5), 476–482.

Shipherd, J. C., & Beck, J. G. (2005). The role of thought suppression in posttraumatic stress disorder. *Behavior Therapy, 36*(3), 277–287.

Teasdale, J. D., Segal, Z. V., Williams, J. M. G., Ridgeway, V. A., Soulsby, J. M., & Lau, M. A. (2000). Prevention of relapse/recurrence in major depression by mindfulness-based cognitive therapy. *Journal of Consulting and Clinical Psychology, 68*(4), 615–623.

Van Dam, N. T., Sheppard, S. C., Forsyth, J. P., & Earleywine, M. (2011). Self-compassion is a better predictor than mindfulness of symptom severity and quality of life in mixed anxiety and depression. *Journal of Anxiety Disorders, 25*(1), 123–130.

Vujanovic, A. A., Niles, B., Pietrefesa, A., Schmertz, S. K., & Potter, C. M. (2011). Mindfulness in the treatment of posttraumatic stress disorder among military veterans. *Professional Psychology: Research and Practice, 42*(1), 24–31.

Williams, I., & Bernstein, K. (2011). Military sexual trauma among U.S. female veterans. *Archives of Psychiatric Nursing, 25*(2), 138–147.

Williams, J. M. G. (2008). Mindfulness, depression and modes of mind. *Cognitive Therapy and Research, 32*(6), 721–733.

18

Treating Childhood Trauma with Mindfulness

Randye J. Semple and Laila A. Madni

Childhood is sometimes characterized in books and movies as being an idyllic and carefree time. However, research suggests that more than two-thirds of all children are exposed to at least one potentially traumatic event prior to adulthood (Copeland, Keeler, Angold, & Costello, 2007). Many are neglected or abused by those they are dependent on the most—parents, caregivers, or other adults in positions of trust (e.g., Finkelhor et al., 2009). Others are bullied and/or physically or sexually assaulted by their peers or older children (e.g., Singer, Anglin, Song, & Lunghofer, 1995) or are exposed to fires, accidents, natural disasters, or life-threatening medical conditions (e.g., Saltzman, Babayan, Lester, Beardslee, Pynoos, et al., 2008; Vogel & Vernberg, 1993).

In many cases, childhood trauma is compounded by adverse social factors, such as parental unemployment, divorce, and neighborhood crime (Twenge, 2000). In the United States, 15.5 million children live in families with incomes below the federal poverty level (Addy & Wight, 2012). Many of these children live in decaying crime- and drug-infested neighborhoods and are regularly exposed to violence or gang activities (Schwab-Stone et al., 1995).

Consequences of Childhood Trauma

Trauma exposure can lead to a wide range of psychiatric, medical, social, academic, occupational, and criminal problems throughout adolescence and adulthood (see Copeland, Miller-Johnson, Keeler, Angold, & Costello, 2007; Dube et al., 2006; Kubak & Salekin, 2009; Ramiro, Madrid, & Brown, 2010). Abused children often develop negative representations of themselves and others, which then influence how they interpret events and interact with others. These children may have trouble with relational problem solving or may be seen by family and friends as being socially immature, unable to trust others, physically aggressive, emotionally overreactive, and generally more difficult than nonabused children (Hildyard & Wolfe, 2002).

One of the most common impacts of trauma in childhood involve symptoms of posttraumatic stress disorder (PTSD; American Psychiatric Association, 2013). Children experiencing posttraumatic stress often present with an array of cognitive, emotional, physiological, and behavioral symptoms. These include trauma-specific fears; fears of recurrence; intrusive trauma-related thoughts or images; nightmares and other sleep disturbances; anxiety, depression, irritability, or anger; and pessimistic attitudes about themselves, others, and the future (Jon A. Shaw, 2000). Behaviorally, children may display age-regressive behaviors such as crying, temper tantrums, separation anxieties, and school refusal. Posttraumatic play reenactments, somatic symptoms, avoidance of traumatic reminders, and social or academic problems are also common (Vogel & Vernberg, 1993). Depersonalization, or disconnecting from emotions and physical sensations, is also not uncommon in traumatized children (Michal et al., 2007). Behavioral avoidance can become a major problem. This has been shown to be true in youth of all ages, although younger children may display more somatic symptoms to avoid daily activities, whereas adolescents are more likely to isolate themselves or to develop alcohol or other substance-related problems (Dube et al., 2006).

Clearly, one of the most important challenges that parents, educators, and mental health professionals face is to help children and adolescents avoid or overcome psychological and behavioral problems in the aftermath of chronic daily stressors, victimization, and other potentially traumatic experiences. As also indicated for adults in other chapters in this volume, there are a number of interventions that may be helpful in the treatment of such children. We suggest that "mindfulness" training may be especially helpful, as described next.

Mindfulness in the Moment and Afterward

One often quoted definition of mindfulness is "paying attention in a particular way: on purpose, in the present moment, and non-judgmentally" (Kabat-Zinn, 1994, p. 4). The effectiveness of structured mindfulness-based interventions in treating a variety of adult mood and anxiety problems is now well established (see recent meta-analyses by Hofmann, Sawyer, Witt, & Oh, 2010; Piet & Hougaard, 2011). Unfortunately, research on the effectiveness of this approach with children is limited, and none has specifically addressed posttraumatic stress symptoms. In our clinical experience, however, and based on existing theoretical perspectives, it is likely that mindful awareness practices parallel many of the components that are known to be effective in treating traumatized children. These include identification of maladaptive trauma-related cognitions, affect regulation skills, decentering from thoughts, and therapeutic exposure to traumatic memories (Briere & Lanktree, 2012).

Anxiety is an emotion that is experienced in response to expectations of anticipated threat or danger. Traumatic events or situations, by definition, are sufficiently powerful to overwhelm the child's existing coping abilities. Physically, cognitively, and emotionally, the child's cope runneth over. During and after a traumatic event, cognitive catastrophizing can further escalate the impacts of what was already a very upsetting experience. High anxiety interferes with problem-solving and decision-making abilities (Bondolfi, 2005). Mindful awareness appears to enhance the individual's ability to stay focused on the most immediate, important, or relevant aspects of a challenging situation. Being able to modulate one's cognitive and emotional experiences and better manage behavioral reactivity allows greater access to situational, cognitive, and emotional information that might then be applied toward creative problem solving posttrauma (Mennin, Heimberg, Turk, & Fresco, 2005). Mindful awareness brings clarity to see what is happening in the moment—including recognizing that catastrophic thinking or intense emotional reactivity interferes with skillful decision making and makes it more difficult to respond appropriately or to choose the best behavioral responses. In this way, being able to decenter from catastrophic cognitions may improve affective self-regulation and increase the child's ability to see whatever choices might present themselves.

Posttraumatic anxieties are often sustained far beyond the precipitating traumatic event. Just as psychological debriefing following trauma may actually impede the natural recovery process (Mayou, Ehlers, & Hobbs, 2000), after the traumatic situation has resolved, repetitive cognitive ruminations about the experience that are maladaptive or distorted by strong emotions may increase the likelihood of developing posttraumatic stress symptoms (Speckens, Ehlers, Hackmann, Ruths, & Clark, 2007). Following the event, therefore, an ability to maintain the same present-focused clarity of thought and affective equanimity that develops with mindfulness practice can offer some protective resiliency and reduce the likelihood of the individual developing posttraumatic stress symptoms. As we discuss, even when posttraumatic stress does develop, mindfulness may serve several functions for the traumatized child, ranging from cognitive restructuring to a form of intrapsychic exposure therapy.

Adapting Mindfulness for Children

Mindful awareness practices are being taught more frequently to children and adolescents in clinic, school, community, and retreat settings. Evaluation of these techniques for developmental appropriateness or effectiveness is in the very early stages, however, and few manualized treatments are currently available. Well-controlled effectiveness studies, although promising, are still limited. In this chapter, we explore how one mindfulness-based therapy for children might be helpful for children suffering from posttraumatic stress symptoms.

Mindfulness-based cognitive therapy for children (MBCT-C; Semple & Lee, 2011) is a child-friendly psychotherapy for anxious children ages 8–12 years old. It was adapted from two well-known adult programs: mindfulness-based stress reduction (MBSR; Kabat-Zinn, 1990) and mindfulness-based cognitive therapy (MBCT; Segal, Williams, & Teasdale, 2002, 2013). Translating an adult therapy for use with children always requires significant practical adaptations, but the theoretical model and broad aims of MBCT-C are consistent with the adult MBSR and MBCT programs.

MBCT-C is a structured 12-week group program of mindfulness training. Each weekly session lasts 90 minutes. Groups generally consist of six to eight children with one or two therapists. Before the children's program begins, parents attend an orientation session, during which they are introduced to some of the children's mindfulness activities and encouraged to practice at home with their children. To facilitate parental participation, all the children receive written summaries at each session with that week's home practice activities described.

Mindfulness is cultivated mainly by practicing mindful awareness activities, which in MBCT-C include a greater variety of activities than do the adult programs. Metacognitive awareness and insights emerge from a process of Socratic inquiry and dialogue that is facilitated by the therapist after each mindfulness activity (Briere & Lanktree, 2012). This is similar to the inquiries conducted in the adult MBSR and MBCT programs but generally includes less abstract explanations and more explicit practice guidance.

Following the introductory session, each session begins with a brief meditation and review of the previous week's home practice activities. In the initial sessions, one therapeutic aim is to help the children discover their own motivations for wanting to practice mindfulness. These are often related to some difficulty the child may be encountering in his or her daily life. Common examples include wanting to deal with debilitating test or social anxieties or to develop better anger-management skills.

Anyone who has tried to make a small child sit still for 45 minutes will immediately understand why significant adaptations from adult mindfulness training activities were necessary. The adaptations in MBCT-C are intended to meet a variety of developmental needs—cognitive, affective, physical, attentional, and relational—appropriate to elementary school-age children. Similar to MBSR and MBCT, the children cultivate mindfulness with seated breath meditations, simple yoga postures, and a technique known as the body scan (Kabat-Zinn, 1990), which is a guided activity of exploring interoceptive body sensations using directed attention. In MBCT-C, however, each of these activities lasts only 3–5 minutes. These basic techniques are practiced multiple times throughout the program by balancing creative repetition with variety. Repetition enhances learning, and the shorter activities make it easier to engage and maintain the children's interest. In addition to these customary adult mindfulness activities, children participate in a wide variety of activities that focus on developing mindful awareness in individual sensory modes (e.g., taste, touch, sight, sound, smell, and body kinesthetics). Each activity is structured to allow the child to practice bringing attention to the moment-by-moment thoughts, feelings, and body sensations that arise with each activity. Mindful eating may involve giving attention to the eating of a single raisin, and mindfulness of touch is cultivated by exploring small objects that are held behind the back, which are selected for their interesting or unusual tactile qualities. Mindful hearing can be receptive (listening to music) or expressive (making music), while noting the internal cognitive commentaries that, as the children soon discover, often consist of rapidly formed judgments about the experience rather than being observations or descriptions of the experience. Children also practice mindful movement activities by mirroring each other's random (often silly) body gestures, mindfully walking very slowly, or pretending to be a flower—mindfully stretching, growing, and opening to the sun. Relevant poems and stories are included in each session that help sustain the children's engagement and deepen their understandings.

In this chapter, we offer only a brief description of MBCT-C because the book *Mindfulness-Based Cognitive Therapy for Anxious Children* (Semple & Lee, 2011) provides a thorough background to the theoretical model, a description of modifications needed when teaching mindfulness to children, a detailed, session-by-session guide to conducting each intervention, and all handouts used in the program. Instead, we discuss the core concepts of MBCT-C and explore some of the issues that clinicians should consider when using mindfulness-based interventions with traumatized children. Although mindfulness is a broad-based resiliency approach, MBCT-C was developed to help children manage stress and anxiety. Children who have been traumatized or abused have distinct needs that must be considered, regardless of the mode of therapy.

Foundations of Mindfulness

Anyone who has had the privilege of working with children knows that effective child psychotherapy generally requires a flexible, creative approach and a healthy dose of patience. Compassionate acceptance and a gentle sense of humor are often useful as well. The MBCT-C model encourages therapists to teach mindfulness from their own experiences of mindfulness. Doing this requires the therapist to cultivate mindfulness in his or her personal life, developing understandings that are grounded in experience. Working in this model can sometimes demand as much of the therapist as the therapist might ask of the child. Perhaps even more so when working with children who have been traumatized or abused. At times, the children's emotional suffering and your own empathic attunement may feel quite intense.

Pain and Suffering

Traumatic experiences produce both pain and suffering. Pain had been defined as "an unpleasant sensory and emotional experience associated with actual or potential tissue damage, or described in terms of such damage" (Merskey & Bogduk, 1994). Suffering is an emotional response to pain. We suggest that suffering is intensified when thoughts and feelings about the traumatic experience are not differentiated from direct perceptions of the experience. For some traumatized children, the thoughts and feelings about the experience dramatically increase their reactions to the traumatic event. However, when we first began teaching mindful awareness practices to children, we learned that some children had found a different way to relate to their own thoughts and feelings. They discovered that what they inferred was not necessarily true, that what they feared was not necessarily real, and that thoughts were "just" thoughts. These are liberating and empowering insights. This "decentering" from thoughts bolster the child's self-compassion and affective equanimity. Suffering might be reduced by strengthening the child's ability to tolerate the intensity and vividness of the traumatic memories—with self-compassion.

Judging and Accepting

In Buddhist psychology, judging our experiences serves to increase suffering (Bhikkhu Bodhi, 1993), particularly when the judgments are grounded in strong emotional memories that are not accurate to the child's present reality. It may be particularly difficult to teach acceptance (nonjudging) when a child has experienced horrific abuse that we all fervently wish had never happened. In the MBCT-C model, acceptance is not an attitude of passive resignation. Nor is it necessarily related to forgiveness of the other, although acceptance of the experience may arouse compassion for the other as well as cultivating compassion for oneself. Rather, acceptance refers to the wholehearted recognition that, difficult though it was, the traumatic experience did actually happen. It was not a dream or a fantasy. It did happen. Really. That's acceptance. Nonetheless, it happened in the past, not in this moment. It is not being judgmental to acknowledge and accept the existence of the traumatic experience and then say, "Okay, so what can we do now?"

"Should-ing" on Oneself and the World

Much of life is unsatisfactory—particularly so when traumatic events occur that are beyond our control. To wish that a traumatic event "shouldn't" have happened is a normal human response. To focus on what one "should" have done during or after the experience is also a common response to feeling helpless in a situation that is typically beyond personal control. Getting stuck in the "shoulds" (or "shouldn'ts") to the exclusion of all else is to reject the reality of what is happening now, as well as what actually happened during the traumatic experience. Emotionally pushing away the reality that did happen may be part of what interferes with emotional healing and learning to move beyond the experience. How do we avoid this natural reaction to push away an unpleasant reality? And what may be done about it now?

Practicing mindful awareness allows us to see what is in the present moment more clearly. In the present moment, the traumatic event is not happening. In the present moment, choices are possible. In order to see those choices, attention must be redirected from the traumatic memories to the present moment. Redirecting attention takes practice. For example, bringing attention to each breath is also practice in letting go of each breath, moment by moment. Over and over again. In order to stay present with this breath, the child must first acknowledge and then let go of the previous one. Breath by breath. Acknowledge and let go of the difficult memory, return to the present. Moment by moment.

Thoughts Are Not Facts

Some mindfulness practices focus on simply observing thoughts as they come and go, learning from repeated observations that thoughts are not facts. Thoughts are events in the mind, or as Kabat-Zinn (1994) has suggested, thoughts are "just thoughts." Learning to relate to one's own thoughts in a different and perhaps more helpful way is known as decentering. Following a traumatic event, a child may feel as if his or her thoughts are compelled to return to the traumatic event, which will likely increase the child's distress. With repetition, these anxious or depressive ruminations become habituated "automatic thoughts." In learning new ways to relate to their thoughts, children may be less inclined to incorporate the thoughts into their self-identities. Defining themselves in terms of repetitive negative or self-judgmental thoughts can further damage these already vulnerable children by limiting their ability to see what choices may be available in the current situation (Frewen, Evans, Maraj, Dozois, & Partridge, 2008). Children can become trapped in self-destructive mind states, which are likely to block the healing process. This is not to suggest that practicing mindfulness meditation will eliminate unwanted thoughts. However, finding a different way to relate to these thoughts may make it easier to let go of them when they do emerge. Mindful awareness can offer children a sense of separation from their own thoughts. Children can learn that they do not need to believe everything they think. By not confusing thoughts with reality, decentering increases the child's opportunities to make clear and conscious choices.

Feelings Are Not Facts, Either

Children often develop strong "emotional memories" following traumatic events, particularly when the trauma is related to chronic neglect or abuse from caregivers (Gilbert & Tirch, 2009). Children may internalize these experiences and grow up feeling unworthy, unlovable, and defective. Traumatic memories are strong and tend to be resistant to extinction. This may have evolved as a survival characteristic, but it also makes trauma processing work more difficult. Traumatic emotional memories can feel overwhelming and may frequently trigger what may be protective dissociative episodes. The habit of dissociating becomes an obstacle to maintaining awareness of what is happening in the present moment. Constant negative self-talk develops into negative self-schemas. The memories influence how the child interprets all of his or her experiences. Negative emotional memories become like a dark filter, distorting the child's interpretations of current experiences. Negative emotional distortions serve to both maintain the negative self-schemas and decrease the likelihood of the child making appropriate or wholesome decisions in the present. Traumatic emotional memories become more real than the current reality. Mindfulness practices may help the child hold these intense emotions without dissociating, develop the resiliency to breathe through the strong emotions, and perhaps learn that feelings are not facts, either.

Choice Points

Children and adolescents make a multitude of choices every day. Some are as minor as choosing what color socks to wear or which way to walk to school. Some may feel weightier, such as choosing to align with one group of peers or another. Others might feel life changing, such as deciding what college to attend. But every choice made—no matter how large or small—contributes something to the course of their lives. Although planning is an essential step in reaching one's goals, the opportunity to make a choice occurs only in the present moment. Have you ever spent a great deal of time weighing a choice, perhaps investigating carefully to decide which car to purchase, and then, when the moment arrived, impulsively made a completely different choice from the one you had spent so much time considering? The actual choice is always made in the moment.

Because choices occur only in the present moment, it seems reasonable to assume that by looking more closely at what is present, we might see more choices. In particular, by looking more closely, children discover that they have internal experiences (thoughts, feelings, and body sensations) that often seem to be independent of external events. With practice, they may notice that sometimes the thoughts and feelings are accurate to the present-moment external event. Much of the time, however, they are not.

Children often cannot choose what happens to them. Many of their daily activities are directed by parents, teachers, or older children. They can, however, choose how to respond to what happens. To see more clearly what those response choices might be, they must attend to the only moment in which a choice can be made. Mindfulness might be defined as a practice of keeping the mind and the body in the same place at the same time. Ruminating about an unchangeable past or worrying about an unknowable future shifts attention from what is happening in the present moment, away from the place where choices can be made. Attention is a limited resource. Becoming "lost in thought," the child has less attention to give to the present. With attention focused on an unchangeable past or straying to an unknowable future, the child may easily miss attending to what choice points may be available in this moment (Semple, Lee, Rosa, & Miller, 2010).

Traumatic events, and particularly those that involve neglect or abuse, also precipitate enduring "emotional memories." Memories associated with feelings of being unloved or unwanted may make it harder for abused children to develop self-compassion and may act as a barrier to maintaining awareness of the present. When children are caught up in negative emotional memories, they may have difficulty making conscious, unbiased choices. Decisions are likely to arise from their reexperienced emotional memories (or body sensations) rather than from events occurring in that moment. Practicing mindful awareness of seeing the emotional memories as memories that are not associated with the current situation may interrupt a maladaptive repetition of emotional memories that can precipitate inappropriate behavioral choices.

Self-Compassion

Self-compassion may buffer the emotional dysregulation that often results from childhood maltreatment (Vettese, Dyer, Li, & Wekerle, 2011). Children with low self-compassion seem to be at increased risk to develop maladaptive coping strategies, such as anxious or depressive rumination and dissociation. Greater self-compassion also appears to be directly related to psychological resilience (Neff & McGehee, 2010). Mindfulness is generally considered one component of self-compassion, along with other emotionally protective factors, such as self-kindness and feelings of common humanity (Vettese et al., 2011). With adults, the practice of mindfulness seems to increase both self-compassion and compassionate empathy for others (Orzech, Shapiro, Brown, & McKay, 2009; Robins, Keng, Ekblad, & Brantley, 2012). Simply redirecting attention by focusing on the breath or body sensations may reduce the frequency, intensity, or duration of self-blaming ruminations. With no cognitive restructuring necessary, decentering may reduce the negative self-talk, increase children's self-esteem, and create a sense of self-empowerment (Semple & Lee, 2011). Paradoxically, increasing awareness of the habituated negative self-talk and understanding how this affects depressed or anxious moods may increase self-compassion.

Mindfulness Interventions with Traumatized Children

Psychoeducation

Mindfulness-based psychotherapies generally include some psychoeducation about psychiatric symptoms. Similar to trauma-focused therapies for adults, it can be helpful for children to learn about common symptoms and reactions to trauma. In educating children about traumatic stress responses, therapists convey understanding and acceptance of possible cognitive, affective, physiological, and behavioral reactions to the event. This can help normalize the posttraumatic stress reactions and reduce the likelihood that the child will internalize the experience as evidence of guilt or worthlessness (Phoenix, 2007). Essentially, psychoeducation may help prevent children from blaming themselves for their own victimization. Psychoeducation also supports the development of resiliency factors, such as identification of emotions, cultivation of empathy, greater self-efficacy, and improved problem-solving abilities (Briere & Lanktree, 2012).

Dissociation versus Decentering

Dissociation and mindful awareness may be conceptualized as being at opposite ends of a continuum and opposite states of mind (Corrigan, 2002). Dissociation is, in some sense, a looking away from difficult thoughts and feelings. This may occur during the traumatic event or afterward, when strong memories of the experience arise. Dissociative episodes can range from brief moments of temporarily losing touch with whatever is happening in the moment to prolonged periods of time for which the child has no memories. Although dissociation has been found to be a risk factor for developing PTSD, it is also a common, and sometimes even helpful, sequelae of trauma. Traumatized children may dissociate from the present moment as a coping strategy to contain what may otherwise feel like overwhelming thoughts and emotions. This can happen during the trauma or afterward. When dissociating, the child disconnects from him- or herself, from the environment, and from those around them.

One aim of mindfulness is to bring clear awareness to the internal and external events that arise in each moment—moment by moment. The central therapeutic change that may emerge from sustained mindfulness practices may be this ability to experience thoughts, feelings, and memories as events in the mind (Segal, Teasdale, & Williams, 2004). Decentering is a metacognitive process of seeing these phenomena clearly—as being "just thoughts" or "just memories." Decentering can shift narrowly focused or ruminative thinking by encouraging changes in how the child relates to his or her internal experiences. Thoughts or feelings begin to be experienced as transient events in the mind, rather than being unquestioned evidence of reality. Decentering appears to strengthen the ability to look toward difficult thoughts and feelings with less emotional reactivity (Taylor et al., 2011). The simple awareness that we have choices in how we respond to our own thoughts may be what underlies the self-empowered feelings associated with decentering.

Intrapsychic Exposure to Life, the Universe, and Everything

Avoidant behaviors can maintain or exacerbate traumatic anxiety (Mowrer, 1960). In adults, mindfulness and acceptance are associated with greater psychological adjustment following exposure to trauma (Smith et al., 2011), whereas persistent dissociation, experiential avoidance, and emotional disengagement as coping strategies are associated with greater PTSD severity (Thompson, Arnkoff, & Glass, 2011). Mindful awareness practices aim to enhance a child's ability to distinguish external events occurring in the present moment from intrapsychic events, which include difficult thoughts or emotion-laden memories of a past traumatic event. To do this, the child must look directly at the difficult thoughts and emotions rather than using avoidant strategies such as dissociation. Essentially, mindful awareness practices can be considered a type of unconditional intrapsychic exposure with response prevention, much as has been described by Briere and Lanktree (2012) and others for adults. The practice of looking toward these difficult intrapsychic events shifts the mental representations that define the child's relationship to his or her own thoughts, feelings, and body sensations (Teasdale, 1999).

Hyperarousal, Desensitization, and Body Awareness

Although physical relaxation is not the aim of mindfulness practices, feeling more relaxed after practicing is a common "side effect." Physiological hyperarousal, agitation, muscular tension, and being overly attentive to body sensations are common responses to trauma. Body sensations are often linked to intense trauma-related emotions. Obvious examples include physical or sexual abuse, but experiences such as medical emergencies or natural disasters can also produce hypersensitive trauma-related body sensations. Children may try to manage some of the intensity of emotions linked to these traumatic events by blocking out both emotions and body awareness—essentially choosing to live in their heads rather than in their bodies. Although this might initially seem protective, the choice to withdraw attention from the body means that the emotional processing of the difficult experiences will be incomplete. Consequently, ongoing efforts are required to suppress these emotion-related body sensations from entering awareness. For some children, intentionally cultivating awareness of body sensations may be very difficult and may bring up intense, seemingly overwhelming emotions. It is important for therapists to be attentive to indications of this during body-focused mindfulness activities. The therapist can help each child find a wholesome balance between shutting out awareness of body sensations entirely and feeling overwhelmed at the intensity of the emotional-sensory experience. Breath meditations can provide a calming foundation that allows the child gently to bring awareness to body sensations present in the moment. Some children may find movement activities such as mindful walking or yoga practices easier than an activity such as the body scan, in which the body is still and attention is focused on internal bodily sensations. Mindfulness may provide a way for children to feel emotionally more stable while reconnecting with their own body sensations.

Distinguishing Past, Present, and Future

To practice mindfulness is to practice seeing clearly what is present in this moment. Some posttraumatic stress symptoms are past-focused. That is, the child's attention is focused on remembering the previous traumatic experience, which likely contributes to repetitive, intrusive thoughts. Other symptoms tend to be future-focused. For example, anticipatory anxiety and behavioral avoidance of places or people associated with the trauma may develop or be exacerbated when the child believes that being in a certain place or near a particular person might somehow invite a recurrence of the trauma. Attention, however, is a limited resource. None of us is able to give full attention to every thought, emotion, perception, sensation, or event that arises in each moment. Given this constraint, cultivating a present-focused awareness necessarily reduces the attention that we have to give to thoughts and feelings about past or future events. Living more fully in the present may help a traumatized child to let go of the past experience and reduce his or her fears of the future.

Home Practice and Home Life

During the 12-week MBCT-C program, children are encouraged to engage in daily, home-based mindfulness practices. The aim is to integrate these practices into the child's everyday life. In ordinary circumstances, the home practice activities themselves raise awareness of obstacles that might interfere with developing a daily practice of mindfulness. For the most part, children are encouraged to simply note these experiences and discuss them at the next group discussion. Attending to the challenges that arise in one's home practice becomes an activity that supports the further cultivation of mindfulness.

Unfortunately, a common source of childhood trauma is familial neglect or abuse (Jennifer A. Shaw, 2010). Living in a chronically unsupportive or abusive environment negatively affects a child's emotional health and increases the likelihood that clinical services will be necessary (Dube, Felitti, Dong, Giles, & Anda, 2003). After learning mindful awareness practices in a clinic (or school-based) program, the child may be returning to the source of the trauma—the neglectful or abusive home. For some children, it will be difficult or impossible to gain support in developing a mindfulness practice from parents or caregivers. When the child is in a high-stress situation, the decision to begin a mindfulness-based treatment program warrants careful consideration. Increasing access to highly charged negative thoughts and feelings while still immersed in an unwholesome environment may emotionally overwhelm some traumatized children (Briere & Lanktree, 2012). In addition, children commonly use dissociative coping strategies to manage what may otherwise be an intolerable environment. This seems likely to interfere with both learning and applying mindful awareness practices. The biggest challenge may be in learning how we can support a child's home practice when the home environment is a big part of the problem. We need to be clear about these and other possible contraindications to beginning mindfulness training with traumatized youth.

Conclusion

Mindfulness-based interventions show considerable promise in the treatment of cognitive, emotional, physiological, and behavioral posttraumatic stress symptoms in children. By practicing mindfulness, children may become more adept at distinguishing traumatic memories and other intrapsychic events from their current realities. Simply because of our limited attentional capacity, practicing mindful awareness of the present may reduce past-oriented traumatic memories and future-oriented anticipatory fears. Mindfulness-based therapies for adults have increasingly focused on specific clinical problems. This approach appears to be effective in enhancing attention and emotion self-regulation while decreasing anxiety and depressive symptoms. A great deal of interest, therefore, is focused on the role of mindfulness in the treatment of posttraumatic stress symptoms with adults and children. Child-friendly mindfulness programs for stress management are being used in schools and community locations, as well as being developed for clinical settings. Given the recent explosion of research supporting the efficacy of mindfulness-based interventions in treating adult mood and anxiety disorders, further developments of mindfulness-based interventions focused on the specific clinical issues of traumatized children seem likely to yield promising results.

References

Addy, S., & Wight, V. R. (2012). *Basic facts about low-income children, 2010.* New York: National Center for Children in Poverty, Columbia University, Mailman School of Public Health.

American Psychiatric Association. (2013). *Diagnostic and statistical manual of mental disorders* (5th ed.). Arlington, VA: Author.

Bhikkhu Bodhi. (Ed.). (1993). *A comprehensive manual of Abhidhamma.* Kandy, Sri Lanka: Buddhist Publication Society.

Bondolfi, G. (2005). Mindfulness and anxiety disorders: Possible developments. *Constructivism in the Human Sciences, 10,* 45–52.

Briere, J. J., & Lanktree, C. B. (2012). *Treating complex trauma in adolescents and young adults.* Thousand Oaks, CA: Sage.

Copeland, W. E., Keeler, G., Angold, A., & Costello, E. J. (2007). Traumatic events and posttraumatic stress in childhood. *Archives of General Psychiatry, 64,* 577–584.

Copeland, W. E., Miller-Johnson, S., Keeler, G., Angold, A., & Costello, E. J. (2007). Childhood psychiatric disorders and young adult crime: A prospective, population-based study. *American Journal of Psychiatry, 164,* 1668–1675.

Corrigan, F. M. (2002). Mindfulness, dissociation, EMDR and the anterior cingulate cortex: A hypothesis. *Contemporary Hypnosis, 19,* 8–17.

Dube, S. R., Felitti, V. J., Dong, M., Giles, W. H., & Anda, R. F. (2003). The impact of adverse childhood experiences on health problems: Evidence from four birth cohorts dating back to 1900. *Preventive Medicine, 37*, 268–277.

Dube, S. R., Miller, J. W., Brown, D. W., Giles, W. H., Felitti, V. J., Dong, M., et al. (2006). Adverse childhood experiences and the association with ever using alcohol and initiating alcohol use during adolescence. *Journal of Adolescent Health, 38*, e1–e10.

Finkelhor, D., Ormrod, R. K., & Turner, H. A. (2009). Lifetime assessment of poly-victimization in a national sample of children and youth. *Child Abuse and Neglect, 33*, 403–411.

Frewen, P., Evans, E., Maraj, N., Dozois, D. A., & Partridge, K. (2008). Letting go: Mindfulness and negative automatic thinking. *Cognitive Therapy and Research, 32*, 758–774.

Gilbert, P., & Tirch, D. (2009). Emotional memory, mindfulness and compassion. In F. Didonna (Ed.), *Clinical handbook of mindfulness* (pp. 99–110). New York: Springer Science.

Hildyard, K. L., & Wolfe, D. A. (2002). Child neglect: Developmental issues and outcomes. *Child Abuse and Neglect, 26*, 679–695.

Hofmann, S. G., Sawyer, A. T., Witt, A. A., & Oh, D. (2010). The effect of mindfulness-based therapy on anxiety and depression: A meta-analytic review. *Journal of Consulting and Clinical Psychology, 78*, 169–183.

Kabat-Zinn, J. (1990). *Full catastrophe living.* New York: Bantam Doubleday Dell.

Kabat-Zinn, J. (1994). *Wherever you go there you are: Mindfulness meditation for everyday life.* New York: Hyperion.

Kubak, F. A., & Salekin, R. T. (2009). Psychopathy and anxiety in children and adolescents: New insights on developmental pathways to offending. *Journal of Psychopathology and Behavioral Assessment, 31*, 271–284.

Mayou, R. A., Ehlers, A., & Hobbs, M. (2000). Psychological debriefing for road traffic accident victims: Three-year follow-up of a randomised controlled trial. *British Journal of Psychiatry, 187*, 589–593.

Mennin, D. S., Heimberg, R. G., Turk, C. L., & Fresco, D. M. (2005). Preliminary evidence for an emotion dysregulation model of generalized anxiety disorder. *Behaviour Research and Therapy, 43*, 1281–1310.

Merskey, H., & Bogduk, N. (Eds.). (1994). *IASP Task Force on Taxonomy: Classifications of chronic pain* (2nd ed.). Seattle, WA: IASP Press.

Michal, M., Beutel, M. E., Jordan, J., Zimmermann, M., Wolters, S., & Heidenreich, T. (2007). Depersonalization, mindfulness, and childhood trauma. *Journal of Nervous and Mental Disease, 195*, 693–696.

Mowrer, O. H. (1960). *Learning theory and behavior.* New York: Wiley.

Neff, K. D., & McGehee, P. (2010). Self-compassion and psychological resilience among adolescents and young adults. *Self and Identity, 9*, 225–240.

Orzech, K. M., Shapiro, S. L., Brown, K. W., & McKay, M. (2009). Intensive mindfulness training-related changes in cognitive and emotional experience. *Journal of Positive Psychology, 4*, 212–222.

Phoenix, B. J. (2007). Psychoeducation for survivors of trauma. *Perspectives in Psychiatric Care, 43*, 123–131.

Piet, J., & Hougaard, E. (2011). The effect of mindfulness-based cognitive therapy for prevention of relapse in recurrent major depressive disorder: A systematic review and meta-analysis. *Clinical Psychology Review, 31*, 1032–1040.

Ramiro, L. S., Madrid, B. J., & Brown, D. W. (2010). Adverse childhood experiences (ACE) and health-risk behaviors among adults in a developing country setting. *Child Abuse and Neglect, 34,* 842–855.

Robins, C. J., Keng, S.-L., Ekblad, A. G., & Brantley, J. G. (2012). Effects of mindfulness-based stress reduction on emotional experience and expression: A randomized controlled trial. *Journal of Clinical Psychology, 68,* 117–131.

Saltzman, W. R., Babayan, T., Lester, P., Beardslee, W. R., Pynoos, R., Brom, D., et al. (2008). Family-based treatment for child traumatic stress: A review and report on current innovations. In D. Brom, R. Pat-Horenczyk, & J. D. Ford (Eds.), *Treating traumatized children: Risk, resilience and recovery* (pp. 240–254). New York: Routledge.

Schwab-Stone, M., Ayers, T., Kasprow, W., Voyce, C., Barone, C., Shriver, T., et al. (1995). No safe haven: A study of violence exposure in an urban community. *Journal of the American Academy of Child and Adolescent Psychiatry, 34,* 1343–1352.

Segal, Z. V., Teasdale, J. D., & Williams, J. M. G. (2004). Mindfulness-based cognitive therapy: Theoretical rationale and empirical status. In S. C. Hayes, V. M. Follette, & M. M. Linehan (Eds.), *Mindfulness and acceptance: Expanding the cognitive-behavioral tradition* (pp. 45–65). New York: Guilford Press.

Segal, Z. V., Williams, J. M. G., & Teasdale, J. D. (2002). *Mindfulness-based cognitive therapy for depression: A new approach to preventing relapse.* New York: Guilford Press.

Segal, Z. V., Williams, J. M. G., & Teasdale, J. D. (2013). *Mindfulness-based cognitive therapy for depression* (2nd ed.). New York: Guilford Press.

Semple, R. J., & Lee, J. (2011). *Mindfulness-based cognitive therapy for anxious children: A manual for treating childhood anxiety.* Oakland, CA: New Harbinger.

Semple, R. J., Lee, J., Rosa, D., & Miller, L. F. (2010). A randomized trial of mindfulness-based cognitive therapy for children: Promoting mindful attention to enhance social-emotional resiliency in children. *Journal of Child and Family Studies, 19,* 218–229.

Shaw, J. A. (2000). Children, adolescents and trauma. *Psychiatric Quarterly, 71,* 227–243.

Shaw, J. A. (2010). A review of current research on the incidence and prevalence of interpersonal childhood trauma. In E. Gil (Ed.), *Working with children to heal interpersonal trauma: The power of play* (pp. 12–25). New York: Guilford Press.

Singer, M. I., Anglin, T. M., yu Song, L., & Lunghofer, L. (1995). Adolescents' exposure to violence and associated symptoms of psychological trauma. *Journal of the American Medical Association, 273,* 477–482.

Smith, B. W., Ortiz, J. A., Steffen, L. E., Tooley, E. M., Wiggins, K. T., Yeater, E. A., et al. (2011). Mindfulness is associated with fewer PTSD symptoms, depressive symptoms, physical symptoms, and alcohol problems in urban firefighters. *Journal of Consulting and Clinical Psychology, 79,* 613–617.

Speckens, A. E. M., Ehlers, A., Hackmann, A., Ruths, F. A., & Clark, D. M. (2007). Intrusive memories and rumination in patients with post-traumatic stress disorder: A phenomenological comparison. *Memory, 15,* 249–257.

Taylor, V. A., Grant, J., Daneault, V., Scavone, G., Breton, E., Roffe-Vidal, S., et al.

(2011). Impact of mindfulness on the neural responses to emotional pictures in experienced and beginner meditators. *NeuroImage*, *57*, 1524–1533.

Teasdale, J. D. (1999). Emotional processing, three modes of mind and the prevention of relapse in depression. *Behaviour Research and Therapy*, *37*(Suppl. 1), S53–S77.

Thompson, R. W., Arnkoff, D. B., & Glass, C. R. (2011). Conceptualizing mindfulness and acceptance as components of psychological resilience to trauma. *Trauma, Violence, and Abuse*, *12*, 220–235.

Twenge, J. M. (2000). The age of anxiety?: Birth cohort change in anxiety and neuroticism, 1952–1993. *Journal of Personality and Social Psychology*, *79*, 1007–1021.

Vettese, L. C., Dyer, C. E., Li, W. L., & Wekerle, C. (2011). Does self-compassion mitigate the association between childhood maltreatment and later emotion regulation difficulties?: A preliminary investigation. *International Journal of Mental Health and Addiction*, *9*, 480–491.

Vogel, J. M., & Vernberg, E. M. (1993). Psychological responses of children to natural and human-made disasters: I. Children's psychological responses to disasters. *Journal of Clinical Child Psychology*, *22*, 464–484.

19

Mindfulness and Meditation for Trauma-Related Dissociation

Lynn C. Waelde

Dissociation is a common reaction to traumatic events. There are many forms of trauma-related dissociation (TRD), but all involve discontinuities of present-moment attention and loss of control of cognitive and other functions. Episodes of TRD are often triggered by reminders of a traumatic event. Trauma triggers and the dissociative episodes they provoke are often difficult for the client and therapist to identify, so careful assessment is crucial. Chronic TRD interferes with recovery from traumatization because, as a form of avoidance, it prevents trauma reactions from being resolved and may interfere with participation in psychotherapy, so it is critical to address dissociation in trauma treatment (Cloitre, Petkova, Wang, & Lu, 2012). Mindfulness and meditation (MM) practices can be used to help traumatized persons maintain the continuity of present-moment attention, even in the face of trauma triggers. As reviewed in this chapter, these powerful and time-tested practices encourage present-moment attention by cultivating capacities for mindfulness, decentering, regulation of physiological arousal, and the ability to let go of trauma reactions as they occur, rather than being overwhelmed by them. This chapter offers some practical suggestions for ways to use MM practices to overcome TRD.

Types of TRD

TRD includes a range of experiences that have the common characteristic of involving incomplete present-moment awareness and control. In the classic definition, dissociation involves a lack of "normal integration of thoughts, feelings, and experiences into the stream of consciousness and memory" (Bernstein & Putnam, 1986, p. 727). A recent review indicates that loss of continuity of present-moment awareness is common to different forms of TRD (Carlson, Dalenberg, & McDade-Montez, 2012). Dissociative gaps in awareness can be accompanied by intrusive reexperiencing symptoms. TRD symptoms involve reexperiencing, including unwanted and involuntary intrusions of trauma-related thoughts, feelings, images, sensory perceptions, and behavior, as well as flashbacks, which constitute TRD because they involve detachment or a sense of separation from everyday experience (Holmes et al., 2005). Carlson and colleagues (2012) pointed out that illusions are a form of TRD when sensory stimuli are misperceived as being related to a traumatic event. TRD also manifests as a sense of disconnectedness or distortions of one's own experience, memory, and perceptions of the self and environment. Common manifestations of disconnectedness with one's experience include "blanking out" or losing track of one's present-moment experience (in the absence of intrusive reexperiencing) and dissociative amnesia. Derealization refers to distortions in events or the environment, such as having the sense that one's experience or surroundings are "unreal," like watching a movie or being in a dream. Depersonalization involves a distorted perception of oneself or one's body, such as the feeling that one body part is exceptionally large, or feeling disconnected from one's body. Carlson and colleagues also pointed out that identity alterations occur in TRD but tend to be less severe than in dissociative disorders. A case example illustrated identity alteration in a military veteran with posttraumatic stress disorder (PTSD), whose "killer self" emerged in response to a trauma trigger (Waelde, 2004).

TRD occurs as a response to extreme stress. Dissociation that arises during or immediately after a traumatic event is called peritraumatic dissociation (Briere, Scott, & Weathers, 2005). Peritraumatic dissociation is a response to fear and other overwhelming emotion, which probably has survival value because it involves automatic behaviors, analgesia, depersonalization, and isolation of the full impact of the trauma (Dalenberg et al., 2012; Lanius, Brand, Vermetten, Frewen, & Spiegel, 2012). Despite any benefits that dissociation might convey in the short term, chronic dissociation is thought to interfere with recovery from the outcomes of trauma exposure, such as PTSD, because it functions as a form of avoidance, distancing the person from distress triggered by trauma reminders and preventing resolution and integration (for a review, see Waelde, Silvern, Carlson, Fairbank, & Kletter, 2009).

Overcoming Dissociation with Mindfulness: A Case Example

Clients can learn to use MM to cope with TRD triggers in daily life by first practicing MM in session with the therapist. For example, one military veteran who had been traumatized by an accident in combat and had severe dissociation sought treatment after he caused his third car accident. By exploring what happened during each of these accidents, he realized that he had dissociated and failed to notice that a car had stopped in front of him, though he was unaware of what had triggered his dissociation. He was eager to try meditation as a way to help maintain the continuity of his present-moment attention. During meditation practice in therapy, he worked on keeping his attention in the present, on the physical sensations of sitting and breathing, and on the sounds in the room. He noted that he could pay attention to himself and his surroundings for only a few minutes before his attention would "slide off," often in response to an intrusive trauma-related memory. The "letting go" practice helped him tolerate the distress associated with these intrusions. As he became distressed, he took a breath right into the place where he felt the distress and visualized a balloon expanding and the sensations of distress and tension dissolving within it. As he exhaled, he visualized the distress flowing out with his breath. After two therapy sessions, feeling confident that he could manage his reexperiencing distress without trying to avoid it or ruminate on it, he was ready to try brief daily practice of meditation. He began to notice that his attention was variable but that he could maintain his attention on the present moment by noting the sensation of his arms on the armrests of the chair. In his daily life, when he was not sitting in a chair, he anchored his attention on his breathing and on the sensation of the fingers of his left hand touching his palm. He found that noticing the flow of his breathing helped to anchor him in the present and provided cues about his level of distress: His breathing speeded up or became irregular and shallow when he was having intrusive thoughts and feelings and becoming more distressed. His increased capacity to stay in the present helped him identify specific triggers for his TRD. For example, the client noted that he was triggered by cars stopping abruptly in front of him in traffic, a reminder of what had preceded his accident in combat. As he became adept at noticing when the flow of his attention was being diverted by triggers, he was better able to maintain his attention on the present by focusing on the flow of his breathing and the sensation of his fingers of his left hand touching his palm. Over time, he learned to tolerate trauma triggers as reminders of past events without dissociating or becoming overly distressed by them.

TRD and Trauma Triggers

As the case example illustrates, reminders of traumatic events can trigger episodes of TRD. Trauma triggers are stimuli that are similar to those present during a traumatic event that provoke posttraumatic symptoms, such as reexperiencing distress or dissociation. They can be internal stimuli, such as a bodily position or pain, or external stimuli, such as sounds, sights, or smells. Trauma triggers are frequently sensory stimuli that were present at the beginning of a traumatic event or when the event suddenly became much worse (Ehlers & Clark, 2000). Trauma memories are often fragmented and not easily verbally accessible (Brewin, Dalgleish, & Joseph, 1996), and trauma triggers may generalize over time, so it may be difficult for therapist and client to understand the connection between circumstances that trigger TRD and past trauma. Because they may be unaware of feelings and situations that trigger dissociation, clients may frequently become extremely distressed and/or dissociate without knowing what provoked these states. Survivors of trauma with these issues may be worried that they are "crazy" or have a panic or psychotic disorder (Waelde, 2012). Careful assessment is necessary to differentiate TRD from these other conditions and to help the client develop the capacity to maintain present-moment awareness and functioning even in the face of trauma reminders.

Assessment of TRD

TRD is often difficult for the client to self-report, and the presentation of dissociation can vary from one therapy session to the next (Briere & Armstrong, 2007). Experiences of TRD are disjunct from the ordinary flow of present-moment awareness, and, as such, it is often difficult for clients to find the words to describe them. TRD may also be difficult to observe in the clinical interaction. It can be difficult to differentiate TRD from normal lapses of attention or serious attentional problems that may stem from a brain injury or insult. Differentiating TRD from attentional problems hinges on whether the discontinuity of attention is a response to a trauma trigger and/or represents a longer term adaptation to distressing emotion. TRD is an automatic response to an overwhelming feeling or memory that is typically trauma-related, though chronically traumatized persons with emotion modulation problems may habitually dissociate in response to a range of difficult emotions (Cloitre, Cohen, & Koenen, 2006). TRD inherently involves a loss of capacities to be fully present and to observe and reflect on one's own actions, feelings, and thoughts in a way that is integrated with a sense of past and future experience (van der Hart, Nijenhuis, & Steele, 2006). Because of the difficulties of both self-report and clinical observation as methods to detect TRD, Briere and Armstrong (2007) recommended structured assessment of TRD so that client and therapist can explore the full range of TRD symptoms and their triggers. They pointed out that therapist and client should explore TRD symptoms in detail, noting when the symptoms occur, how they are experienced, and what situations and feelings trigger the TRD. Engaging in structured assessment will help therapist and client identify the types and triggers of TRD and should aid in identification of TRD as it occurs during therapy sessions. Information about how TRD manifests for the client will help the therapist assess the effects of MM practice during the session. As described below, careful monitoring will ensure that the client is using MM effectively rather than dissociating during practice periods.

TRD and Mindfulness Meditation

The use of mindfulness and related meditation practices for TRD may seem counterintuitive. Many clients may believe that meditation involves absorption, trance-like or disconnected states, or an escape into fantasy. Clinicians may also wonder whether meditation involves cognitive avoidance and/or loss of continuity of present-moment awareness and therefore is inappropriate or even dangerous for trauma clients. Although MM and dissociation both affect the nature of present-moment attention and awareness, the states are quite distinct (Lau et al., 2006; Waelde, 2004). Mindfulness involves at least two components: self-regulation of attention to maintain the continuity of present-moment experience, including awareness of thoughts, feelings, and sensory experiences; and an orientation of acceptance, curiosity, and openness to present-moment experience (Bishop et al., 2004). The mindful orientation to experience encourages decentering, which is the ability to be self-reflective about thoughts and feelings as transient mental events in a wider field of awareness, rather than overly identifying with them and accepting them as reality (Teasdale et al., 2002). MM practitioners learn to experience, but then let go of, mental contents as they arise, rather than elaborating, analyzing, reacting to, and ruminating on them. The breath focus entailed in meditation practice may also help to regulate physiological arousal (Ospina et al., 2007; Waelde, 2008) and encourage emotion regulation (Arch & Craske, 2006), which are clearly beneficial for persons with TRD and other trauma symptoms.

These components of MM practice make it well suited for developing the necessary capacities to overcome TRD. As discussed by van der Hart and colleagues (2006), skills for TRD include accurately perceiving reality, including the mindful capacity to be present in the moment; regulating and tolerating emotions and impulses; and managing hyperarousal. The foregoing review indicates that all of these domains might be directly improved by MM practices. MM practices might also support the development of other skill domains mentioned by van der Hart and colleagues (2006). For example, MM may enhance the capacity to symbolize experience in words, because paying attention to and accepting experience seem fundamental to verbal expression. Further, capacities for time management, organization, and problem solving may be supported by MM because these more complex functions would be well served by the capacity to regulate attention. As discussed below, the ability to attend to present-moment experience is also a core component of cognitive and exposure treatments for PTSD.

Considerations for Using MM in Trauma Therapy

MM can be integrated into trauma-focused therapies that aim to help clients identify trauma triggers and maintain present-moment attention when they are exposed to the triggers. From the perspective of cognitive theory, exposure to trauma reminders helps resolve traumatization because it helps the survivor accept that the traumatic event is in the past and because it decreases the ongoing sense of vulnerability and danger (Ehlers & Clark, 2000). MM practices may support the ability to tolerate exposure to trauma reminders. Recent empirical work found that nonjudgmental mindfulness of experiences was associated with lower levels of PTSD avoidance symptoms in a study of traumatized college students (Thompson & Waltz, 2010). In exposure therapy, mindfulness training may promote the ability to maintain awareness and tolerance of conditioned stimuli and thus promote extinction (Treanor, 2011). In daily life, the maintenance of present-moment attention may foster opportunities for natural exposure to trauma reminders. Natural exposure, like exposure procedures in therapy, helps to restructure cognitions about current vulnerability and danger (Nemeroff et al., 2006). In addition to the benefits of attention regulation, breath awareness may improve emotion regulation and increase relaxation (Arch & Craske, 2006; Nemeroff et al., 2006), which in turn may promote tolerance for natural exposure to trauma reminders. In sum, mindfulness training may aid in treatment of TRD because it interferes with avoidance by promoting acceptance of distressing thoughts and feelings (Follette, Palm, & Pearson, 2006).

What types of MM practices are helpful? Although many writers have placed great emphasis on the distinction between mindfulness and concentrative meditation practices, recent work recognizes that mindfulness meditation begins with a period of focused attention (FA), such as focus on the breath, and progresses to open monitoring (OM), which involves nonreactive and nonselective attention to the flow of experience (e. g., Lutz, Slagter, Dunne, & Davidson, 2008). Recent research also indicates that forms of meditation usually thought of as concentrative can increase mindfulness (Tanner et al., 2009), so mindfulness (or a related construct) may be common to multiple forms of meditation. It is likely that the transition from FA to OM states is common to many forms of meditation. For example, breath-focused mantra repetition (i.e., the silent recitation of words or syllables in a manner synchronized with breathing) is designed to provide a more concrete and structured way to maintain breath-focused attention for clients who need additional cognitive structure beyond that provided by simple mindful awareness of breathing. After attention is stabilized with mantra repetition, practitioners can typically transition to a practice of open awareness (e. g., Waelde, 2005). As described below, for those with more severe symptoms, a focus on breathing may trigger symptoms, so mindful awareness of more peripheral bodily sensations, such as on the hands or arms, is preferable at the beginning stages (Germer, 2005).

However, many clients with TRD are not motivated to overcome avoidance. TRD functions to keep the full impact of overwhelming distress from present-moment awareness. Exposure to reminders of the trauma in therapy can be intensely painful for survivors and can provoke TRD. The rationale for using MM in TRD treatment is to help the client develop the capacity to tolerate the traumatic material without dissociating. MM practices can promote the experience of trauma triggers for what they are, that is, experiences in the present moment that are reminders of past experiences, rather than as indications of vulnerability and danger. For example, survivors of trauma are often numb to their own bodily sensations, which may act as triggers for trauma-related reexperiencing and dissociation. MM promotes awareness of bodily states, so that physical sensations can be experienced as they occur in the present moment, rather than as trauma triggers. Mindful awareness of bodily sensations provides the client with a sense of being safe and grounded in his or her own physical body, which may in turn promote tolerance for distressing thoughts and feelings. On a cognitive level, MM encourages decentering, which supports the client in taking a perspective about the traumatic event as an event that occurred in the past, rather than representing a current threat. Decentering can also aid in correcting unhelpful trauma-related cognitions as the client learns that thoughts are just thoughts, rather than facts. To the extent that practice of breath-focused awareness improves regulation of physiological arousal and negative emotions, the client should become better able to tolerate trauma triggers without TRD or overwhelming distress.

Clients with TRD are often reluctant to attempt MM practice because they are afraid that if they suspend their usual patterns of avoidance, they will be overwhelmed by reexperiencing distress. Indeed, there is some risk that clients who are unprepared for MM practice will experience painful and intrusive thoughts, bodily sensations, or TRD. There are three essential procedures for using MM in TRD therapy. The therapist must (1) provide a rationale for MM in treatment, (2) provide adequate structure to the MM practice, and (3) monitor the response to MM and make adjustments to the practice recommendations as needed.

The therapist must begin with a clear rationale for using MM in the therapy. As with other forms of trauma therapy, the client should understand that there is a risk that trauma symptoms will be temporarily exacerbated but that the distress and discomfort should abate with practice. Trauma survivors may fear exposure to trauma-related thoughts and feelings (van der Hart, Nijenhuis, & Steele, 2005), so the issue of control of exposure to trauma-related material is important to many survivors. Therapist and client should discuss the issue of control as it relates to MM practice, because practicing MM techniques involves using new ways of relating to the trauma material, replacing avoidance and dissociation with awareness and openness to experience. Because trauma survivors can be easily overwhelmed by distressing trauma-related thoughts and feelings early in psychotherapy, it is important to explain that the treatment includes "mindfulness titration"—that is, the client will be guided in ways to gradually increase present-moment awareness at a pace and in ways that are tolerable. The rationale should include a clear statement of the specific practices that the therapist will teach and how they are expected to alleviate the client's presenting issues. For example, a client who frequently dissociates in response to interactions with a coworker who resembles her past abuser may find it helpful to know that she can maintain her present-moment awareness by learning to follow the flow of her breathing to reduce the hyperarousal and distress that triggers her TRD at work.

For many clients with TRD, simply sitting and watching the flow of the breath may seem like an abstract exercise because they are so removed from their own felt bodily experience; or, worse, it may seem that it does not provide enough structure to cope with reexperiencing distress and the resulting TRD. It is important for the therapist to provide adequate structure to meditation sessions to scaffold the client's ability to maintain present-focused awareness and to interfere with avoidance. The therapist can offer additional structure by providing (1) verbal guidance for the meditation practice and (2) highly structured types of MM practice. In early sessions, the therapist may provide verbal guidance for the meditation very frequently, with only brief pauses between instructions to allow the client time to complete the instruction. These clients also benefit from having audio recordings of guided meditation practice so that they can structure their between-session practice adequately. With practice, clients learn that they are able to tolerate trauma-related cues, even though they may always have some reaction to them. As their capacity to tolerate distress increases, the therapist can gradually provide less structure to meditation practice in the session by providing longer pauses between instructions until the client is able to meditate without verbal guidance from another source. Offering more structured types of practice is helpful for clients with TRD. Early in treatment, many clients cannot tolerate breath-focused awareness and may benefit from focusing attention on the body periphery, such as noticing sensations in hands (Germer, 2005). As the client's ability to tolerate bodily sensations increases, breath-focused mantra repetition, such as repeating "Hum Sah" with each cycle of breath, can provide cognitive structure to mindfulness practice by redirecting the practitioner's attention from ruminative thoughts to the breath and present moment (Waelde, 2005). Breath-focused imagery, such as picturing the lungs filling with air like two balloons, also adds structure to focused-attention forms of MM.[1] The *Inner Resources for Stress* manualized meditation protocol (Waelde, 2005) has an active technique called "Letting Go," which encourages the practitioner to note distress or tension as it arises and then use breath-focused imagery to watch it pass, without attempting to engage or avoid the material. These diverse types of MM practice, such as watching the flow of the breath, mantra repetition, and breath-focused imagery, allow the therapist to match practice recommendations to the client's needs and capacities. For example, clients differ in their capacities to use visualization or to experience sensations of breath. The practice recommendations can be adjusted to fit the client, rather than trying to make the client adapt him- or herself to a particular technique. Knowing how and when to adapt practice recommendations depends on careful monitoring of the client's responses to the different practices.

The therapist should monitor response to MM by asking about what the client experienced during the practice. The therapist can consider the client's typical manifestations of dissociation (as discovered during the assessment) to be sure that the practice is not encouraging TRD. Simple questions such as "How did that go?" and "What did you experience?" will aid in understanding how the client is using the practices. It is especially important to understand the client's experience when he or she reports difficulty or discomfort. Often, the therapist's first impulse is to clarify the instructions, based on the assumption that the client, as a beginner, "isn't doing it right." It is usually more helpful to clarify what occurred for the client, so it will be clear whether the client is having an expected or an unexpected experience of the practice. For example, many clients may believe that MM entails the cessation of thoughts so they can enjoy simple and blissful present-moment awareness, and they may be chagrined to realize that their thoughts were persisting or even increasing during meditation. In

---

[1]Note that breath-focused imagery is distinct from escape imagery, such as picturing oneself on the beach. To the extent that escape imagery distracts the practitioner from the present moment, there is a risk that it promotes avoidance.

this instance, the therapist can normalize the experience and note the client's ability to attend to the flow of his or her experience. In other cases, the client may actually be dissociating during the practice. Some clients have developed the ability to use dissociation in a deliberate way that may bear some resemblance to meditation experiences (Waelde, 2004). Dissociating clients may say that they "had a wonderful experience," that they were "floating on a cloud" or "lost in space," or they may have no recollection of the meditation period. As a form of escape and avoidance, dissociation can feel rewarding to the client, so it is important to distinguish helpful from unhelpful forms of engagement with the practice. It is useful to have dissociating clients keep their eyes open during MM practice, perhaps with eyelids relaxed and gaze lowered. MM periods can also be kept very brief until the client is able to maintain present focus for longer periods of time.

Implementing MM in Trauma Therapy

Broadly speaking, mindfulness practice involves techniques designed to develop stable, nonreactive, nonjudgmental, present-moment awareness (Kabat-Zinn, 2005), and meditation practices are designed to regulate attention and awareness to bring mental processes under voluntary control (Walsh & Shapiro, 2006). Mindfulness practice is not synonymous with seated meditation practice. For example, dialectical behavior therapy involves mindfulness practices designed to promote self-monitoring, but does not involve sitting meditation (Linehan, 1993). There are several ways that MM can be applied in trauma therapy. It can be incorporated into standard trauma therapy or used as an adjunct or even as a second-line treatment after completion of trauma treatment. A recent survey of trauma therapists indicated that most therapists integrate MM into standard treatment, rather than offering MM instruction in an adjunctive format (Waelde, Thompson, Robinson, & Iwanicki, 2014). However, integrating MM into individual therapy rather than presenting it in a group-based skill-building format should not mean dispensing with between-session practice. Across studies, time spent in between-session meditation practice is associated with better treatment outcomes (Carmody & Baer, 2008; Kukreja et al., 2007), so establishing a regular practice of meditation may support using mindfulness in daily life to cope with TRD.

   In the course of trauma therapy, brief periods of MM practice can be used to ease the transition into exposure to the trauma material. Therapist and client can spend the first 5–10 minutes of each therapy session practicing breath- or body-focused awareness. Persons with TRD have often learned to numb awareness of their bodies and physical sensations, and these brief guided meditation periods can encourage active awareness of bodily states. In the initial stages of treatment, clients with TRD may use a "grounding" practice, such as the sensation of fingertips touching the palm of the hand, to reorient to the present moment when trauma triggers provoke an episode of TRD. As the client can tolerate mindful awareness of breathing, the simple practice of noticing each part of the breath, as it comes in through the nose, past the throat, and expands the diaphragm on the inhalation and watching each part of the expiration, from the diaphragm, past the throat and past the nose, can be beneficial. The therapist can encourage the client to be aware of all of the physical sensations of the breath, including the movement of the inhalation and exhalation, temperature, and sound of the breath. Keeping the periods of meditation brief is important during the beginning stage of therapy, when the client may have very limited ability to tolerate mindful awareness. These mini-meditations are especially useful in the context of therapies that require self-ratings of distress during the session.

Successful in-session practice can provide the necessary foundation for practice outside of sessions. Many therapists recommend between-session practice and provide materials, such as audio recordings of guided practice, to enhance regular daily practice. Between-session practice should include recommendations for using MM techniques to cope with presenting issues.

Conclusion

MM techniques hold great promise for helping clients with dissociation maintain their attention on the present moment, even in the face of distressing trauma reminders. As the foregoing review indicates, although definitive indication of its effectiveness for TRD awaits future clinical trials, MM may address trauma symptoms through attention training, cognitive mechanisms such as decentering, and beneficial effects on hyperarousal and emotion regulation.

References

Arch, J. J., & Craske, M. G. (2006). Mechanisms of mindfulness: Emotion regulation following a focused breathing induction. *Behaviour Research and Therapy, 44,* 1849–1858.

Bernstein, E. M., & Putnam, F. W. (1986). Development, reliability, and validity of a dissociation scale. *Journal of Nervous and Mental Disease, 174,* 727–735.

Bishop, S. R., Lau, M., Shapiro, S., Carlson, L., Anderson, N. D., Carmody, J., et al. (2004). Mindfulness: A proposed operational definition. *Clinical Psychology: Science and Practice, 11,* 230–241.

Brewin, C. R., Dalgleish, T., & Joseph, S. (1996). A dual representation theory of posttraumatic stress disorder. *Psychological Review, 103,* 670–686.

Briere, J., & Armstrong, J. (2007). Psychological assessment of posttraumatic dissociation. In E. Vermetten, M. Dorahy, & D. Spiegel (Eds.), *Traumatic dissociation: Neurobiology and treatment* (pp. 259–274). Arlington, VA: American Psychiatric Publishing.

Briere, J., Scott, C., & Weathers, F. (2005). Peritraumatic and persistent dissociation in the presumed etiology of PTSD. *American Journal of Psychiatry, 162,* 2295–2301.

Carlson, E. B., Dalenberg, C., & McDade-Montez, E. (2012). Dissociation in posttraumatic stress disorder: Part I. Definitions and review of research. *Psychological Trauma: Theory, Research, Practice, and Policy, 4,* 479–489.

Carmody, J., & Baer, R. A. (2008). Relationships between mindfulness practice and levels of mindfulness, medical and psychological symptoms and well-being in a mindfulness-based stress reduction program. *Journal of Behavioral Medicine, 31,* 23–33.

Cloitre, M., Cohen, L. R., & Koenen, K. C. (2006). *Treating survivors of childhood abuse: Psychotherapy for the interrupted life.* New York: Guilford Press.

Cloitre, M., Petkova, E., Wang, J., & Lu, F. (2012). An examination of the influence of a sequential treatment on the course and impact of dissociation among women with PTSD related to childhood abuse. *Depression and Anxiety, 29,* 709–717.

Dalenberg, C. J., Brand, B. L., Gleaves, D. H., Dorahy, M. J., Loewenstein, R. J., Cardeña, E., et al. (2012). Evaluation of the evidence for the trauma and fantasy models of dissociation. *Psychological Bulletin, 138,* 550–588.

Ehlers, A., & Clark, D. M. (2000). A cognitive model of posttraumatic stress disorder. *Behaviour Research and Therapy, 38,* 319–345.

Follette, V., Palm, K. M., & Pearson, A. N. (2006). Mindfulness and trauma: Implications for treatment. *Journal of Rational-Emotive and Cognitive-Behavior Therapy, 24,* 45–61.

Germer, C. K. (2005). Teaching mindfulness in therapy. In C. K. Germer, R. D. Siegel, & P. R. Fulton (Eds.), *Mindfulness and psychotherapy* (pp. 113–129). New York: Guilford Press.

Holmes, E. A., Brown, R. J., Mansell, W., Fearon, R. P., Hunter, E. C. M., Frasquilho, F., et al. (2005). Are there two qualitatively distinct forms of dissociation?: A review and some clinical implications. *Clinical Psychology Review, 25,* 1–23.

Kabat-Zinn, J. (2005). *Full catastrophe living: Using the wisdom of your body and mind to face stress, pain, and illness.* New York: Delta Trade Paperback/ Bantam Dell.

Kukreja, S., Carr, M., Estupinian, G., Mortensen, M. J., Penner, A., Gallagher-Thompson, D., et al. (2007, August). *Meditation homework adherence among family dementia caregivers.* Poster session presented at the 115th annual convention of the American Psychological Association, San Francisco, CA.

Lanius, R. A., Brand, B., Vermetten, E., Frewen, P. A., & Spiegel, D. (2012). The dissociative subtype of posttraumatic stress disorder: Rationale, clinical and neurobiological evidence, and implications. *Depression and Anxiety, 29,* 701–708.

Lau, M. A., Bishop, S. R., Segal, Z. V., Buis, T., Anderson, N. D., Carlson, L., et al. (2006). The Toronto Mindfulness Scale: Development and validation. *Journal of Clinical Psychology, 62*(12), 1445–1467.

Linehan, M. M. (1993). *Skills training manual for treating borderline personality disorder.* New York: Guilford Press.

Lutz, A., Slagter, H. A., Dunne, J. D., & Davidson, R. J. (2008). Attention regulation and monitoring in meditation. *Trends in Cognitive Sciences, 12,* 163–169.

Nemeroff, C. B., Bremner, J. D., Foa, E. B., Mayberg, H. S., North, C. S., & Stein, M. B. (2006). Posttraumatic stress disorder: A state-of-the-science review. *Journal of Psychiatric Research, 40*(1), 1–21.

Ospina, M. B., Bond, T. K., Karkhaneh, M., Tjosvold, L., Vandermeer, B., Liang, Y., et al. (2007). *Meditation practices for health: State of the research. Evidence Report/Technology Assessment No. 155* (AHRQ Publication No. 07-E010). Rockville, MD: Agency for Healthcare Research and Quality.

Tanner, M. A., Travis, F., Gaylord-King, C., Haaga, D. A. F., Grosswald, S., & Schneider, R. H. (2009). The effects of the transcendental meditation program on mindfulness. *Journal of Clinical Psychology, 65,* 574–589.

Teasdale, J. D., Moore, R. G., Hayhurst, H., Pope, M., Williams, S., & Segal, Z. V. (2002). Metacognitive awareness and prevention of relapse in depression: Empirical evidence. *Journal of Consulting and Clinical Psychology, 70,* 275–287.

Thompson, B. L., & Waltz, J. (2010). Mindfulness and experiential avoidance as predictors of posttraumatic stress disorder avoidance symptom severity. *Journal of Anxiety Disorders, 24,* 409–415.

Treanor, M. (2011). The potential impact of mindfulness on exposure and extinction learning in anxiety disorders. *Clinical Psychology Review, 31,* 617–625.

van der Hart, O., Nijenhuis, E. R. S., & Steele, K. (2005). Dissociation: An insufficiently recognized major feature of complex posttraumatic stress disorder. *Journal of Traumatic Stress, 18,* 413–423.

van der Hart, O., Nijenhuis, E. R. S., & Steele, K. (2006). *The haunted self: Structural dissociation and the treatment of chronic traumatization.* New York: Norton.

Waelde, L. C. (2004). Dissociation and meditation. *Journal of Trauma and Dissociation, 5,* 147–162.

Waelde, L. C. (2005). *Inner resources for stress.* Palo Alto, CA: Palo Alto University.

Waelde, L. C. (2008). Meditation. In G. Reyes, J. Elhai, & J. Ford (Eds.), *The encyclopedia of psychological trauma* (pp. 419–421). Hoboken, NJ: Wiley.

Waelde, L. C. (2012). Trauma triggers. In C. R. Figley (Ed.), *Encyclopedia of trauma: An interdisciplinary guide* (pp. 738–741). Thousand Oaks, CA: Sage.

Waelde, L. C., Silvern, L., Carlson, E., Fairbank, J. A., & Kletter, H. (2009). Dissociation in PTSD. In P. F. Dell & J. A. O'Neil (Eds.), *Dissociation and the dissociative disorders: DSM-V and beyond* (pp. 447–456). New York: Routledge.

Walsh, R., & Shapiro, S. L. (2006). The meeting of meditative disciplines and Western psychology: A mutually enriching dialogue. *American Psychologist, 61,* 227–239.

Waelde, L. C., Thompson, J. M., Robinson, A., & Iwanicki, S. (2014). *Trauma therapists' training, personal practice, and clinical applications of mindfulness and meditation.* Manuscript submitted for publication.

20

Focusing-Oriented Therapy with an Adolescent Sex Offender

Robert A. Parker

In this chapter, I show how focusing-oriented therapy (Gendlin, 1996) as modified for complex trauma (Centre for Focusing Oriented Therapy, 2012; Turcotte, 2012) can be a useful part of the treatment program for an adolescent sex offender. I briefly explain what focusing is, how it works, how it has been adapted for treating complex trauma, and how it can be used to help adolescent sex offenders whether or not they suffer from complex trauma. I conclude by discussing three characteristics of this approach: (1) its precision, both in process and in outcome; (2) the speed with which growth can take place; and (3) the pervasiveness and durability of the resulting change.

Focusing

Focusing is a way of attending to the body's implicit knowing of situations (Gendlin, 1991). It was developed by philosopher Eugene Gendlin (Gendlin, 1997b; Gendlin, Beebe, Cassens, Klein, & Oberlander, 1968) as part of an investigation into the relation between implicit and explicit knowing.

Implicit knowing might sound exotic, but it is an everyday fact of life. For example, you might notice your experience as you read this paragraph. You probably don't think about the meaning of each word. Instead, you probably have an implicit sense of the meaning of the words, while you focus your attention on the explicit meaning of the sentences. Of course, you could explicitly define any single word, *sentence*, for example. But notice what happens: You start with the implicit sense of meaningfulness, and you gradually find words and concepts that go with that sensing, until you formulate an explicit definition of *sentence*. And your definition is formulated with words whose meaning is implicit. This illustrates a basic relationship between explicit and implicit knowing: Explicit knowing is never alone but always in a context or background of implicit knowing (Gendlin, 2012).

Implicit knowing is, by definition, outside of awareness, but it is possible to bring it into awareness by paying attention to how a problem or situation "feels." William James described this "feel" in his *Principles of Psychology*:

> Suppose we try to recall a forgotten name. The state of our consciousness is peculiar. There is a gap therein; but no mere gap. It is a gap that is intensely active. A sort of wraith of the name is in it, beckoning us in a given direction. . . . If wrong names are proposed to us, this singularly definite gap acts immediately so as to negate them. . . . And the gap of one word does not feel like the gap of another, all empty of content as both might seem necessarily to be when described as gaps. When I vainly try to recall the name of Spalding, my consciousness is far removed from what it is when I vainly try to recall the name of Bowles. . . . (1890/2009, p. 251)

When it becomes the focus of attention, implicit knowing is called a *felt sense*. Without going into a detailed discussion of Gendlin's philosophy (see Gendlin, 2003, for a summary, or Gendlin 1997a and 1997b for more detail), we can note two things about the felt sense that are not immediately obvious.

First, implicit knowing (and therefore the felt sense, when it comes) is a sense of what is needed. Our bodies know implicitly how to breathe; but if we try to hold our breath for 60 seconds, we feel in our bodies something like a "needing" or "wanting" to breathe. So we see that implicit knowing includes something like "needing" or "wanting." Gendlin calls this *implying*; our bodies *imply* breathing. Another example is feeling uncomfortable if someone is standing too close. Most people do not even know what the right distance is for them until someone stands too close. Our bodies know and *imply* the right distance.

How can this be? Our living bodies *are* in ongoing interaction with our environments, including our social environments. Thus it should not be surprising that our bodies sense and implicitly know our situation and what it needs; or that, as James noted, what we are calling the felt sense is "intensely active . . . beckoning us in a given direction . . . [acting] immediately so as to negate [a bad suggestion]."

Another important thing about the felt sense is that, if we pay attention to it in a certain way, some of the body's implicit knowing can be formulated explicitly in words, so that James, for example, could have used his felt sense to recover the name he had forgotten. This is interesting because a felt sense initially feels frustratingly vague, ephemeral, and impossible to describe. It can also be remarkably helpful, because in situations in which one feels "stuck" (i.e., currently available explicit understanding is not adequate), the felt sense often leads to a deeper understanding of the problem that includes a way forward.

The key to listening to the felt sense is to protect it from already-formed concepts by attending to it with a gentle and supportive attitude, gently and tentatively trying out different words that might describe the feel of it. We can tell when we have found the right words, because there is a feeling of resonance (the words feel right) and because the felt sense responds by bringing out more of what is implicit. Then we can attend to the new felt sense by finding new words to describe it. Again, the felt sense brings out more, and we attend to that and find new words to describe it, and so on. If we continue the process, always gently allowing the felt sense to choose its own words, it will often (not always) lead to a *felt shift* that includes a solution to the problem at hand but often has implications far beyond the original problem. This way of interacting with the felt sense, including the felt shift, is called *focusing* (Gendlin, 1982).

Focusing is not psychotherapy, but it is useful in therapy. For example, a considerable body of research has used the Experiencing Scale (Klein, Mathieu, Gendlin, & Kiesler, 1970), a measure of client focusing in psychotherapy, to study the process of psychotherapy. The resulting studies, spanning more than four decades, suggest that clients who interact with their felt sense during therapy have significantly better outcomes in many forms of therapy, including cognitive-behavioral therapy, process experiential therapy, and client-centered psychotherapy (e.g., Watson & Bedard, 2006; for summaries of this research, see Elliott, Greenberg, & Lietaer, 2004; Elliott, Watson, Greenberg, Timulak, & Freire, 2013; Greenberg, Elliott, & Lietaer, 1994; and Parker, 2014).

Frozen Structures

The felt sense is a kind of awareness, but it can be experienced as an object that one "stands apart from" and "interacts with," just as one might figuratively stand apart from and interact with (e.g., describe) an emotion or idea. This standing apart requires a clear sense of self, separate from the felt sense. Sometimes, however, the client's sense of self is merged with an implicit knowing and is thus unable to stand apart from it and interact with it. Then, instead of experiencing the present moment freshly in all its details, the client notices primarily what was relevant at some earlier time, finding aspects of the present situation that seem overwhelming and thus implicitly *reliving* the earlier experience. This reliving is called *regression* (Turcotte, 2012). With no interaction between explicit conceptual knowing and implicit knowing, neither can change. We call this a *frozen structure* (Gendlin, 1964). Psychological trauma is an example of frozen structure but the "small-t" traumas of everyday life can also produce frozen structures, reliving, and regression.

The signs of a frozen structure can be subtle, but with practice they are easily recognized; for example, the client may display a repetitive behavior or gesture, or the gaze may briefly shift into space as if seeing something in the room that is not actually there. These are signs that the client could be reliving something. It is important to recognize these signs, because if reliving becomes too vivid, it will become retraumatizing and will reinforce the frozen structure.

Shirley Turcotte (Centre for Focusing Oriented Therapy, 2012; Turcotte, 2012) has addressed this problem by developing focusing-oriented therapy for complex trauma (FOT-CT). Like focusing, FOT-CT is *client centered* (it is based on the client's implicit knowing), but it is *therapist driven* (the therapist must actively look for and follow signs of regression). Because a frozen structure does not interact with explicit conceptual knowing, the client cannot verbalize it, and the therapist must actively look for it in the client's body language and reflect it back to the client. The therapist carefully regulates this process, ensuring that the client always has a strong enough sense of self to observe and interact with the frozen structure, so that it can change (i.e., become a felt sense). If more comes than the client can handle, the client will lose his or her sense of self and begin reliving the frozen structure. There are specific ways to avoid this by helping clients strengthen sense of self before starting the focusing phase of therapy and by helping them maintain sense of self during each therapy session.

Working with Sex Offenders

Sexual offending, by its nature, often involves a rigid way of experiencing that is insensitive to details of the present moment, such as a victim's expressions of suffering. Therefore, an awareness of frozen structures, focusing, and FOT-CT is often useful in the treatment of adolescent sex offenders.

FOT-CT is not appropriate in all situations, but the requirements are relatively simple. The therapist, of course, must be experienced in working with this population. Clients must be able and willing to explore their inner experience, at least introspectively. It is not absolutely necessary that they share their inner experience with the therapist, because the therapist can respond to body language during the first few sessions while the client builds trust. However, clients who externalize their problems and/or are relatively unaware of their inner experience may need some preparatory work focused on those issues. Generally, clients who can benefit from individual therapy can benefit from FOT-CT.

For those who can benefit, FOT-CT can be a remarkably rapid and effective intervention. The following vignette (a composite of several actual therapy sessions) illustrates some of the key characteristics of FOT-CT and also the process of focusing.

Case Example

John is a 14-year-old boy who was adopted at age 6. He had adapted easily to his new home; everyone liked him, and he seemed to excel at everything he tried. About a year before he was seen, John's foster mother began babysitting her sister's 4-year-old daughter for several hours a day on weekdays. After about 4 months, she went into John's bedroom one day to discover the girl performing fellatio on him. Investigation suggested that the sexual behavior had started with roughhousing and wrestling shortly after the girl moved in and had escalated over several weeks to more or less daily sexual touching with rewards such as candy and attention.

John was adjudicated and sentenced, in lieu of detention, to a residential treatment program for adolescent sex offenders. He followed his treatment program diligently and was well liked by staff and peers. He quickly understood why his behavior was wrong, and he appeared to be sincerely remorseful. But his reason for molesting a 4-year-old remained unclear. He did not appear to be sexually attracted to children, and he was popular at school and had many female same-age friends, so there was no apparent reason for him to do this.

There were some clues. John was very good at almost everything he tried. He usually handled this gracefully, but there were signs that he was putting himself under pressure; for example, he avoided activities he felt he might not be good at, and he could be quite hard on himself if he lost a game or got a bad grade at school. A fear of failure and a need to always be in control and to always succeed could have been a factor in his offense; perhaps he could not risk a relationship with a female peer but could with a 4-year-old child.

The following session took place after about 4 months of individual, group, and milieu therapy.

THERAPIST: What would you like to work on today?

CLIENT: My anger.

THERAPIST: OK, tell me about a time when you were angry.

[Anger is a label that we put on certain emotional experiences. It is not a felt sense, but it can be a way in, if John can go beyond the label and open himself to the actual experience. John tells me about starting a fight when somebody "messed with" him on the basketball court, causing him to miss a shot. His description is filled with self-justification (it was the other boy's fault, etc.). But we're not here to discuss whether starting a fight was a good or bad thing to do. We need to go beyond labels and preconceptions, to the actual experience.]

THERAPIST: So, can you remember that feeling? Can you feel it inside, right now?

CLIENT: (*pause*) Yes.

THERAPIST: Where inside do you feel it?

CLIENT: (*pause*) In my chest . . .

THERAPIST: In your chest. . . . What is that feeling like? . . . How heavy is it, what color is it?

[Asking him to describe his feeling as if it were an object is a way of inviting him to encounter it freshly, without his usual concepts and labels. Surprisingly, most people will answer such "nonsense questions" with certainty and precision, after only a few moments of reflection.]

CLIENT: It's heavy . . . and red. . . . It has jagged sharp edges, and it explodes.

THERAPIST: So it's heavy and red . . . it has jagged sharp edges . . . and it explodes.

[We are going beyond the culturally defined concept of "anger." Saying John's words back slowly helps him to compare the words with his actual experience. This typically leads to a new and more differentiated description (the reflection-correction process described earlier).]

CLIENT: Well . . . sometimes it's gray . . . but it turns red when I start feeling angry.

THERAPIST: So it's gray sometimes . . . and it turns red when you start feeling angry. . . .

CLIENT: That's right.

[I try a few more reflections, but nothing more comes. This could be a frozen structure, and he may need help finding it. It could be my imagination, but the way he sits makes him seem younger than his actual age; and even though he's talking about anger, his eyes look sad.]

THERAPIST: . . . What can you call that part? Could you give it a name?

CLIENT: (*after several attempts to name it*) "Bad news."

THERAPIST: OK, how does "bad news" feel, what's he like?

[Personifying the experience is another way of encountering it freshly, without the conceptual and cultural baggage that a label such as "anger" would carry.]

CLIENT: He's angry.

[John reverts to the old label; I want to help him away from the label and back to what he is actually experiencing.]

THERAPIST: What bothers him? What makes him angry?

CLIENT: It's people messing with me.

[The look of sadness is still there, and for a few moments his eyes are focused several feet in front of him, as if he's looking at something that I can't see. This is a sign of regression. John is on the edge of reliving something but is still clearly present in the room, so he is OK so far. We can begin tracking the regression, to see where it leads.]

THERAPIST: . . . and part of you feels angry about that, and also maybe sad, is that right?

CLIENT: Kind of sad, but more angry. . . . It's like they're criticizing me for no reason.

THERAPIST: What's it like to be criticized?

CLIENT: It's like, I'm already doing badly, I've missed the basket, and I already feel bad, and they're trying to make me feel worse. . . .

[After a series of reflections from me and corrections from John, John realizes that it is not so much a feeling that they are criticizing him, but more a feeling that he has failed. As he says this, he again appears to be looking at something in front of him, with sadness in his eyes; and he is still clearly in the room and relating to me. So we can continue following the regression; and to do that we need to find out more about how he experiences failure.]

THERAPIST: What does it feel like inside when you fail?

CLIENT: I feel like a failure, sad, depressed, frustrated. . . .

[John kept himself "separate" from his anger, personifying it with the name "bad news." In contrast, "I feel like a failure" suggests he's beginning to identify with something. The next reflection aims to help him get some distance so he can *observe* the experience of failure instead of identifying with it.]

THERAPIST: . . . So there's a place inside of you that feels sad . . . depressed . . . and frustrated . . . about failing; what's that like?

CLIENT: I don't know. . . .

[We go back and forth a few times, but he can't say anything more about the feeling of failure. John sits in his chair like a small child, looking at me, and sometimes at the space in front of him, with sad eyes. He appears to be reliving something, but he has no words for it. This is probably a frozen structure, which will require a different kind of reflection. We start by making sure he is maintaining an observing self, separate from the frozen structure.]

THERAPIST: Can you feel that in your body, that feeling of being a failure?

CLIENT: Yes.

THERAPIST: OK, where inside do you feel it?

CLIENT: In my chest.

THERAPIST: How old does that place feel?

[The question works on two levels. First, I want to learn something about how old he is and what he is looking at. But at the same time, it is a process intervention. A frozen structure is like wallpaper; it's a context that we take for granted. If this is a frozen structure, imagining how old it is will help John maintain his own identity separate from it and simultaneously connect it to some period in his life, helping him experience it freshly and with more detail, so that he and it can begin to change.]

CLIENT: It feels like when I was little. . . .

THERAPIST: What was going on in your life when you were that age?

[We are now looking for something in his history that may connect with the feel of the frozen structure. John describes his family. His mother was verbally and physically abusive. I explore for feelings of failure about pleasing his mother, but nothing comes. Her abuse was like getting caught in a thunderstorm; it had nothing to do with him. It is the same with his father, who was more distant, would disappear for days a time, and basically had very little to do with him. Again, John has no sense of failure about this.]

THERAPIST: Who did you look to for approval? Who did you try to please?

CLIENT: My brother and sisters . . . and maybe one teacher at school.

[There appear to be no significant feelings of failure with any of these individuals. But as he talks, his body language reminds me of a small child, maybe 4 or 5 years old. He looks very sad, and although he is still clearly present in the room, for brief moments he appears to gaze at something several feet in front of him. These signs of reliving are subtle but unmistakable. He is on the edge of something. But what?]

THERAPIST: OK, imagine you're a child again, living with your mother and father, and look for that feeling of failure. Back in those days, when you were living at home, when did you experience that feeling?

CLIENT: (long pause) It was when my mother died.

[The immediate, felt certainty shows that John is speaking from a felt sense. The frozen structure is shifting from an implicit, pervasive mood that fills his life to *this* feeling, related to *this* event. The frozen structure is beginning to melt.

But we still do not know very much. John has already described, in earlier sessions, fragmented memories of his mother's illness and death from cancer when he was about 5. We could speculate that this was traumatic for John, but such speculation would be irrelevant. John's regression is telling us that he is reliving something about failure. We need to follow the regression.]

THERAPIST: So you had that feeling of failure when your mother died, like it was your fault in some way?

CLIENT: No, it wasn't my fault, I just had that feeling of failure.

[This is interesting: if it wasn't his fault, why is there a feeling of failure? But further exploration goes nowhere.]

THERAPIST: Let's try an experiment, OK? (*John agrees.*) Suppose I say to you "It's your fault that your mother died." How do those words feel inside?

[We have done this exercise before in other contexts, and John understands that the words have nothing to do with what I believe; it is an experiment, a therapist-driven reflection, to see if anything inside of him responds to those words.]

CLIENT: I don't feel anything inside, because it's not true. It's not my fault that she died . . . (*long pause*). It's just that when she died, I felt like I should have done something to save her; I should have gotten her to change the way she was living, maybe spoken to her and gotten her to take better care of herself. . . . I should have done something.

[Of course! Five-year-old John had wanted to save his mother.]

THERAPIST: So your failure was that you failed to do something to keep her from dying, you failed to help her.

CLIENT: Right.

[Again, the felt certainty and the new perspective indicate that this is his felt sense speaking.]

THERAPIST: And you've carried that feeling with you ever since?

CLIENT: Yes.

THERAPIST: And how strong is that feeling, the feeling that you failed to save your mother, on a scale of 1 to 10?

CLIENT: It's a 10.

[We've found the frozen structure; now we need to connect it to the present. As John learns to recognize the frozen structure functioning in different areas of his life, it will become a felt sense.]

THERAPIST: How close is this feeling to the feeling of failure that you sometimes have these days?

CLIENT: Not close at all, they're different feelings; if I fail to make a basket, that has nothing to do with my mother dying.

[People often confuse the magnitude of a felt sense with the qualitative aspect, so this is worth going over again. A felt sense is very precise. If we're on the right track, the felt senses will be exactly the same; if they're only close, we're missing something and may have to start over.]

THERAPIST: OK, get the two feelings. . . . Can you feel them now?

CLIENT: Yes.

THERAPIST: OK, how are they different?

CLIENT: Well, the feeling of my mother dying is much bigger than the feeling of failure if I miss a basket.

THERAPIST: . . . so one feeling is much bigger than the other feeling; but apart from that, how are they different?

CLIENT: (*Pause*) Apart from that, they're not different at all, they're the same.

THERAPIST: OK . . . do you mean they're exactly the same, or just very close?

CLIENT: They're exactly the same, except that one is much bigger than the other.

THERAPIST: OK, now how are they related to each other?

CLIENT: The two feelings aren't related, my mother dying has nothing to do with me missing a basket.

[I try to explore this further, but get unclear answers and a tendency to go off on tangents. I'm not sure what he means, he is becoming unfocused, and I'm afraid he'll lose his connection with the felt sense.]

THERAPIST: OK, now I'm going to say something to you, and I want you to check it inside, you know what I mean? Not in your head, but inside your body, see how these words feel.

CLIENT: OK.

THERAPIST: So, you're not saying this exactly, but what I'm hearing is that you're carrying around this big burden, that it's your fault that you didn't save your mother, and that this weighs down on you all the time. How does that feel inside?

CLIENT: Right (*with some release of tension, visible in the face*).

THERAPIST: So, whenever anything goes wrong, if you miss a basket, or you do bad in school, or whatever, you feel like a failure, and that feeling of being a failure goes right to the big feeling of being a failure because of your mother. So whenever a small thing gets touched off, the big thing gets touched off at the same time. How close is that to what you feel?

[This is not an interpretation, it is a kind of reflection. I'm not asking for agreement, I'm asking how the words feel inside, and I know from experience that John will tell me if they don't feel right. John's body language and his description of his childhood situation have given me a sense of his frozen structure, but neither John nor I can know for sure if my sense is right. Only his body can tell us. As I listen to and reflect his frozen structure, I am teaching John to do the same. In doing this exercise, he is learning to stand outside the frozen structure and look at it, so that it becomes a felt sense he can interact with and learn from.]

CLIENT: That's it, that's what happens (*enormous release of tension, visible in face and body posture*).

[We go over this a few times, making sure that it feels right to John.]

THERAPIST: So there is a feeling that you failed to save your mother, and that's a very important feeling in your life. I think we both know that you couldn't have done anything to save your mother at age 5, but can the place inside hear that and take that in?

[This is a real question. As I noted earlier, the felt sense is experienced as an active agent; it is a "still small voice" that one can ignore but cannot control. There is no guarantee that John's felt sense will agree with us. His felt sense might say "no," which would mean we are missing something and have to do some more listening.]

CLIENT: Yes (*with visible relaxation and apparent relief*).

[The body shift (not the verbal "yes") indicates that John has received an accurate reflection, meaning that he can recognize it as a reflection of himself at a deep level. And as he takes it in, both implicitly and explicitly, he will begin to know himself and the world in a new way.]

THERAPIST: So, it seems that where we're at is [*I summarize*]. Does this feel like a good place to stop?

CLIENT: Yes.

THERAPIST: So, how is that failure place feeling right now?

CLIENT: It's feeling gratitude (*looking at me with moist eyes, as if the gratitude is for me*).

THERAPIST: Who is it grateful to?

CLIENT: It's grateful to both of us, to me for recognizing it, and to you for helping me recognize it.

Because John was able to interact with it, the frozen structure had "melted" and become a felt sense, able to change with experience. In a sense, John forgave himself for letting his mother die.

We had gone into this session with the hypothesis that John's motive for offending might have involved a fear of failure that prevented him from relating to girls his own age. By the end of the session, we had a clear confirmation of the fear of failure. The sense of relief was immediate, but there were also deep changes in his self-concept and social relationships that manifested more gradually and suggested that the fear of failure had indeed shaped his life and motivated him to molest a child.

In therapy, John realized that his relationship with the 4-year-old girl had indeed given him a feeling of safety by protecting him from feelings of rejection and failure. He was struck by the absurdity of seeking safety with a child, when there was no need to be so afraid of failure in the first place.

More important, over the following weeks John developed a new attitude, as well as new body language and behavior. His attitude toward sports and schoolwork changed; instead of treating each new activity as a test of his competence, he began enjoying things for their own sake and because he enjoyed being with people. He became interested in girls his own age, immersed himself in extracurricular activities, and in general became more relaxed and playful, like a normal teenager. In our last session together, he spoke excitedly about his activities on the school choir, which was about to go on tour out of state, and he asked to end our session early so he could meet a female classmate.

During a 2-year follow-up period, there was no evidence of any inappropriate sexual behavior or inappropriate interest in younger children.

Discussion

This clinical vignette illustrates three characteristics of FOT-CT mentioned in the introduction: (1) its precision, both in process and in outcome; (2) the speed with which growth can take place; and (3) the pervasiveness and durability of the resulting change.

We can now see why this is possible. FOT-CT allows a youthful offender to engage directly with his own implicit knowing, with the therapist acting as a coach or facilitator. However, this requires a particular kind of listening that can be problematic for both therapist and client.

Listening

To understand where the offense came from, both offender and therapist must be open to the offender's experience, which means listening to and accepting who he is so that he can grow from his own center in a way that has integrity for him. Teaching him to follow rules is sometimes the best we can do, but it is not the same as helping him grow from the inside.

Listening to a sex offender can be difficult for both the therapist and the offender, for a number of reasons. The offense itself is difficult to accept. The therapist may have feelings about what the offender did and probably wants the offending to stop, whereas the offender wants to convince everyone that he is cured and should go home. Both want the offense to go away, and this agenda makes it difficult for both to accept and listen to the offender. A related problem is that listening to oneself requires an attitude of openness, curiosity, and kindness toward oneself. This can be difficult and frightening for a kid who was emotionally abused and is especially difficult for an offender who feels stigmatized by his family and society (Gilbert, McEwan, Gibbons, Chotai, Duarte, & Matos, 2012). Offenders often do not want to look inside for fear of what they will find.

Listening means surrendering preconceptions and opening to the possibility of something new that one hasn't considered before, something for which one might not even have words. In the preceding example, John initially did not have words for his sense of failure; it was a pervasive background feeling, like wallpaper. His conscious formulation was not about failure at all; it was about people picking on him. The therapist's job was to help him notice the murky inchoate background feeling, his implicit knowing, and to notice and find words for different aspects of it. As John noticed and named different aspects, it changed from a murky unknown to something with more and more qualities; so that "It's heavy, and red . . . sometimes it's gray" became "I feel like a failure, sad, depressed, frustrated. . . . " This is a radical kind of listening. The therapist is teaching John to listen to himself, and neither knows where it is going to lead. It takes a lot of trust.

But this radical listening is in some ways easier than normal listening. It tends to bypass hidden agendas; neither client nor therapist needs to persuade the other of anything. The client is less likely to feel evaluated because the process is descriptive and whatever he says is honored and appreciated. Thus, although listening presents difficulties, FOT-CT cuts through many of these difficulties, allowing growth to come from the inside.

Speed and Precision of Therapy

When therapist and client are both able to listen in this way, then FOT-CT can proceed with considerable speed and precision. As the therapist looks for and reflects nonverbal signs of regression, the client's body immediately shows how accurate the reflection was, so the next reflection can be more precise. With each reflection, more of what was implicit tends to emerge, so the back-and-forth process tracks the regression and leads directly to the frozen structure. The client learns from inside, not from the therapist. Situations that have been frozen structures, relived implicitly for years, become explicit and can be reevaluated.

In John's case, for example, a 5-year-old boy *implied* (needed . . . wanted . . .) a mother, so his mother's illness *implied* that he should save her. When she died, that implying had no way forward, no resolution, so he continued to live it as a frozen structure. When he finally experienced the implying explicitly, he finally could live it forward and resolve it, simply by realizing that a 5-year-old cannot change things like that and that his failure then does not make him a failure now.

No amount of brilliant clinical insight or client introspection could have achieved this, and both John and his therapist were equally surprised by it. The therapist carefully tracked the regression and did some reflecting in order to clarify issues, but the actual change came from John's implicit knowing and, in the end, from his felt sense.

Pervasiveness and Durability of Change

There are many ways to do therapy, but there is an advantage in working "from the inside out" rather than "from the outside in." We can encourage sex offenders to memorize offense cycles and relapse prevention plans, but none of that is likely to change their way of experiencing the world, which is where the offense often comes from. If the offense is related to a frozen structure, then real change is more likely to come from the inside, when the frozen structure becomes a felt sense and the offender wants to change because he has discovered a better way to live. In that case, change tends to be pervasive and durable, as we saw with John.

Conclusion

FOT-CT can be thought of as a guided mindfulness practice. Normally, when we experience frozen structures, there is a tendency to become disoriented; we lose track of who we are and implicitly identify with the frozen, blocked implyings from some earlier, formative time. In FOT-CT, the therapist provides steady, accurate reflections of the client's experience, so clients can stay oriented and remember who they are as they walk through this disorienting passageway.

Adolescents commit sexual offenses for many reasons, and no single approach will help everyone. FOT-CT is most likely to be helpful for offenders like John who are able and willing (with the necessary support) to attend to and describe their felt experience. By helping youth like John to remember who they are, we can free them to form healthy relationships and find or return to a positive developmental path.

References

Centre for Focusing Oriented Therapy. (2012). *Treatment and training for complex trauma.* Retrieved February 23, 2012, from *www.fotcomplextrauma.com.*

Elliott, R., Greenberg, L. S., & Lietaer, G. (2004). Research on experiential psychotherapies. In M. J. Lambert (Ed.), *Bergin and Garfield's handbook of psychotherapy and behavior change* (5th ed., pp. 493–540). New York: Wiley.

Elliott, R., Watson, J., Greenberg, L. S., Timulak, L., & Freire, E. (2013). Research on humanistic-experiential psychotherapies. In M. J. Lambert (Ed.), *Bergin and Garfield's handbook of psychotherapy and behavior change* (6th ed., pp. 495–538). New York: Wiley.

Gendlin, E. (1964). A theory of personality change. In P. Worchel & D. Byrne (Eds.), *Personality change* (pp. 100–148). New York: Wiley.

Gendlin, E. T. (1982). *Focusing* (2nd ed.). New York: Bantam Books.

Gendlin, E. T. (1991). On emotion in therapy. In J. D. Safran & L. S. Greenberg (Eds.), *Emotion, psychotherapy and change* (pp. 255–279). New York: Guilford Press.

Gendlin, E. T. (1996). *Focusing-oriented psychotherapy: A manual of the experiential method.* New York: Guilford Press.

Gendlin, E. T. (1997a). *A process model.* Spring Valley, NY: Focusing Institute.

Gendlin, E. T. (1997b). *Experiencing and the creation of meaning: A philosophical and psychological approach to the subjective.* Evanston, IL: Northwestern University Press.

Gendlin, E. T. (2003). Beyond postmodernism: From concepts through experiencing. In R. Frie (Ed.), *Understanding experience: Psychotherapy and postmodernism* (pp. 100–115). London: Routledge.

Gendlin, E. T. (2012). Implicit precision. In Z. Radman (Ed.), *Knowing without thinking: The theory of the background in philosophy of mind* (pp. 141–166). New York: Palgrave Macmillan.

Gendlin, E. T., Beebe, J., Cassens, J., Klein, M., & Oberlander, M. (1968). Focusing ability in psychotherapy, personality and creativity. In J. M. Shlien (Ed.), *Research in psychotherapy research in psychotherapy* (Vol. 3, pp. 217–241). Washington, DC: American Psychological Association.

Gilbert, P., McEwan, K., Gibbons, L., Chotai, S., Duarte, J., & Matos, M. (2012). Fears of compassion and happiness in relation to alexithymia, mindfulness, and self-criticism. *Psychology and Psychotherapy: Theory, Research and Practice, 85*(4), 374–390.

Greenberg, L. S., Elliott, R., & Lietaer, G. (1994). Research on humanistic and experiential psychotherapies. In A. E. Bergin & S. L. Garfield (Eds.), *Handbook of psychotherapy and behavior change* (4th ed., pp. 509–539). New York: Wiley.

James, W. (1890). *The principles of psychology* (Vol. 1). New York: Henry Holt. Retrieved July 11, 2014, from *https://archive.org/stream/theprinciplesofp01jameuoft#page/n5/mode/2up.*

Klein, M., Mathieu, P., Gendlin, E. T., & Kiesler, D. J. (1970). *The experiencing scale: A research and training manual* (Vols. 1–2). Madison: Wisconsin Psychiatric Institute, Bureau of Audio Visual Instruction.

Parker, R. A. (2014). Focusing oriented therapy: The message from research. In G. Madison (Ed.), *Theory and practice of focusing oriented psychotherapy: Beyond the talking cure* (pp. 259–272). London: Jessica Kingsley.

Turcotte, S. (2012). [Course handout.] Retrieved February 23, 2012, from *www.focusing.org/turcotte_handout.html.*

Watson, J. C., & Bedard, D. L. (2006). Clients' emotional processing in psychotherapy: A comparison between cognitive-behavioral and process–experiential therapies. *Journal of Consulting and Clinical Psychology, 74*(1), 152–159.

21

Intensive Vipassana
Meditation Practice
for Traumatized Prisoners

Jenny Phillips and James W. Hopper

The United States has the highest rate of incarceration in the world. According to the Bureau of Justice Statistics (2012), 2,266,800 adults were incarcerated in U.S. federal and state prisons and county jails at the end of 2010—about 0.7% of the resident adult population. Childhood trauma increases the likelihood of criminal justice involvement in adulthood (Wolf & Shi, 2010). A high percentage of prisoners are survivors of childhood abuse and other traumas before they are imprisoned (Wallace, Connor, & Dass-Brailsford, 2011), and prisons are notoriously violent and traumatic places for inmates. In a survey of inmates in Midwestern prisons, 54% of men and 28% of women reported having been raped in their current facilities (Struckman-Johnson & Struckman-Johnson, 2000). In short, prisons are veritable warehouses of traumatized adults.

Very few prisons have mental health treatment programs, and the few that are available—which range from educational to cognitive and behavioral in nature—do not have the capacity to treat chronic trauma and posttraumatic stress disorder (PTSD). The daily environment of prisons—aggressive and often violent, in which any indication of vulnerability or weakness is potentially life threatening—means that such programs cannot fulfill the requirements of safe and effective trauma treatment, especially for processing and integrating memories (Herman, 1992). Similarly, mindfulness and meditation programs cannot provide safe and effective trauma treatment in prisons, although evidence suggests they can reduce inmates' stress and anxiety and increase their self-regulation capacities (Casarjian, Phillips, & Wolman, 2005; Samuelson, Carmody, Kabat-Zinn, & Bratt, 2007).

Here we present an approach that, although new to prison-based trauma intervention, is over 2,000 years old: an intensive, 10-day vipassana meditation course that has been conducted inside a maximum-security prison since 2002. We briefly make the case that intensive, traditional, and communal vipassana practice makes good sense and holds great promise as a short-term prison-based trauma treatment that can provide stabilization, skills development, and safe and effective opportunities to process traumatic memories.

Prison Culture: Hypermasculinity and Violence

Imprisoned men live in an environment rife with deprivation, subordination, and danger. They are stripped of all the external, worldly trappings of status and power and are on a daily basis confronted with realities of degradation and humiliation that can cause crippling shame. Many feel there is nothing left to lose but their manhood. The constricted male role and ever-present sense of danger further contribute to extreme displays of manhood, including emotional "hardening" and acts of violence. In their intense and unrelenting battles over manhood and "respect," there are small but significant spoils. A can of soup borrowed but not replaced can lead opposing groups of "homeboys" and close associates into battle. They may not know exactly what they are fighting for, but it is acutely understood that the fight is about respect, honor, and the preservation of their manhood (Phillips, 2001).

Stages of Recovery and Treatment

In *Trauma and Recovery*, Judith Herman (1992) articulates a three-stage model of recovery from trauma. The central task of the first stage is the establishment of safety, which must begin with safety of the body and reduction of hyperarousal and intrusive symptoms. Safety next refers to gaining some control over one's environment, with the provision of a safe refuge and nurturing relationships. As Herman observes, "Recovery can take place only within the context of relationships; it cannot occur in isolation" (1992, p. 133).

Stage 2 of trauma recovery, if pursued, involves working directly with traumatic material, typically via formal exposure therapy or trauma-informed "talk therapy." As Herman notes, this work "actually transforms the traumatic memory, so that it can be integrated into the survivor's life story" (1992, p. 175). Indeed, a "narrative that does not include the traumatic imagery and bodily sensations is barren and incomplete" (Herman, 1992, p. 177). Finally, Stage 3 is described as a process of moving into the future and "reclaiming the world."

With respect to the second stage of recovery, van der Kolk and colleagues (van der Kolk, McFarlane, & van der Hart, 1996) write that the aims include helping clients "move from being haunted by the past and interpreting subsequent emotionally arousing stimuli as a return of the trauma, to being fully engaged in the present and becoming capable of responding to current exigencies . . . learning to tolerate the memories of intense emotional experiences is a critical part of recovery" (1996, p. 419). The stage model of trauma treatment is key to a central question posed in this chapter: Is it beneficial—even possible—to offer prisoners interventions that involve directly engaging with traumatic memories?

Trauma-Informed Correctional Care

The institutional focus of prisons is typically maintenance of order and control. With scarce resources, little attention can be directed to treatment of mental illness and trauma (Kupers, 1999). Until recently, the literature on prison treatment rarely even discussed trauma treatment (Wallace et al., 2011). Clearly prisons and jails are challenging settings for treating acute trauma and PTSD. Yet there is a great need for accessible and effective mental health services. Without treatment, incarcerated men and women with PTSD are more likely to relapse into substance use and return to criminal behavior (Kubiak, 2004).

In response to these realities, Wallace and colleagues (2011) have called for an integrated approach to trauma treatment in correctional health, one that is multimodal and concurrent (e.g., one that addresses substance abuse, trauma, and other psychiatric symptoms at the same time, rather than incompletely or only sequentially). This approach draws from a menu of evidence-based treatments, including cognitive-behavioral therapy, motivational interviewing, relapse prevention, and 12-step programs (Wallace et al., 2011), and is consistent with National Institute on Drug Abuse (1999) guidelines for the treatment of drug addiction.

Given the culture of most prisons—institutions governed by systems of control and norms of punishment and violence—we contend that merely inserting trauma-focused treatment, even the best empirically validated and integrated approach, will always be inadequate. Given the need for safety in trauma treatment, "trauma-informed correctional care" has been advanced as a model of staff and administration involvement in changing prison cultures to promote safety, recovery, and rehabilitation. Trauma-informed correctional care, a relatively recent concept, has the following primary goals, articulated by Harris and Fallot (2001): "accurate identification of trauma and related symptoms, training all staff to be aware of the impact of trauma, minimizing re-traumatization, and a fundamental 'do no harm' approach that is sensitive to how institutions may inadvertently reenact traumatic dynamics" (2001, p. 1).

Cognitive-behavioral interventions have been viewed as central components of a broad and integrated trauma-informed care approach (Miller & Najavits, 2012). Meta-analyses have shown that such interventions reduce substance use, mental health symptoms, and recidivism (Andrews, Bonta, & Hoge, 1990; Landenberger & Lipsey, 2005). Yet as Miller and Najavits (2012) have noted, "There is sometimes great reluctance to open the trauma 'can of worms' given the prison environment and the limited clinical resources available" (p. 6). This is particularly the case with respect to Stage 2 treatments involving exposure to and processing of traumatic memories. Indeed, thoughtful clinicians and researchers have been dubious about the prospects in today's prisons:

> Past-focused models, such as exposure therapy (Foa, Hembree & Rothbaum, 2007), may be evidence-based models for PTSD, but have a real risk of emotionally destabilizing inmates who are already vulnerable. The security response to such destabilization can set the cycle of re-traumatization in motion. In the current climate, prison environments are likely best suited to present-focused approaches, given the unmet need for more mental health training, staffing limitations, and the typical lack of funding for additional formally trained and supervised staff required for past-focused PTSD treatments such as exposure therapy. (Miller & Najavits, 2012, p. 6)

As described in this chapter, our experience and preliminary empirical data suggest that intensive vipassana meditation practice, specifically a well-designed 10-day group retreat within prison walls, can be a safe and potentially effective Stage 1 and Stage 2 trauma treatment. Before addressing our experience and findings, however, it is necessary to provide theoretical and practical knowledge about vipassana meditation and its potential as a trauma-specific intervention in correctional settings.

Contemplative Practices as Trauma Treatment: Implications for Prisoners

The English word *mindfulness* is derived from the Pali term *sati* and its Sanskrit counterpart *smṛti*. These terms refer to deliberately and knowingly keeping one's attention on a desired object without having attention become captured by proliferating mental phenomena that normally arise following the brain's automatic assignment of positive, negative, or neutral feeling tones to passing sensations, including mental sensations, that is, thoughts (Grabovac, Lau, & Willett, 2011). This concept and its application in meditation practice lie at the heart of 2,500-year-old Buddhist psychology and underlie contemporary definitions of mindfulness such as that of Kabat-Zinn (2003, p. 145): "the awareness that emerges through paying attention on purpose, in the present moment, and non-judgmentally to the unfolding of experience moment to moment."

A detailed and technical discussion of mindfulness and the traditional Buddhist practices for its cultivation and application to yield transformative "insight" into the moment-to-moment causes of suffering, liberation, and lasting happiness is beyond the scope of this chapter. In brief, a mindful approach to trauma treatment values direct experience of post-traumatic phenomena more than recounting or processing trauma narratives. Painful memories and feelings (especially passing interoceptive sensations) are directly experienced, in great detail, with an observing or witnessing awareness. A combined focus on present experiences and memories—as both continually arise into and pass out of awareness—allows several healing processes to unfold. These include the awareness and recognition of previously unattended bodily sensations and emotional processes (e.g., extremely brief yet powerful links in chains of fear and addictive conditioning). Another healing process involves accessing and associatively linking together memory representations, including previously consciously unavailable or dissociated ones, which can foster the spontaneous emergence of transformative insights and wise, healing personal narratives.

Consistent with this perspective, Simpson and colleagues (2007) contend that intensive mindfulness-based meditation practice targets and can reduce "experiential avoidance." This is particularly relevant for those who suffer from PTSD and substance dependence, as experiential avoidance may be a driver of substance use in that population (Orsillo & Roemer, 2005; Walser & Westrup. 2007). That is, mindfulness interventions "seek to limit efforts to avoid internal and external experience by fostering non-judgmental acceptance of moment-to-moment experiences" (Simpson et al., 2007, p. 240), and mindfulness training has the potential to reduce substance abuse relapse by providing skills for tolerating unpleasant and painful emotions. Indeed, in their pilot study of a 10-day Vipassana program in a minimum security jail, Simpson and colleagues (2007) found comparable improvements in illicit drug use and drinking outcomes for those both with and without PTSD. The researchers concluded that those with PTSD benefited from having "a new way of dealing with painful affect and thoughts, including those that are trauma related" (Simpson et al., 2007, p. 246). This preliminary finding suggests that intensive vipassana meditation could be an effective treatment for both trauma and substance abuse among prisoners.

Buddhist Psychology and Vipassana Meditation

Grabovac and colleagues (2011, p. 220) focus on three essential tenets of Buddhist psychology, traditionally referred to as the "three characteristics":

1. "Sense impressions and mental events are transient (they arise and pass away)."
2. "Habitual reactions (i.e., attachment and aversion) to the feelings of a sense impression or mental event [i.e., basic hedonic attributions as positive, negative, or neutral], and a lack of awareness of this process, lead to suffering."
3. "Sense impressions and mental events do not contain or constitute any lasting separate entity that could be called a self."

A core insight of Buddhist psychology is that suffering and symptoms can be reduced, even eliminated, through disciplined practices. Dispassionately observing the unfolding stream of sensations (including mental events) without attempting manipulation or control is central to the approach. Eventually, this can greatly reduce or eliminate the typical proliferation of mental phenomena (including maladaptive appraisals, thoughts, and emotions) that follow the brain's automatic attributions of salience to passing sensations. (These attributions of positive, negative, or neutral salience are largely based in prior conditioning, including prior traumatic and addictive experiences.) This, in turn, allows unexplored, rejected, and suppressed experiences and emotions to surface and become part of the (therapeutic) process of mindful attending. In essence, equanimity in the presence of one's suffering is the path to freedom from that suffering—and to a truly satisfying happiness that is not fleetingly dependent on grasping what is wanted and rejecting what is unwanted.

In Pali, one of the ancient languages of earliest Buddhist texts, *vipassana* means "seeing things as they actually are." The Burmese vipassana tradition derives from the original training techniques of the Buddha, and a version founded by S. N. Goenka is followed in the prison course described in this chapter.[1] *Anapana sati*, the Pali phrase meaning awareness of respiration, is an important skill taught and practiced during the first 3 days of a Goenka vipassana course. For a total of 30 hours, a student sits and focuses on the upper lip below the nostrils, noticing sensations of the breath coming in and going out. This is known as moment-to-moment "bare

---

[1]Over the past 10 years, Goenka 10-day vipassana programs have been offered in prisons in India, Israel, Mongolia, New Zealand, Taiwan, Thailand, the United Kingdom, and the United States. Other vipassana traditions and practices, brought to the West by Jack Kornfield, Joseph Goldstein, Sharon Salzberg, Thanisarro Bhikkhu, and others, may be equally appropriate in prison settings.

attention" to the natural breath. For 15 minutes after every sitting meditation throughout the course, students are taught and practice metta (or loving-kindness) meditation, in which they concentrate on visual images, bodily sensations, and thoughts associated with wishing happiness, health, and the freedom from suffering for themselves and others (Salzberg, 1995). Students reported that this practice helped them calm their minds to effectively engage in the other practices, as well as providing experiences of love, compassion, and happiness that were found to be profound, healing, and transformative in their own right.

As one sits, hour after hour, the mind may go wild with thoughts, emotions, memories, and other distractions. Students learn that the breath is an important bridge between body and mind. *Anapana sati* trains mind, brain, and body to become calm, still, and sharply focused. To the extent that attentional resources are focused on breathing sensations and away from the automatically arising proliferation of mental events and the "default activity" of the wandering mind, habitual reactions and patterns of aversion and craving progressively lose their intensity and dominance of mental processes. *Anapana sati* also allows students to gradually develop an anchoring skill that can help with facing deeper emotional storms that will likely emerge later in the course.

On the 4th day and over the following 6 days, the core skill of Goenka vipassana is practiced: systematically directing one's awareness, refined by *anapana sati*, throughout the body, from the top of the head to the toes and back again, observing bodily sensations as they manifest themselves. After 3 days of *anapana sati*, this shift to the whole body can be liberating, but it can also uncover and release strong emotions, and traumatic memories and experiences may rise to the surface. Eventually, if the practice goes well, whatever arises—including vivid traumatic memories or intense experiences of grief, shame, and guilt—can be observed dispassionately as arising and passing events, without generating or feeding one's typical proliferation of emotional, cognitive, and behavioral responses associated with aversion and craving.

Vipassana meditation can be understood as offering elements of both Stage 1 and Stage 2 trauma treatment. Although it may seem strange, given the prison context, a safe refuge is created by a supportive environment, set apart from the rest of the prison, with guidance and constant support of course teachers. Stabilization and regulation of mind and body are achieved through the practice of *anapana sati*. With that stabilization in place, the practice of vipassana facilitates a spontaneous and simple yet deep processing of traumatic material. In essence, long-avoided and previously unavailable memories, emotions, and other posttraumatic experiences are brought to the surface and—in an observant, stable, and present-focused state—become available for understanding and integration that are transformative and healing.

In the words of meditation teacher Bruce Stewart, who has led 10-day programs for prisoners:

The unlocking of these memories, physical sensations and emotions produces what we refer to as 'storms,' or waves, of reactivity. We guide the student through these storms so they can discover experientially that, regardless of how deep and horrible and painful a storm might be—mentally, physically and emotionally—everything is constantly changing, arising and passing away. (as quoted in Phillips, 2008, p. 28)

Bringing Vipassana Inside: The Case of a Maximum-Security Prison in Alabama

The William E. Donaldson Correctional Facility is a maximum-security Alabama prison known as the "house of pain," which houses approximately 1,500 prisoners, mostly those with the worst crimes and longest sentences. In 2002, the Alabama Department of Corrections began conducting 10-day Goenka vipassana meditation courses at Donaldson. This was the first time a vipassana program was brought into a state prison within the United States.[2] A detailed account of how the vipassana program was brought to Donaldson is found in *The Dhamma Brothers: East Meets West in the Deep South*, an award-winning documentary film (Phillips, Stein, & Kukura, 2008), and in Phillips (2008).

After more than a year of meetings between the Donaldson staff and the North American Vipassana Prison Trust and of orientation meetings with the prisoners who signed up for the program, the warden and administrative staff at Donaldson were ready to take a highly unusual step: They agreed to allow three skilled and experienced vipassana teachers to move into the prison and live in close quarters with the inmates during the 10-day vipassana program. The continual presence and guidance of the teachers, a normal requirement of all vipassana courses, was an essential aspect of the prison program. The teachers were a constant, calm presence, meditating among the prisoners and quietly overseeing their daily lives—sorting their laundry, serving their vegetarian food, and offering encouragement and instruction. This nurturing atmosphere, highly unusual within prison, helped create a secure and supportive refuge in which safety, stabilization, and the work of encountering traumatic material could take place.

Another requirement of the North American Vipassana Prison Trust for prison-based courses is that some prison staff members themselves first take a 10-day vipassana course. Six members of Donaldson's treatment and security staffs did so, which enabled them to understand personally and deeply the experience of vipassana and its potential benefits in the prison environment.

---

[2]The first vipassana course in a North American correctional facility was conducted in 1997 at the North Rehabilitation Facility, a minimum-security adult jail in Seattle, Washington (Meijer, 1999). The first in the world took place in India in the 1970s, as documented in the 1997 film, *Doing Time, Doing Vipassana* (Ariel & Manahemi, 1997).

In January of 2002, the three vipassana teachers and 20 prisoners moved into a gym at Donaldson, forming a meditating community that spent the next 10 days locked in together, meditating for over 100 hours. There was much apprehension; both teachers and prisoners feared each other. Some prisoners were from rival gangs, and correction officers placed bets on whether they could last even 1 day. The 20 prisoners made a pact: "Twenty in, twenty out, twenty strong." The teachers quickly overcame their fear of the prisoners, and within an atmosphere of hushed tranquility and safety, a deep sense of shared purpose and mutual respect developed.

The teachers recognized the prisoners as exceptional vipassana students who brought high levels of commitment, fortitude, and dedication to meditating and facing their inner demons. They witnessed the prisoners' collective desire to cultivate equanimity and wisdom. Most of the prisoners had no background in formal meditation, yet the teachers noticed that they worked harder than students in courses outside prison. At times, the prisoners had to be encouraged to back off and to take breaks. As described by teacher Bruce Stewart:

> These guys already knew suffering so profoundly and blatantly. They were under no illusion that they were happy. They knew from the start that they were miserable. But they didn't yet know why they were miserable. Now through meditation they . . . learned to be in the present, to face the present moment at the level of sensations and to accept that moment. Vipassana gave them the tools to face, at a deep level, all that misery inside." (as quoted in Phillip. 2008, p. 29)

Preliminary Outcome Research

Since 2006, the 10-day vipassana course has been offered four times a year at Donaldson, and a 3-day course is offered twice a year. By fall of 2012, 19 courses had been held, and 550 inmates had completed the 10-day program. Collecting data in a prison setting presents many challenges, particularly over longer time periods, because prisoners may be transferred to other facilities. Only limited research has been conducted and published thus far, though limited preliminary results have been reported in a peer-reviewed publication (Perelman et al., 2012). The authors report on data collected immediately before the program (111 participants: 50 in vipassana meditation and 61 in a comparison group), immediately after completion (74 total, 45 vipassana meditation), and at 1-year follow-up (56 total, 35 vipassana meditation). The comparison condition was Houses of Healing (HOH; Casarjian, 1995), a 10-week small-group program based in principles of mindfulness and emotional awareness that provides guidance in taking responsibility for oneself via healthy stress management, in brief meditation and coping strategies, and in forgiving oneself and others.

Around 80% of study participants were incarcerated for a violent offense, with one-third serving life sentences. Over 90% reported belonging to a Western religion, and the vipassana meditation and comparison groups did not differ demographically, with the exception that more vipassana meditation participants identified their race as "other." The vipassana meditation group had also served more time (12.4 vs. 8.6 years), though neither group had more prison infractions (controlling for time served). Both groups had much lower rates of substance abuse diagnoses (12.6%) than have been found among state and federal inmates (53% and 45%, respectively; Mumola & Karberg, 2007). History of trauma, as well as current and past PTSD and other psychiatric diagnoses, was not assessed.

The major dependent variables in the first wave of research included self-reported mindfulness (Cognitive and Affective Mindfulness Scale [CAMS-R]; Feldman, Hayes, Kumar, Greeson, & Laurenceau, 2007), anger (Novaco Anger Inventory—Short Form [NAI-25]; Mills, Kroner, & Forth, 1998), overall mood disturbance (Profile of Mood States—Short Form [POMS-SF]; Shacham, 1983), and emotional intelligence (Trait Meta-Mood Scale [TMMS]; Salovey, Mayer, Goldman, Turvey, & Palfai, 1995), as well as documented infractions. Given missing data due to attrition and other factors, analyses employed linear mixed modeling followed by pairwise comparisons.

For self-reported mindfulness, vipassana meditation participants had higher scores overall (due to some vipassana meditation participants having completed a prior intensive vipassana meditation program), but using conservative (analysis of variance) statistical analyses, there were no changes over time, including as a function of intervention. More liberal statistical methods (pairwise comparisons) revealed higher postintervention mindfulness in the vipassana meditation group and an increase in pre- to postretreat mindfulness scores among vipassana meditation but not HOH participants. For emotional intelligence, the conservative analysis found improvements over time across both groups but no differences between groups or effects of intervention; the more liberal analysis indicated increases in the vipassana meditation group over the postretreat year. For overall mood disturbance, there was a group difference, with the vipassana meditation group having lower disturbance overall, but no effects of the intervention, even as assessed with less conservative statistics. For self-reported anger, no effects were found. Finally, with respect to documented institutional infractions, no effects of group or intervention were found; these findings could have been due to range restriction in the data, as 54% of participants across both groups had no infractions in the year after the course.

These preliminary findings suggest that vipassana meditation participants had, at least on self-report, (1) generally greater mindfulness than comparison participants, perhaps due to meditation experience, including prior 10-day programs; (2) immediate postretreat improvements in mindfulness; and (3) greater levels of emotional awareness 1 year after the retreat. This preliminary research has several limitations, however, including small sample size, lack of random assignment to group, substantial missing data, and assessment with a limited number of measures, none of which addressed posttraumatic symptoms.

Future research should assess for effects of this intensive prison vipassana program on PTSD, depression, and other posttraumatic symptoms and problems (e.g., difficulties with emotion regulation), as well as behavioral indicators associated with prison conduct and recidivism. In addition to other design and analysis refinements, future studies should assess and control for prior retreat experience and extent of regular vipassana meditation practice, both before and after the 10-day program.

Whereas the quantitative findings to date are quite limited, the qualitative data are very rich and compelling. As noted earlier, one particular 10-day program and several of its participants are subjects of the acclaimed documentary *The Dhamma Brothers: East Meets West in the Deep South* (Phillips et al., 2008), and a companion book, *Letters from the Dhamma Brothers: Meditation behind Bars* (Phillips, 2008). There are many stories of Donaldson prisoners learning to concentrate and calm their minds, observe their internal experiences with bare attention, and, in exquisite detail, process and integrate past traumas and develop transformative new capacities for self-reflection, insight, and understanding. Many tell of taking responsibility for their lives, including their crimes and the great harms they have caused others.

Conclusion and Implications

Given the right conditions, it appears that a prison can be a place for successfully implementing a traditional contemplative meditation retreat—one that constitutes a brief, intensive, and potentially transformative mental health intervention. A 10-day vipassana meditation program is appropriate for some prisoners, has been used in several jails and prisons in India and the United States, and has begun to produce empirical evidence of its potential benefits.

Although prisons can be harsh, hypermasculine, and often violent places for traumatized inmates (and staff), they can also be places in which there can arise—thanks in part to the acute and undeniable suffering inmates confront within themselves every day—profound yearnings for inner freedom and powerful commitments to self-transformation. Vipassana programs like that offered at maximum-security Donaldson Correctional Facility have the potential to harness those yearnings and commitments to a disciplined practice that can bring calm, clarity, insight, and healing to traumatized prisoners. The current quantitative evidence is limited but growing, while the personal stories of inmates and testimony of staff members have been compellingly documented in films, books, and other publications (e.g., Phillips et al., 2008; Phillips, 2008). It is important evidence and testimony as well that Donaldson has offered four 10-day Vipassana retreats every year since 2006.

Certainly not every inmate is ready or willing to engage in such intensive contemplative work, and other interventions and skills are needed to complement disciplined traditional meditation practice. But for those who are able, it appears that vipassana retreats can facilitate both the first and second stages of trauma recovery—including processing and integration of memories, typically regarded as impossible or simply too risky to attempt in today's prison environments. Again, more research is needed, including how best to select and prepare prisoners for intensive practice and how to help them maintain and integrate its benefits.

Increasingly, prison mental health staff and administrators are seeking interventions that can address prisoners' posttraumatic suffering—and their deficits of empathy, conscience, self-respect, and self-control—that can be so destructive to prisoners, prison staff, and the families and communities into which many prisoners are released. The 2,500-year-old practice of intensive vipassana meditation is now an available and promising option, both for prisoners who will be released someday and those who never will.

Notable Resources

The Dhamma Brothers: East meets West in the deep South. (2007). Award-winning documentary film by J. Phillips, A. M. Stein, and A. Kukura. *www.dhammabrothers.com*

The Dhamma Brothers on Facebook. Creating a national conversation and call to action about the need for effective prison treatment programs. *www.facebook.com/DhammaBrothers*

Letters from the Dhamma Brothers: Meditation Behind Bars (2008). Jenny Phillips tells the story of how the Vipassana course came to Donaldson Correctional Facility, introduces many of the "Dhamma brothers," and shares their letters of testimony about their initial and ongoing experiences of the practice and its transformation of their lives.

Vipassana Prison Trust. Website on S. N. Goenka vipassana meditation courses offered at Donaldson and other prisons and correctional environments, including information about how to bring courses to a particular facility. *www.prison.dhamma.org*

References

Andrews, D. A., Bonta, J., & Hoge, R. D. (1990). Classification for effective rehabilitation: Rediscovering psychology. *Criminal Justice and Behavior, 17,* 19–52.

Ariel, E., & Menahemi, A. (1997). *Doing time, doing vipassana* [Motion picture]. Tel Aviv: Karuna Films.

Begley, S. (2007). *Train your mind, change your brain.* New York: Ballantine.

Bureau of Justice Statistics. (2012). *Correctional population in the United States.* Washington, DC: U.S. Department of Justice.

Casarjian, R. (1995) *Houses of healing: A prisoner's guide to inner power and freedom.* Boston: Lionheart Foundation.

Casarjian, R., Phillips, J., & Wolman, R. (2005). An emotional literacy intervention with incarcerated individuals. *American Journal of Forensic Psychiatry, 26,* 65–85.

Feldman, G., Hayes, A., Kumar, S., Greeson, J., & Laurenceau, J.-P. (2007). Mindfulness and emotion regulation: The development and initial validation of the Cognitive and Affective Mindfulness Scale—Revised (CAMS-R). *Journal of Psychopathology and Behavioral Assessment, 29,* 177–190.

Foa, E. B., Hembree, E. A., & Rothbaum, B. O. (2007). *Prolonged exposure therapy for PTSD: Emotional processing of traumatic experiences—Therapist guide.* New York: Oxford University Press.

Germer, C. (2005). Mindfulness: What is it? What does it matter? In C. K. Germer, R. D. Siegel, & P. R. Fulton (Eds.), *Mindfulness and psychotherapy* (pp. 3–27). New York: Guilford Press.

Grabovac, A. D., Lau, M. A., & Willett, B. R. (2011). Mechanisms of mindfulness: A Buddhist psychological model. *Mindfulness, 2,* 154–166.

Harris, M., & Fallot, R. D. (2001). *Using trauma theory to design service systems.* San Francisco: Jossey-Bass.

Harrison, P. M., & Beck, A. J. (2005). *Prison and jail inmates at mid-year.* Washington, DC: U.S. Department of Justice, Bureau of Justice Statistics. Retrieved from *www.ncjrs.gov/app/publications/abstract.aspx?ID=234627.*

Herman, J. (1992). *Trauma and recovery.* New York: Basic Books.

Kabat-Zinn, J. (2003). Mindfulness-based interventions in context: Past, present, and future. *Clinical Psychology: Science and Practice, 10*(2), 144–156.

Kubiak, S. P. (2004). The effects of PTSD on treatment adherence, drug relapse and criminal recidivism in a sample of incarcerated men and women. *Research on Social Work Practice, 14,* 424–433.

Kupers, T. (1999). *Prison madness: The mental health crisis behind bars and what we must do about it.* San Francisco: Jossey Bass.

Landenberger, N. A., & Lipsey, M. W. (2005). The positive effects of cognitive-behavioral programs for offenders: A meta-analysis of factors associated with effective treatment. *Journal of Experimental Criminology, 1,* 451–476.

Langan, P. A., & Levin, D. J. (2002, June 2). *Recidivism of prisoners released in 1994.* Washington, DC: U.S. Department of Justice, Bureau of Justice Statistics.

Liptak, A. (2008, February 28). 1 in 100 U.S. adults behind bars, new study says. *New York Times.* Available at *www.nytimes.com.*

Meijer, L. (1999). Vipassana meditation at the North Rehabilitation Facility. *American Jails Magazine, 4,* 9–13.

Miller, N., & Najavits, L. (2012). Creating trauma-informed correctional care: A balance of goals and environment. *European Journal of Psychotraumatology, 3.* Available at *www.readcube.com/articles/10.3402/ejpt.v3i0.17246.*

Mills, J. F., Kroner, D. G., & Forth, A. E. (1998). Novaco Anger Scale: Reliability and validity within an adult criminal sample. *Assessment, 5,* 237–248.

Mumola, C. J., & Karberg, J. C. (2007, January 19). *Drug use and dependence, state and federal prisoners, 2004.* Washington, DC: U.S. Department of

Justice, Bureau of Justice Statistics. Retrieved from *http://bjs.ojp.usdoj.gov/content/pub/pdf/dudsfp04.pdf.*

National Institute on Drug Abuse. (1999). *Principles of drug abuse treatment: A research based guide* (NIH Publication No. 09-4180). Rockville, MD: Author.

Orsillo, S. M., & Roemer, L. (Eds.). (2005). *Acceptance and mindfulness-based approaches to anxiety: New directions in conceptualization and treatment.* New York: Kluwer Academic/Plenum.

Perelman, A. M., Miller, S. L., Clements, C. B., Rodriguez, A., Allen, K., & Cavanaugh, R. (2012). Meditation in a Deep South prison: A longitudinal study of the effects of Vipassana. *Journal of Offender Rehabilitation, 51,* 176–198.

Phillips, J. (2001). Cultural construction of manhood in prison. *Psychology of Men and Masculinity, 2,* 13–23.

Phillips, J. (2008). *Letters from the Dhamma brothers: Meditation behind bars.* Onalaska, WA: Pariyatti Press.

Phillips, J., Stein, A. M., & Kukura, A. (2008). *The Dhamma brothers: East meets West in the deep South* [Motion picture]. Concord, MA: Freedom Behind Bars Productions.

Samuelson, M., Carmody, J., Kabat-Zinn, J., & Bratt M. A. (2007). Mindfulness-based stress reduction in Massachusetts correctional facilities. *Prison Journal, 87,* 254.

Salovey, P., Mayer, J. D., Goldman, S. L., Turvey, C., & Palfai, T. P. (1995). Emotional attention, clarity, and repair: Exploring emotional intelligence using the Trait Meta Mood Scale. In J. W. Pennebaker (Ed.), *Emotion, disclosure, and health* (pp. 125–154). Washington, DC: American Psychological Association.

Salzberg, S. (1995). *Lovingkindness: The revolutionary art of happiness.* Boston: Shambhala.

Shacham, S. (1983). A shortened version of the Profile of Mood States. *Journal of Personality Assessment, 47,* 305–306.

Simpson, T. L., Kaysen, D., Bowen, S., MacPherson, L. M., Chawla, N., Blume, A., et al. (2007). PTSD symptoms, substance use, and vipassana meditation among incarcerated individuals. *Journal of Traumatic Stress, 20,* 239–249.

Struckman-Johnson, C., & Struckman-Johnson, D. (2000). Sexual coercion rates in seven midwestern prisons for men. *Prison Journal, 80,* 379–390.

van der Kolk, B., McFarlane, A. C., & van der Hart, O. (1996). A general approach to treatment of posttraumatic stress disorder. In B. A. van der Kolk, A. C. McFarlane, & L. Weisaeth (Eds.), *Traumatic stress* (pp. 417–440). New York: Guilford Press.

Wallace, B., Connor, L., & Dass-Brailsford, P. (2011). Integrated trauma treatment in correctional health care and community-based treatment upon reentry. *Journal of Correctional Health Care, 17,* 329–343.

Walser, R., & Westrup, D. (2007). *Acceptance and commitment therapy for the treatment of post-traumatic stress disorder and trauma-related problems: A practitioner's guide to using mindfulness and acceptance strategies.* Oakland, CA: New Harbinger.

Wolf, N. L., & Shi, J. (2010). Trauma and incarcerated persons. In C. L. Scott (Ed.), *Handbook of correctional mental health.* Arlington, VA: American Psychiatric Publishing.

22

Cognitively Based
Compassion Training
for Adolescents

Brooke Dodson-Lavelle, Brendan Ozawa-de Silva,
Geshe Lobsang Tenzin Negi, and Charles L. Raison

Cognitively based compassion training (CBCT) is a systematic, secular program for enhancing emotional intelligence, social connectedness, empathy, and compassion. The program was originally developed in 2005 by Geshe Lobsang Tenzin Negi at Emory University to investigate whether a compassion-meditation-based program might help address the rising rate of depression among undergraduate students. In subsequent years, the program has been adapted for use with healthy adults, elementary school-children, adolescents in foster care, and survivors of trauma as a means of promoting prosocial skills, resiliency, health, and well-being. Though it incorporates certain elements of mindfulness practice, it differs substantially from mindfulness-based programs in that it relies heavily on analytical meditation practices drawn from the Tibetan Buddhist *lojong* (Tibetan: *blo sbyong*) or "mind training" tradition (Negi, 2009). The *lojong* tradition offers systematic methods to help practitioners progressively cultivate other-centered, altruistic thoughts and behaviors while overcoming maladaptive, self-focused thoughts and behaviors, which are understood to be the cause of suffering for oneself and others (Jinpa, 2006). In this chapter we outline the theory and practice of CBCT and provide an overview of our current research programs. We then discuss potential applications for the treatment of trauma in the context of our experience in adapting CBCT for adolescents in foster care.

Cognitively Based Compassion Training

Increasing evidence suggests that positive emotions, including compassion and feelings of social connection, have demonstrable effects on psychological and physiological health and well-being (Cacioppo & Hawkley, 2009; Pace et al., 2009, 2010). Moreover, research suggests that a seemingly innate capacity for compassion can be trained (Lutz, Slagter, Dunne, & Davidson, 2008; Pace et al., 2009, 2010). Though there are many methods for cultivating compassion, there are at present only a few programs selected for scientific research that focus primarily on the systematic cultivation of compassion.

In the CBCT model, compassion is understood as the heartfelt wish that others be free from suffering and the readiness to act on their behalf. It arises from a deep sense of affection for others, coupled with the recognition that their suffering can be alleviated. This sensitivity arises from both a sense of closeness or connectedness to others and a recognition of the causes of their suffering.

Generally, a person is able to empathize readily with members of his or her own family or social group but generally finds it more difficult to empathize with strangers or members of other social groups, especially those who have harmed or who threaten to harm oneself in some way. To generate this closeness to others and expand his or her capacity for empathy, a person works through a series of analytical meditations aimed at deconstructing in-group and out-group categories. To generate affection and gratitude, an individual reflects on the kindness of others and the ways in which he or she depends on others in countless ways to survive. The person also reflects on the ways in which all people are alike in their wish to experience happiness and avoid suffering. To understand this last crucial point, which is central to the success of the program, the individual reflects upon his or her own desire for happiness and carefully examines the habits of mind that lead to happiness and those that lead to further suffering.

This is the basic conceptual framework of the CBCT program. These components are taught systematically in the following eight ordered steps, typically over the course of 8 weeks: (1) developing attention and stability of mind; (2) cultivating insight into the nature of mental experience; (3) cultivating self-compassion; (4) developing impartiality; (5) developing appreciation and gratitude; (6) developing affection and empathy; (7) generating aspirational compassion; and (8) realizing active compassion. These steps build sequentially upon one another in a logical manner, and thus we move systematically through each step in the protocol, providing a brief description of the key theoretical and pedagogical points, as well as the potential implications for the treatment of trauma contained within each step.

Developing Attention and Stability of Mind

The foundation for the practice of compassion is the cultivation of a basic degree of refined attention and mental stability. In this step, practitioners are instructed to attend to their breath moment by moment. When distractions arise, they are instructed to simply note them and then to return attention to the breath. Basic training in attention is necessary for practitioners to gain awareness into thoughts, feelings, and emotions. Without gaining this awareness, one cannot interrupt and transform habitual, maladaptive reactions. Focused meditation is also necessary in order for one to learn to stabilize and incorporate the understanding that results from the analytical meditations that follow. Research has shown that attention training is associated with a decrease in habitual patterns of reaction in general and also to emotionally reactive behaviors, which may be one effect of the ability to disengage from distractions (Lutz et al., 2008). Thus this initial training stage may not only serve as a support for additional stages but may also have additional salutary effects.

Cultivating Insight into the Nature of Mental Experience

After cultivating a degree of stable attention, practitioners are taught to turn their attention to the inner processes of thoughts, feelings, emotions, and reactions in order to gain insight into their mental experience. In this step, practitioners are instructed to simply attend to whatever arises within one's field of awareness, without judgment, and without getting caught up or carried away by thoughts, images, or emotions that may arise. This style of practice is not object-focused but instead encourages one to monitor the content of experience, without rejecting or suppressing any particular thoughts or feelings. Practitioners therefore learn to attend to their experience without judgment, thereby building up an openness or tolerance to all experiences.

Research suggests that mental noting or affect labeling may inhibit automatic emotional responses, thereby interrupting or diminishing their duration (Lutz et al., 2008). This style of practice can help practitioners avoid getting caught up in various conceptual schemes or simulations, including emotionally aversive or ruminative ones. It may also buffer against a potential negative consequence of focused attention training that is especially relevant to the treatment of trauma: in some cases, if practiced incorrectly, focused attention training may actually condition one to become averse to distracting, and especially negative, stimuli. Thus an objectless style of practice that promotes an openness to all experience may be particularly useful in this context.

Cultivating Self-Compassion

In this step, the practitioner explores his or her innate desire for happiness and well-being and investigates the mental states and habits that contribute to well-being and those that contribute to suffering. With this insight, the practitioner resolves to overcome these negative and harmful mental and emotional states and cultivate those that promote and increase happiness and well-being. Taken together, (1) the recognition of the source of one's suffering, together with (2) the understanding that one can change one's mental habits and (3) the commitment to do so are understood as self-compassion.

Although we incorporate more common conceptions of self-compassion as being kind and understanding toward oneself, this model assumes that without insight into the causes of suffering, one cannot effect the radical transformation necessary to overcome that suffering. We believe that this additional step, coupled with practices that help one develop a firm conviction to overcome suffering, further engenders emotional balance and intelligence, inner strength, determination, and resilience. This is the most difficult—and most crucial—step in the protocol.

Developing Impartiality

In this protocol, impartiality refers to specific analytical training aimed at helping practitioners overcome bias and develop equanimity toward others. Normally one tends to cling to categories such as friends, strangers, and adversaries and to react unevenly to people, based on those categories, with overattachment, indifference, and dislike. In this step, the practitioner is instructed to visualize a friend, a stranger, and a person whom they have difficulties with and to note the different and uneven feelings that arise as they imagine these three individuals undergoing positive or negative experiences. The practitioner is then encouraged to investigate these responses and examine whether the categories of friend, stranger, and adversary are fixed and rigid or superficial. For example, one may reflect upon whether an adversary has become a friend and vice versa. Upon recognizing that these categories are flexible and that they are not based on any inherent differences, one generates the intention to relate to people from an equal perspective and also works to recognize that all people are alike in wanting to be happy and to avoid suffering.

This step helps the practitioner facilitate an openness to others not normally considered as part of his or her in-group. He or she also learns to recognize the social dangers inherent in biased thinking and works to correct these imbalances. By reducing the strong boundaries that seem to exist between these groups, an individual can also slowly learn to expand his or her own social circle and feel more connected to others. Studies have shown that social connectivity has a protective effect against a wide range of factors, including stress, depression, and posttraumatic stress disorder (PTSD; Cacioppo & Hawkley, 2009). Psychosocial stress, including depression or a perceived sense of social isolation, can also trigger the production of proinflammatory cytokines, which have been implicated in a host of chronic disorders (Raison, Capuron, & Miller, 2006).

Developing Appreciation and Gratitude for Others

In this step, one reflects on all the ways in which one's very survival is dependent on the support and kindness of countless others. For example, a practitioner is instructed to visualize someone in his or her life who has been kind or generous and to reflect on the various ways in which this person has helped him or her. He or she then considers the various ways in which this kindness could be repaid. The practitioner is then encouraged to reflect upon the interdependent web of individuals that people rely upon for basic needs like food, clothing, or shelter. A deep recognition of this fundamental interdependence can facilitate a sense of appreciation and gratitude for others. Researchers have found that simply listing or recalling others' kind acts can increase one's subjective happiness (Otake, Shimai, Tanaka-Matsumi, & Otsui, 2006). Further, research suggests that reflecting on things one is grateful for has protective health benefits (Emmons & McCullough, 2003).

Developing Affection and Empathy

This step involves deeper contemplation and insight into the ways in which benefits are derived from countless others. As mentioned before, these reflections are said to induce a natural inclination or wish to repay the kindness of others. By again focusing on the similarities between people rather than their differences, one also works to increase a sense of connectedness and affection. By relating to others with a profound sense of affection and endearment, one is able to empathize more deeply with them and be unable to bear to see them suffer.

Though research suggests that we are "wired" for empathy, so to speak, our ability to empathize with others seems to depend on our degree of closeness and affection toward them (Singer & Lamm, 2009). For example, researchers have found that observing pictures of disgusted faces and experiencing disgust oneself activates the same neural responses in the anterior insula (AI) (and the anterior cingulate cortex to a lesser extent; Wicker et al., 2003). Singer et al. (2004) also found that these areas were activated both when participants received a painful stimulation and when they observed or anticipated a loved one receiving the same stimulus, yet these responses were dampened when people observed strangers receiving the same stimulus. In another study, Singer et al. (2006) found that empathic responses are modulated by participants' like or dislike for others and, further, that some males exhibit increased activity in reward-related areas, which correlated with an expressed desire for revenge, when they observe people they dislike receiving the same stimuli. The researchers concluded that empathic responses are shaped by the evaluation of other's social behavior. In short, our empathic responses seem to be regulated by our sense of closeness to others but also by their perceived social behavior (or, to put it another way, whether or not they "deserve" empathy).

The modulation of our empathic response can have significant social implications. Empathy can both prevent us from harming and enable us to help others. We all perceive the world from our own particular vantage point, yet when we take our vantage point to be the correct or most important one, we sacrifice the ability to truly understand others' perspectives. This practice works to help us develop equanimity toward others and also to continually remember that all beings are similar in wanting happiness. This is further emphasized by the work of Batson, Eklund, Chermok, Hoyt, and Ortiz (2007), who have suggested that our empathic response is based on assessment of need rather than perception of similarity or closeness. For example, in a controlled study Batson and colleagues (2007) found that college students feel more empathy toward seemingly helpless beings (small children or injured animals) than toward very sick college students. Though this does not necessarily override the importance that similarity or "in-group" perception plays in our empathic response, it does seem that the recognition of others' suffering—regardless of similarity—is also crucial. Thus another important key to this practice is the constant reflection that others constantly suffer, much in the same way one does oneself.

Realizing Wishing and Aspirational Compassion

This step encourages enhanced empathy for others, coupled with intimate awareness of their suffering and its causes, which naturally gives rise to compassion. As one further develops one's empathy, one naturally becomes more aware of the suffering of others. In this step, the practitioner is instructed to visualize and reflect upon the suffering of three people—a loved one, a stranger, and an adversary. One then is encouraged to recognize how difficult it is to witness another's suffering and to allow one's heart to resonate with the wish for this person to be free from suffering.

Realizing Active Compassion for Others

In the final step, the participant is guided through a meditation designed to move from simply wishing others to be free of unhappiness to actively committing to assistance in their pursuit of happiness and freedom from suffering. Further, in these final sessions the practitioner works to overcome potential distress he or she might feel in contemplating the suffering of others by recognizing that others' suffering can be overcome and by constructively thinking about ways he or she might helpfully engage and support them. Without a recognition that others' suffering can be transformed, the practitioner is prone to feel helpless or overwhelmed and thus could eventually experience burnout or "compassion fatigue." This recognition is therefore an important step in the program.

Cultivating Compassion and Mindfulness: Important Distinctions

Though CBCT incorporates key practices, such as focused attention and awareness, that form the basis of many popular mindfulness-based programs such as mindfulness-based stress reduction (MBSR), CBCT and mindfulness programs differ in approach. In general, mindfulness-based programs help practitioners learn how to re-perceive stressful situations and thought patterns by attending to each moment with open, nonjudgmental awareness (Shapiro, Carlson, Astin, & Freedman, 2006; Kabat-Zinn, 1994). A key aspect of mindfulness-based practices in general, therefore, involves changing one's relationship to thoughts rather than altering the content of thoughts themselves. A growing body of evidence supports the idea that mindfulness practices have significant potential to reduce stress, likely by breaking the seemingly automatic habitual tendencies that individuals have to react, rather than respond, to stressful situations and by reducing the negative impact of recurring distressing thoughts. In other words, mindfulness practice may work by interrupting automatic simulations of past or future events and encourage one to be fully present (Williams, 2010).

CBCT, on the other hand, relies on systematic analytical meditations that encourage practitioners to gain insight into their thoughts, feelings, and emotions and to actively simulate alternative ways of relating to oneself and others. Whereas mindfulness programs encourage the reduction of cognitive simulations, CBCT programs actively encourage the construction or production of cognitive and emotional simulations that reorient, or rehabituate, oneself to healthier and more constructive modes of being. Rather than learning simply to change one's relationship to thoughts, CBCT training requires practitioners to actively work with their emotions and cognitive appraisals in order to release hostility and indifference toward others and develop a deep feeling of affection and gratitude for, and positive connection with, others. This marks an important distinction between the two models. In the CBCT model, which can be described as an "antidote model," the practitioner runs through a series of analytical contemplations concerning, for example, the fact that irrational anger leads to suffering and does not bring happiness. It is important to note that analytical meditation does not refer to simply thinking about something in a purely intellectual or detached way. The point of these reflections is to gain insight, or to arrive at what one might call an "a-ha moment," which is then deepened through repeated analysis and through sitting with this insight once it has been arrived at. One then constructs the antidote to irrational anger, in this case love and compassion, and then repeatedly familiarizes oneself with this feeling through meditation until it becomes vivid and felt. Through repeated practice, one's feeling of love or compassion becomes stronger and more refined and, importantly, more integrated into one's way of being.

CBCT practices are not opposed to less analytically oriented practices such as mindfulness but, as outlined earlier, incorporate elements of mindfulness training, recognizing its importance for subsequent analytical practices. Further, it is important to note that although some mindfulness-based programs incorporate loving-kindness practice, there are important distinctions between CBCT and loving-kindness practice. Loving-kindness meditation, as typically taught, involves the generation of an affective state (love and affection), which is then extended outwardly to encompass broadening circles of individuals. Many loving-kindness practice instructions do not explicitly provide instructions for examining or transforming the cognitive mechanisms that underlie feelings of hostility or instances of judgment and bias. Finally, the related Tibetan Buddhist practice of *tonglen* ("sending and receiving"), in which one imagines taking on the suffering of others and endowing them with happiness, can be extremely beneficial. Though the practice of *tonglen* is embedded in our protocol, we emphasize the "sending" aspect of this practice by encouraging practitioners to allow the compassionate desire to alleviate others' suffering to arise in their hearts and to imagine sending others the source of happiness and well-being in the form of white light. We do not explicitly encourage practitioners to imagine taking on the suffering of others, for we feel it may be too difficult for beginners to do this in a meaningful way, and moreover it may very well be too overwhelming for those who have experienced abuse or trauma.

CBCT Research Programs and Potential Implications for Trauma Treatment

The CBCT program is an 8-week group intervention that meets once per week for 2 hours. Classes include presentations of pedagogical material, discussion, and guided meditation. Participants are asked to meditate daily throughout the course of the program. The results of the first study to employ CBCT demonstrated that college students who were taught and practiced CBCT exhibited reduced emotional upset in response to psychosocial stress, as well as less activation of autonomic and immune pathways that have been implicated in the development of a host of chronic, stress-related illnesses, including depression, heart disease, obesity, diabetes, and dementia (Pace et al., 2009; Pace et al., 2010). The promising results of this project encouraged us to explore means of adapting and delivering CBCT to a variety of other populations. We are currently conducting a follow-up study, funded by the National Institutes of Health, evaluating the efficacy of CBCT compared with both an attentional training intervention and a health education group in healthy adults.

In addition to employing CBCT as a means of reducing stress and enhancing immune function, we have begun to conceive of ways in which CBCT could promote prosociality and mental flourishing. Members of our team adapted the CBCT program for use with elementary schoolchildren (ages 5–9). Relative to a mindfulness control, children who received CBCT developed more inclusive social networks that were characterized by increased peer friendships. They also demonstrated greater prosocial reasoning (e.g., greater compassion, more consideration for others' beliefs and desires) when asked how to best resolve a social conflict. Published data from this work are forthcoming, and the preliminary pilot study with these young children is described in Ozawa-de Silva and Dodson-Lavelle (2011).

In 2008, we piloted a CBCT program for adolescent girls in foster care (ages 13–16). This particular adaptation was designed to help girls develop inner resilience and build stronger, healthier relationships. The success of this pilot program, described in Ozawa-de Silva and Dodson-Lavelle (2011), has led to ongoing studies investigating the effects of compassion training in this population. In 2010 the Georgia Department of Health and Human Services in Atlanta, Georgia, funded a randomized, wait-list control trial of CBCT for 72 foster children. This study, which we describe in greater detail subsequently, examined the impact of this training on immune and neuroendocrine biomarkers linked to the development of both mental and medical illness, as well as its effectiveness in reducing emotional reactivity, psychosocial stress, and behavioral problems.

Though CBCT was not designed to treat trauma specifically, we believe the training offers practitioners a set of strategies and skills that may ameliorate or protect against the effects of trauma. Similar to mindfulness-based interventions, CBCT may hold promise as an adjunctive therapy to empirically supported therapies, such as prolonged exposure therapy, by helping participants increase their capacity to attend to thoughts and feelings in the present moment, thereby gaining some psychological flexibility and reducing suppression or avoidance of intrusive thoughts and emotions (Foa, Hembree, & Rothbaum, 2007; Follette, Palm, & Pearson, 2006). A recent study suggests that a mindfulness-based intervention may also help reduce symptoms of PTSD and depression (Kearney et al., 2012), although more work remains to be done in this area.

CBCT may provide therapeutic benefits over and above those offered by mindfulness-based interventions alone in that the compassion practices contained within this program aim to prime secure attachment, increase positive emotions, and enhance social connectedness. PTSD can negatively affect interpersonal relationships and can potentially trigger or exacerbate avoidant or ambivalent attachment styles. CBCT aims to prime secure attachment through reflections on the kindness of others, including mentors, and through the practice of self-compassion described earlier. Research also suggests that self-compassion is a predictor of reduced symptom severity among patients with depression and anxiety (Van Dam, Sheppard, Forsyth, & Earleywine, 2011). CBCT also fosters the development of positive emotions, including love and compassion, which may counteract the deleterious effects of negative emotions and enhance coping and resilience (Frederickson 2001, Frederickson, Tugade, Waugh, & Larkin, 2003). Further, CBCT aims to enhance social connectedness through practices of equanimity and empathy. As mentioned, social connectedness has a protective effect against stress, depression, and PTSD (Cacioppo & Hawkley, 2009). Studies have also suggested that perceived social isolation may be the strongest predictor of suicidal thoughts and behavior (Van Orden et al., 2010).

These considerations must be taken to reflect nothing more than a working hypothesis on the potential efficacy of CBCT for the treatment of trauma and related symptoms. Members of our research team and colleagues from the U. S. Centers for Disease Control and Prevention field-tested CBCT in Kosovo to investigate its potential to heal war-related trauma, and others on our team at Emory University are also investigating the efficacy of CBCT among suicide attempters at a local hospital in Atlanta. Our work with adolescents in Atlanta's foster system involves ongoing studies with many survivors of trauma, yet we have not, to date, explicitly evaluated the efficacy of CBCT for trauma. This is an important next step.

CBCT for Adolescents in Foster Care

Youth in foster care generally suffer from exposure to traumas known to negatively affect one's ability to deal with stressful life events. Most significantly, foster youth often suffer from abuse or neglect, both of which have been shown to produce lifelong maladaptive physiological and psychological changes (Committee on Early Childhood, Adoption, and Dependent Care, 2002). Even in the context of abusive or neglectful parents, parental separation itself is a risk factor for poor adult emotional and physical health outcomes (Pesonen et al., 2007).

Childhood trauma has also been shown to predict reduced academic performance and to increase the likelihood of dropping out of school. Youth in foster care are four to five times more likely than peers in the general population to be hospitalized for suicide attempts and are many times more likely to be hospitalized for serious psychiatric disorders in their teens and young adulthood (Vinnerljung, 2006).

Taken together, these data suggest that an intervention designed to enhance emotional resilience and promote prosocial behavior might be of benefit to adolescents in foster care. Our team hypothesized that CBCT could help foster youth learn to connect more deeply with others and learn to develop nurturing relationships with adults who can provide the guidance and support missing from relationships with their biological parents. Children in foster care tend to be guarded and to "shut down" in order to avoid the threat of future pain, rejection, or trauma. This approach, however, exacerbates feelings of loneliness and social isolation. Compassion training builds strength and an openness and willingness to face fears of rejection and trauma. It also helps participants reconnect with their natural tendency to want to feel loved and connected. CBCT further offers adolescents strategies for regulating emotion, reducing stress, and reframing life experience in more constructive ways. It encourages participants to face their habitual ways of being in and relating to the world that further contribute to suffering and helps them aspire to overcome them. The program also aims to build self-confidence and self-worth and to promote optimism, gratitude, and connectedness.

As mentioned earlier, although the CBCT program was not designed to treat trauma specifically, we adapted this program for adolescents in foster care with these issues in mind. The program begins with mindfulness training, framed as a means of reducing stress and noticing triggers that cause us to react rather than respond to situations. We quickly realized, however, that these adolescents had tremendous difficulty settling in and feeling comfortable in their bodies. Thus we began incorporating yoga practice into our classes and selected poses and sequences that would enhance balance and strength while promoting calm and stability, including tree pose, chair pose, and child's pose. Though the adolescents initially had difficulty practicing sitting meditation for more than a few minutes at a time without feeling agitated, yoga practice afforded them an alternate means of accessing stability, calm, and relaxation and helped them begin to "settle" into meditation practice during the program. This type of body-oriented work additionally offers participants alternate ways of tapping into and sustaining awareness of their emotional experiences.

For some, physical movement and body-directed attentional practices also seem to be a more direct or tangible way of learning to attend to the present moment.

Some of the adolescents struggled at first with the practice of self-compassion. Though they could more easily recognize and appreciate the ways in which their own perceptions, judgments, and patterns of reactivity contributed to or exacerbated their stress and suffering, some found it difficult to believe that they could find happiness or that they deserved to be happy and loved. One girl said that her greatest fear in life was not finding someone to love her, as she felt worthless and damaged. As some of these anxieties were worked through in the class, many found comfort in the recognition that they were not alone in sharing this fear but could understand where it came from. We worked to empower the youth to recognize that they are responsible for and capable of transforming their own minds and also that they, like all other beings, are worthy of receiving love and care. This was a crucial step in the process.

Extending this love and compassion to others also proved difficult, for various reasons. Many adolescents exhibited significant in-group biases and found it tremendously difficult at first to understand the notion of impartiality. Further, many found it difficult to feel a sense of connectedness to others. Working through a series of reflections and analytical meditations helped cultivate perspective taking and a willingness to open to and be sensitive to the pain of others. One example of this emerged during one of our sessions on impartiality. During this session, participants are invited to play an empathy game in which the instructor reads out a scenario describing another person in a somewhat difficult situation. Participants are asked to stand along an "empathy scale" depending on how strongly they both relate to and care about the individual described in the situation. Individuals in each scenario were varied based on gender, race, and social circle, as well as by categories such as "friend," "stranger," and "enemy," to demonstrate how our capacity to empathize is in large part shaped by our in-group biases and judgments as well as by our own life experiences. In one powerful session, drawing on a recent news story that had become the focus of the class, students were presented with the situation of a girl who had been assaulted outside of a school event. The event had drawn significant news attention because many people stood by and witnessed the horrific event, yet no one contacted the police or school authorities or tried to stop the assault. When the scenario was first read, many students stood on the no-empathy end of the scale, labeled "I don't care." When asked about their reactions, some explained that they felt little or no empathy because they did not know the girl or the circumstance that precipitated the event (perhaps suggesting that she may have deserved it). Students were then asked to imagine that the girl in the scenario was their best friend or sister. Immediately they moved to the opposite end of the scale. When probing for justifications for the switch, many said that their empathic response should be obvious, that of course one should empathize with one's sister. Then one boy, after some reflection, said, "But that girl from the news was someone's sister. Everyone is someone's sister or friend. . . . " This insight seemed to be deeply felt by many in the room and seemed to mark a shift in the students' thinking about not only their willingness to empathize and connect with others but also their interest in doing so.

This shift also helped students begin to work to generate compassion toward difficult people in their lives. Students were explicitly instructed not to choose a person who had caused them significant harm but rather someone who had treated them unkindly. Nevertheless, we believe that working through these analytical investigations could enable students to draw parallels with trauma-related situations in their lives and prepare them to work through these more difficult traumatic experiences with the help of their primary therapists. Many of these children also suffer from dysfunctional attachment styles, and thus we also found it essential to prime secure attachment by asking children to recall the kindness, compassion, and support of a mentor and, from this basis, begin to work to extend compassion to others. Over the course of the program, students seemed to become more skilled at perspective taking and also displayed more concern for others. Students in general became more understanding and were able to articulate the idea that people cause harm—intentionally or unintentionally—out of ignorance. This insight seemed critical to the healing process.

Results from this study showed that participation in a 6-week CBCT program was associated with increased hopefulness and a trend in decreased general anxiety (Reddy et al., 2012). Based on measures collected from saliva prior to and following CBCT or the wait-list control condition, CBCT also reduced markers for stress and immune system hyperactivity that have been associated with the development of psychiatric and medical illnesses (Pace et al., 2012). Qualitative results indicated that adolescents found CBCT helpful for dealing with life stressors, and nearly all participants reported that they would recommend this training to a friend. This is consistent with our anecdotal data. At the end of training, participants were asked to name one positive thing they learned about themselves and one thing they wanted to work on. One girl said, "I learned that I am a great friend. I'm loyal. And I'm reliable." She then said, "And I want to learn how to trust people more, because I see how good it feels." We believe this openness and willingness to connect with and trust others is also critical to the healing process.

This anecdote is also consistent with our experience from an early pilot program conducted in 2008. After completion of this program, which was delivered to six girls living together in a group home, one girl said the training transformed her relationship with her estranged adoptive mother. She noted that due to her past experiences she tended to repress or hide her emotions and keep others at a distance. Through the program, she came to realize that such behavior would only harm herself and prevent her from having meaningful relationships with others, including her adoptive mother. She also shared that following the end of the program, she continued to practice compassion meditation on a daily basis.

Future Directions

The success of this research program has led to ongoing studies investigating the effects of compassion training in foster care populations. In addition to its profound potential for foster children themselves, we also recognize the importance of providing training and support to foster parents, caregivers, and other providers. Such training could have a greater impact on interpersonal dynamics and may also begin to effect institutional change, as well. To this end, we have begun to develop a training program for foster providers and are looking for ways to deliver this training in foster care group homes for maximum effect. Last year we designed and piloted a peer-training program for students who had completed at least one round of the CBCT program and who showed promise to cofacilitate CBCT courses with one of our instructors. This program aimed not only to help develop a group of well-trained peer-leaders but also to help empower these adolescents to recognize and embody their strength and leadership potential. There is tremendous potential for CBCT, as well as compassion- and mindfulness-based programs in general, for addressing trauma and suffering. Given this, we are eager to continue research in this area.

References

Batson, C. D., Eklund, J. H., Chermok, V. L., Hoyt, J. L., & Ortiz, B. G. (2007). An additional antecedent of empathic concern: Valuing the welfare of the person in need. *Journal of Personality and Social Psychology, 93*, 65–74.

Cacioppo, J. T., & Hawkley, L. C. (2009). Perceived social isolation and cognition. *Trends in Cognitive Sciences, 13*(10), 447–454.

Committee on Early Childhood, Adoption, and Dependent Care. (2002). Health care of young children in foster care. *Pediatrics, 109*(3), 536–541.

Emmons, R. A., & McCullough, M. E. (2003). Counting blessings versus burdens: An experimental investigation of gratitude and subjective well-being in daily life. *Journal of Personality and Social Psychology, 84*(2), 377–389.

Foa, E. B., Hembree, E. A., & Rothbaum, B. O. (2007). *Prolonged exposure therapy for PTSD: Emotional processing of traumatic experiences: Therapist guide.* New York: Oxford University Press.

Follette, V., Palm, K. M., & Pearson, A. N. (2006). Mindfulness and trauma: Implications for treatment. *Journal of Rational-Emotive and Cognitive-Behavior Therapy, 24*(1), 45–61.

Frederickson, B. L. (2001). The role of positive emotions in positive psychology: The broaden-and-build theory of positive emotions. *American Psychologist*, 56(3), 218–226.

Frederickson, B. L., Tugade, M., Waugh, C. E., & Larkin, G. R. (2003). What good are positive emotions in crises?: A prospective study of resilience and emotions following the terrorist attacks on the United States on September 11th, 2001. *Journal of Personality and Social Psychology*, 84(2), 365–376.

Jinpa, T. (2006). *Mind training: The great collection*. Boston: Wisdom.

Kabat-Zinn, J. (1994). *Wherever you go, there you are: Mindfulness meditation in everyday life*. New York: Hyperion.

Kearney, D. J., McDermott, K., Malte, C., Martinez, M., & Simpson, T. L. (2012). Association of participation in a mindfulness program with measures of PTSD, depression and quality of life in a veteran sample. *Journal of Clinical Psychology*, 68(1), 101–115.

Lutz, A., Brefczynski-Lewis, J., Johnstone, T., & Davidson, R. J. (2008). Regulation of the neural circuitry of emotion by compassion meditation: Effects of meditative expertise. *PLoS ONE*, 3(3), e1897. Available at *www.plosone.org/article/info%3Adoi%2F10.1371%2Fjournal.pone.0001897*.

Lutz, A., Slagter, H. A., Dunne, J. D., & Davidson, R. J. (2008). Cognitive-emotional interactions: Attention regulation and monitoring in meditation. *Trends in Cognitive Sciences*, 12, 163–169.

Negi, L. T. (2009). *Cognitively-based compassion training manual*. Unpublished manuscript.

Otake, K., Shimai, S., Tanaka-Matsumi, J., & Otsui, K. (2006). Happy people become happier through kindness: A counting kindnesses intervention. *Journal of Happiness Studies*, 7(3), 361–375.

Ozawa-de Silva, B., & Dodson-Lavelle, B. (2011, Spring). An education of heart and mind: Practical and theoretical issues in teaching cognitive-based compassion training to children. *Practical Matters*, 4, 1–28.

Ozawa-de Silva, B., Dodson-Lavelle, B., Raison, C. L., & Negi, L. T. (2011). Compassion and ethics: Scientific and practical approaches to the cultivation of compassion as a foundation for ethical subjectivity and well-being. *Journal of Healthcare, Science and the Humanities*, 2, 145–161.

Pace, T. W., Negi, L. T., Dodson-Lavelle B., Ozawa de-Silva B., Reddy S., Cole, S. W., et al. (2012). Engagement with cognitively-based compassion training is associated with reduced salivary C-reactive protein from before to after training in foster care program adolescents. *Psychoneuroendocrinology*, 38(2), 294–299.

Pace, T. W. W., Negi, L. T., Adame, D. D., Cole, S. P., Sivilli, T. I., Brown, T. D., et al. (2009). Effect of compassion meditation on neuroendocrine, innate immune and behavioral responses to psychosocial stress. *Psychoneuroendocrinology*, 34(1), 87–98.

Pace, T. W. W., Negi L. T., Sivilli, T. I., Issa, M. J., Cole, S. P., Adame, D. D., et al. (2010). Innate immune, neuroendocrine and behavioral responses to psychosocial stress do not predict subsequent compassion meditation practice time. *Psychoneuroendocrinology*, 35(2), 310–315.

Pesonen, A. K., Räikkönen, K., Heinonen, K., Kajantie, E., Forsén, T., & Eriksson, J. G. (2007). Depressive symptoms in adults separated from their parents as children: A natural experiment during World War II. *American Journal of Epidemiology, 166*(10), 1126–1133.

Raison, C. L., Capuron, L., & Miller, A. H. (2006). Cytokines sing the blues: Inflammation and the pathogenesis of depression. *Trends in Immunology, 27,* 24–31.

Reddy, S., Negi, L. T., Dodson-Lavelle, B., Ozawa-de Silva, B., Pace, T. W., Cole, S. P., et al. (2012). Cognitive-based compassion training: A promising prevention strategy for at-risk adolescents. *Journal of Child and Family Studies, 22*(2), 219.

Shapiro, S. L., Carlson, L. E., Astin, J. A., & Freedman, B. (2006). Mechanisms of mindfulness. *Journal of Clinical Psychology, 62,* 373–386.

Singer, T., & Lamm, C. (2009). The social neuroscience of empathy. *Annals of the New York Academy of Sciences, 1156,* 81–96.

Singer, T., Seymour, B., O'Doherty, J., Kaube, H., Dolan, R. J., & Frith, C. D. (2004). Empathy for pain involves the affective but not sensory components of pain. *Science, 303*(5661), 1157–1162.

Singer, T., Seymour, B., O'Doherty, J., Stephan, K. E., Dolan, R. J., & Frith, C. D. (2006). Empathic neural responses are modulated by the perceived fairness of others. *Nature, 439,* 466–469.

Van Dam, N. T., Sheppard, S. C., Forsyth, J. P., & Earleywine, M. (2011). Self-compassion is a better predictor than mindfulness of symptom severity and quality of life in mixed anxiety and depression. *Journal of Anxiety Disorders, 25,* 123–130.

Van Orden, K. A., Witte, T. K., Cukrowicz, K. C., Braithwaite, S., Selby, E. A., & Joiner, T. E. (2010). The interpersonal theory of suicide. *Psychological Review, 117*(2), 575–600.

Vinnerljung, B. (2006). Suicide attempts and severe psychiatric morbidity among former child welfare clients: A national cohort study. *Journal of Child Psychology and Psychiatry, 47*(7), 723–733.

Wicker, B., Keysers, C., Plailly, J., Royet, J. P., Gallese, V., & Rizzolatti, G. (2003). Both of us disgusted in my insula: The common neural basis of seeing and feeling disgust. *Neuron, 40,* 655–664.

Williams, M. J. (2010). Mindfulness and psychological process. *Emotion, 10*(1), 1–7.

Conclusion

John Briere, Victoria M. Follette, Deborah Rozelle,
James W. Hopper, and David I. Rome

As the chapters of this book attest, one of the more exciting developments in the psychotherapy field is the growing application of mindfulness and related practices in the specific treatment of trauma effects. This burgeoning awareness also has reinforced and expanded earlier psychological notions of compassion, acceptance, and posttraumatic growth. The fact that science is finding contemplative perspectives and procedures relevant to the suffering of trauma survivors should not be surprising. Many early spiritual traditions were developed, in part, as pathways out of suffering, whether the results of deprivation, oppression, loss, or hurtful events. When these perspectives and methodologies are combined with effective Western therapies, the result can be a wealth of new opportunities to assist those whose lives have been affected by adversity and painful life events.

The chapters of this book suggest that there may be at least two broad pathways through which contemplative approaches can ameliorate trauma-related suffering. Some writers described theoretical or philosophical applications to psychotherapy, wherein the client is intentionally affected by the clinician's voiced and implied contemplative perspective and responses. For other writers, such as those describing trauma-informed mindfulness-based stress reduction (MBSR) or yoga, the focus is often less on the clinician's or facilitator's ability to transmit or facilitate knowledge and understanding (although those things still pertain) and more directly on the actual teaching of skills, such as meditation, mindfulness, movements (e.g., *asanas*) that increase embodiment, and the expansion of loving-kindness. These two general approaches intersect and overlap, of course. Interventions that foster self-awareness and self-acceptance during psychotherapy often teach cognitive skills associated with mindfulness, for example, and mindfulness training frequently leads to reevaluation of previously tightly held assumptions about self and others that were formed in the context of adverse experiences.

Interestingly, certain themes tended to recur across the various perspectives and interventions presented in this book. Whether focused on skills or insight, chapter writers generally described opportunities for the trauma survivor to develop:

- A broader perspective on past experiences, such that he or she is less personally "identified" with what happened to him or her, potentially leading to reduced self-blame, anger, and hopelessness.
- Metacognitive awareness, so that emerging trauma-related cognitions, memories, and triggered emotions are seen as just that— remnants of the past as opposed to actual data about the present.
- Greater self-acceptance, self-knowledge, and appreciation of internal experience, whether wanted and pleasurable or unwanted and painful.
- Emotional regulation skills, so that activated memories and current stressors are less overwhelming and produce less extreme reactions or "impulsive" behavior.
- The capacity to live more in the present moment, rather than excessively ruminating about the past or worrying about the future.
- A greater likelihood of well-being and fulfillment.

Because the goals and activities of mindfulness and contemplation outlined in this book run, to some extent, against the stream of currently dominant psychotherapeutic perspectives, it is important to ask whether there are good data to support these "new" ideas. Fortunately, as reported by the various authors here, as well as in a number of meta-analyses (e.g., Grossman, Neimann, Schmidt, & Walach, 2004; Hoffman, Sawyer, Witt, & Oh, 2010), the news thus far is good. Many of these interventions have been found in controlled studies to be effective in reducing a range of psychological symptoms, problems, and disorders, including those associated with trauma. As might be predicted, however, the outcome variables examined in these studies tend to be of immediately observable or reportable phenomena, such as anxiety, depression, low self-esteem, or posttraumatic stress. Less studied are more existential and spiritual concerns, for example, those involving demoralization, alienation, a sense of meaninglessness, fear of death, and an inability to experience loving-kindness and compassion toward oneself and others, although some chapters refer anecdotally to positive outcomes in these areas as well. We strongly support empirical research on these less easily measured phenomena, because many contemplative approaches explicitly address such outcomes and may be, in fact, specifically helpful in this area relative to other current therapies.

Although research to date is encouraging, we also recommend empirical examination of additional issues as contemplative/mindfulness interventions become more widely accepted and the field matures. These include, for example, the following:

• Can mindfulness skills development (e.g., MBSR groups) alone address some of the "deeper" or more complex sequelae of severe trauma? Or is a therapeutic relationship in the context of trauma-informed psychotherapy also required for resolution at this level? And, if these are necessary, how, specifically, might contemplative methods such as mindfulness and trauma-informed relational psychotherapy coexist or be sequenced?

• What should the standards of care be for teaching mindfulness, meditation, and/or other contemplative activities? Because inwardly directed awareness implies greater exposure to internal states and processes—including potentially painful or even overwhelming memories, thoughts, and emotions—how can we ensure safety for those who are most traumatized? Certainly, as indicated in this volume, screening for suicidality, severe depression, mania, psychosis, chronic affect dysregulation, and extreme posttraumatic stress is a first step. But are there ways to modify mindfulness training or contemplation-informed therapies so that they might be helpful and safe for even these otherwise excluded client groups?

• To what extent is it critical that the therapist be mindful, compassionate, and wise, above and beyond teaching mindfulness, self-compassion, or related skills to the client? In a related vein, what is sufficient training or experience for the therapist to ethically provide mindfulness-based treatment? And is it essential that the clinician have his or her own ongoing meditation practice in order to apply meditation-based or -informed interventions? If so, what constitutes necessary and sufficient ongoing practice?

Although writing has been done in each of these domains, research data are lacking, and consensus regarding standards of care has yet to be reached on these and other central issues. Given the current rate of development in this area, however, we expect that our knowledge base will expand in the near future to address such gaps in the literature.

The wide range and rich content of the chapters of this volume served as a constant reminder to the editors of the tremendous breadth and vibrancy of the work being done in this area. It is likely that the next decade will witness even more innovation, research, and writing on the intersection of psychotherapy, skills development, and contemplative approaches as they apply to trauma-related suffering. We are thankful for the opportunity to bring these wonderful expositions to you and hope that they have bestowed upon you, as they did us, excitement and optimism for the future of trauma treatment and the well-being of trauma survivors.

References

Grossman, P., Neimann, L., Schmidt, S., & Walach, H. (2004). Mindfulness-based stress reduction and health benefits: A meta-analysis. *Journal of Psychosomatic Research, 57*, 35–43.

Hofmann, S. G., Sawyer, A. T., Witt, A. A., & Oh, D. (2010). The effect of mindfulness-based therapy on anxiety and depression: A meta-analytic review. *Journal of Consulting and Clinical Psychology, 78*(2), 169–183.

Index

The letter *f* following a page number indicates figure; the letter *t* indicates table; the letter *n* indicates note.

Abusive behavior; *see also* Childhood trauma
  antecedent phenomena and, 22–23
Acceptance
  in ACT model, 65
  children and, 289–290
  client internalization of, 34–38
  therapist, 33–34
Acceptance and commitment therapy (ACT),
  4–5, 15, 61–74
  assessment in, 68
  Buddhism and, 64
  central goal in, 62
  mindfulness and, 70–71
  outcome data on, 62–63
  practice of, 68–71
  processes in, 64–68, 65*f*
  psychological flexibility and, 62
  and seeking true goods, 196
  targeting avoidance with, 63–64
  therapist's role in, 69–70
Acupuncture and Meditation for Wellness
  (AMWELL) studies, 143
Addiction
  seeking circuitry and, 187–188
  special help for, 200
Adolescent(s)
  cognitively based compassion training
    for (*see* Cognitively based compassion
    training (CBCT))
  in foster care, 7, 352–356
Adolescent sex offenders, 7; *see also* Focusing-
  oriented therapy, with adolescent sex
  offenders
Affect regulation, MBSR and, 143
Allies, calling on, 36–39
Allostatic load, 259
Amygdala, function of, 186–187
Analytical meditation, 112
Anapana sati practice, 335
Anxiety
  childhood trauma and, 286
  illness, mindfulness practices for, 262–263

Assagioli, Roberto, 126–127
Attachment
  defined, 22
  developing brain and, 211–212
  disorganized, impaired integration and,
    214–216
  to MBSR instructor, 250
Attention
  versus awareness, 217
  in CBCT, 343
  DBT and, 77
  functions of, 216–217
  mindfulness training and, 218
Autobiographical memory, overgeneralized; *see*
  Overgeneralized memory
Autonomic system, reactivity of, chronic pain
  and, 258–259
Avoidance; *see also* Pain paradox
  ACT and, 63–64
  cultural support of, 14
  development of, 62
  effects of, 13
  mindfulness and, 19
  mindfulness meditation and, 333
  persistence of, 307–308
  in PTSD, 104, 104n1, 146
  therapist approach to, 147–148
Awareness, *versus* attention, 217

B

Backdraft, compassion and, 52–53
Barnhofer, Thorsten, 5
Bilateral stimulation (BLS), in EMDR,
  106–109, 115–116
Blanking out, in TRD, 302
Bodhisattva, ideal of, 132–133
Bodhisattva vow, IFS and, 133–135, 137
Bodily awareness
  childhood trauma and, 295
  and transformation of suffering, 198–
    199

Body
  befriending, 177
  developing toleration of, 172–175
Body scan
  for children, 288
  MBSR guidelines for, 153–155
Body wisdom, talk therapy and, 158
Borderline personality disorder (BPD), PTSD
      and, 75
Brach, Tara, 4, 202
Brain
  cortisol damage to, 211
  default mode of, 189
  impaired integration in (see Integration,
      impaired)
  meditation-related changes in, 219–220
  PTSD and, 158
Brain circuitries, 185–209
  Buddhist psychology and, 196n2
  cycles of suffering and, 191–193
  defined, 185
  embodiment, 190–191
  fear, 186–187
  healing, 193–197, 195f, 197f
  satisfaction, 189–190
  seeking, 187–189
Brain development, attachment relationships
      and, 211–212
Brain dynamics, overview of, 6
Breathing
  awareness of, 33–34, 41–42, 54, 154
  chronic pain and, 268
  dissociation and, 303, 307–308, 311
  fear response and, 187, 234
  in focusing-oriented therapy, 315
  mindfulness and, 219
  trauma-sensitive yoga and, 175–176
  in vipassana meditation, 335
  yoga practice and, 170–171, 175–176, 178
Briere, John, 4, 142–143
Buddha Nature, 133, 133n1
Buddhism
  ACT and, 64
  disidentification in, 114
  eightfold path of, 67
  existential insight and, 20–21
  Four Noble Truths of, 21
  and law of impermanence, 118
  and law of opposing states, 117–118
  Mahayana, internal family systems model
      and (see Internal family systems [IFS]
      model)
  and metatheory of change, 117–118
  suffering and, 42, 104–105
  Tibetan
    CBCT and, 343
    IFS and, 128
Buddhist meditation
  aspects of, 110
  IFS and, 130–132
Buddhist practice
  versus EMDR, 103, 105
  PTSD and, 104–105
  Vajriyana, 116

Buddhist psychology, 4
  brain circuitries and, 196n2
  compassion in, 47
  cycles of suffering and, 191n1
  essential tenets of, 334
  suffering and, 334
  vipassana meditation and, 334–336
  versus Western psychology, 16

C

Change, in EMDR and Buddhism, 117–118
Childhood trauma, 284–300
  adverse social factors and, 284
  children's choice points, 292–293
  consequences of, 284–285
  emotional memories and, 292–293
  impacts of, 214–215, 353
  and mindfulness adaptations for children,
      287–293
  mindfulness interventions for, 293–296
    and dissociation versus decentering, 294
    and distinguishing past, present, future,
      295–296
    and home practice, 296
    hyperarousal, desensitization, body
      awareness and, 295
    intrapsychic exposures and, 294–295
    psychoeducation, 293
  prevalence of, 140
  self-criticism and, 46
  therapies helpful for, 16
Children
  choice points for, 292–293
  interventions for, 7
  mindfulness-based cognitive therapy
      (MBCT-C) for, 287–289
Chronic depression, 91–101
  characteristics of, 93
  defined, 92
  long-term studies of, 92
  overgeneralized memory and, 93–96
  prevalence of, 92
  trauma-related, MBCT and, 96–98
  treatment-resistant, 97
Cognitive processing therapy (CPT), limitations
      of, 244–245
Cognitive-behavioral therapy (CBT)
  in prisons, 332
  PTSD and, 12
Cognitively based compassion training (CBCT),
      343–358
  active compassion and, 349
  for adolescents in foster care, 7, 352–356
    future directions for, 356
  aspirational compassion and, 348
  attention and stability of mind in, 345
  background and characteristics of, 344–349
  conceptual framework of, 344–345
  and development of affection and empathy,
      347–348
  and development of appreciation and
      gratitude, 347
  and impartiality, 346–347

and insight into mental experience, 345–346
versus mindfulness practice, 343, 349–350
research programs on, 350–352
and self-compassion, 346
structure of, 350–352
Collaborative Depression Study of NIMH, 92
Combat veterans, needs of, 6–7
Common humanity, sense of, 44
Compassion
active, 349
aspirational, 348
backdraft and, 52–53
in Buddhist psychology, 47
versus loving-kindness, 47
seeking circuitry and, 203
Compassion-focused therapy (CFT), child abuse survivors and, 46
Concentration meditation, 198*n*3
Consciousness, integration of, 216
Confidentiality, MBSR and, 148
Contemplative approaches
definitions of, 2
evidence supporting, 360–361
needed research on, 361
neuroscience of, 6
pathways of, 359–360
for seeking true goods, 200–205
Coping strategies, normalizing, 150
Core values; *see* Values
Correctional institutions; *see* Prisons; Traumatized prisoners
Cortisol, impacts of, 211
Countertransference, mindfulness and, 25

D

Dalai Lama, 6, 44, 201, 203
Decentering
childhood trauma and, 294
mindfulness and, 305
Defense mechanisms, seeking circuitry and, 188
Defusion
in ACT model, 65–66
defined, 66
Dependent origination, 22–23
Depersonalization, in TRD, 302
Depression; *see also* Chronic depression; Major depression
MBCT and, 5
mindfulness-based cognitive therapy and, 47
prevalence of, 91
and risk of recurrence, 91
Depression/defeat circuitry, cycle of suffering and, 192–193, 192*f*
Depressive thinking, 97–98, 98f
Derealization, in TRD, 302
Desensitization, childhood trauma and, 295
De-shaming, 34–35
Developmental trauma; *see* Interpersonal neurobiology
Dhamma Brothers: East Meets West in the Deep South, 336, 339

Dialectical behavior therapy (DBT), 5, 15–16, 55, 75–90
borderline personality disorder and, 75
change-based strategies in, 82–84
mindfulness and, 75, 76–88
case example of, 84–88
as "core" skill, 77–81
definitions of, 77
"how" skills in, 80–81
in session, 82–84
"what" skills in, 78–79
opposite action in, 82–83
overview of, 76
therapist relationship mindfulness and, 81–82
Disidentification process, in EMDR and Buddhism, 114
Dissociation, 32; *see also* Trauma-related dissociation (TRD)
childhood trauma and, 294
definitions of, 302
and failure to notice pain, 259
impaired integration and, 214–216
peritraumatic, 302
special help for, 200
trauma-sensitive yoga and, 175
Dissociative identity disorder (DID), 126–127
Dodson-Lavelle, Brooke, 7
Donaldson Correctional Facility, *vipassana* meditation program in, 336–339
Dutton, Mary Ann, 6

E

Embedded relational mindfulness, 227–239
case example of, 234–237
and mindfulness definitions, 228–229
and mindfulness in clinical practice, 229–231
safety and risks and, 231–232
therapeutic skills and, 232–234
Embodiment circuitry, 190–191
healing cycle and, 194
Emerson, David, 5
Emotion
negative, avoidance of, 260–261
positive, health and, 344
Emotional flooding, reduced risk of, with MSBR, 251
Emotional regulation, as therapy commonality, 360
Empathy, developing, in CBCT, 346–347
Empathy fatigue, 51–52
Engle, Jessica, 4
Existential insight, 17
supporting, 20–24
Exposure therapy; *see also* Intrinsic therapeutic exposure
client responses to, 61–62
EMDR and, 109–110
and emphasis on symptoms, 61
evidence supporting, 61
intrapsychic, childhood trauma and, 294–295
limitations of, 244–245

Exposure therapy (*continued*)
  versus mindfulness meditation, 307
  risks of, for prisoners, 332
Eye movement desensitization and reprocessing
    (EMDR), 5
  bilateral stimulation in, 106–109, 115–116
  Buddhist practice and, 103, 105
  case example of, 103–104, 106–109,
    111–113, 118–119
  change in, 117–118
  crucial processing episode in, 112–113
  disidentification in, 114
  exposure and, 109–110
  free association in, 111–113
  insight and realization in, 114
  insight and sudden gains in, 115
  Interweave intervention in, 109
  as meditation, 110
  metatheory of, 117–118
  versus other mindfulness-based therapies,
    115
  positive pole of, 110–111
  positive/preferred cognition in, 108,
    110–111, 119
  PTSD and, 102–103
  research on, 102–103
  safe place phase of, 106–107
  stability phase of, 107
  studies of, 115–116
  trauma processing phase of, 107–109

F

Fear; *see also* Healing traumatic fear
  pain and, 260
  without solution, 214
Fear circuitry, 186–187
  cycles of suffering and, 191–192, 192*f*
Feelings
  children's relationship with, 289
  nonfactual nature of, 291
Felt sense
  attending to, 316
  characteristics of, 315–316
  precision of, 322–323
Fight–freeze–flight response, 12, 43, 258
Fiorillo, Devika R., 5
Focusing
  felt sense and, 316
  versus psychotherapy, 316
Focusing-oriented psychotherapy, 5, 157–169
  with adolescent sex offenders, 314–328
    case example of, 318–325
    change and, 327
    listening and, 325–326
    therapy speed and precision and,
      326–327
  applications of, 168
  case example of, 162–168
  and characteristics of focusing, 314–316
  context of, 158–160
  and *felt* sense of trauma, 158–162
  frozen structures and, 316–317
  inner relationship in, 166–167

  as living-body approach, 157–158
  spiritual transformation in, 167–168
  theory of, 160–162
Focusing-oriented therapy for complex trauma
    (FOT-CT), 317
Follette, Victoria M., 4
Foster care, adolescents in, CBCT for, 352–
    356
Four Noble Truths, 21
Free association, in EMDR, 106–107, 111–113
Freud, Sigmund, 126
Frozen structures
  focusing-oriented therapy and, 316–317
  sex offenders and, 317–318
  signs of, 317
Fruzzetti, Alan E., 5
Fusion, defined, 65–66

G

Galton cue-word paradigm, 93
Gandhi, Mahatma, 48
Garrison Institute conference, 3
Gendlin, Eugene, 314–315; *see also* Focusing-
    oriented psychotherapy
  theory of, 160–162
Germer, Christopher K., 4
Geshe Lobsang Tenzin Negi, 7
Goenka, S. N., 334–335
Gottman, Moriah, 6
Gratitude, in CBCT, 343

H

Habits of mind, MBSR and, 151–152
Hatha yoga; *see also* Trauma-sensitive yoga;
    Yoga
  trauma-sensitive, 5–6
Hayes, Steven, 64
Healing
  backdraft and, 52–53
  brain circuitries and, 186
  versus escape, 193–194
  seeking circuitry and, 193–197, 195f, 197f
Healing circuitry, 186, 193–197, 195f, 197f
  and seeking to transform suffering, 194–195,
    195f
  and seeking true goods, 195–197, 197f
Healing traumatic fear, 31–42
  and cultivation of inner refuge, 35–38
  de-shaming and, 34–35
  progression in, 32
  supportive context for, 31
  and wing of mindfulness, 40–42
Health
  loving-kindness (*metta*) meditation and,
    279–280
  positive emotions and, 344
  self-compassion and, 279–280
  spirituality and, 159
  yoga and, 170
Herman, Judith, 330
Hesse, Erik, 214
Homeostasis
  see Psychological homeostasis, 13

Hopper, Elizabeth K., 5
Hopper, James W., 6, 7
Houses of Healing, 338
Hyperarousal, childhood trauma and, 295

I

Identity issues
    MBSR and, 142
    in TRD, 302
Illness anxiety
    chronic pain and, 259
    mindfulness practices for, 262–263
Impartiality, developing, in CBCT, 346–347,
        354–355
Impermanence, 22
    Buddhist law of, 118
Incarceration; see also Traumatized prisoners,
        vipassana meditation for
    US rate of, 329
Inner refuge
    cultivation of, 35–38
    deepening, 38–40
Integration, impaired
    disorganized attachment and dissociation
        and, 214–216
    and Interpersonal neurobiology, 213
    mindfulness, trauma treatment, and,
        218–220
    mindfulness and, 216–218, 219–220
Internal family systems (IFS) model
    Buddha wisdom and, 132–133
    case example of, 127–129
    Mahayana Buddhism and, 125–139
    multiplicity of mind and, 125–127
    paradigms of, 125
    Self and mindfulness in, 130–132
    Self of therapist and, 135–136
    Self-to-Self connectedness and, 136–137
    submind concept of, 125–127
Interpersonal neurobiology, 210–226
    and impaired integration in trauma, 213
        disorganized attachment and dissociation
            and, 214–216
        mindfulness, trauma treatment, and,
            218–220
        mindfulness and, 216–218
    left shift and, 217–218
    view of developmental trauma, 210–
        213
Interweave intervention, in EMDR, 109
Intimate partner violence
    prevalence of, 243
    therapies helpful in, 16
Intrinsic therapeutic exposure, 19
Intrusive thoughts
    fear of, trauma-related chronic pain and,
        260–261
    mindfulness practice and, 276

J

James, William, 159–160, 315–316
Jha, Amishi, 218
Jungian psychology, 126–127

K

Kabat-Zinn, Jon, 6, 216, 245–246
Karma, 23
Katonah, Doralee Grindler, 5
Kearney, David J., 6–7
Kindness; see also Compassion; Self-compassion
    seeking circuitry and, 203
King, Martin Luther, Jr., 48
Klein, Melanie, 126
Knowing, implicit versus explicit, 314–315; see
        also Focusing-oriented psychotherapy
Kornfield, Jack, 17, 43

L

LeDoux, Joseph, 187
Letters from the Dhamma Brothers: Meditation
        behind Bars, 339
Lewis, David J., 5
Listening, in focusing-oriented therapy,
        325–326
Lobsang Tenzin Negi, 343
Lojong (mind training) tradition, 343
Love, seeking circuitry and, 203–204, 204n6
Loving-kindness, versus compassion, 47
Loving-kindness (metta) meditation, 18, 203
    brain impacts of, 35–36
    Buddha's talk on, 44
    for chronic pain, 263–264
    healthy psychological functioning and,
        279–280
    for traumatized veterans (see Traumatized
        veterans)
    in vipassana prison program, 335

M

Madni, Laila A., 7
Magyari, Trish, 5
Mahayana Buddhism; see also Buddhism;
        Buddhist practice; Buddhist psychology
    IFS and, 132–133
Main, Mary, 214
Major depression, diagnosis and duration of,
        92
Meditation; see also Loving-kindness (metta)
        meditation; Mindfulness meditation
    analytical, 112
    appropriateness of, 17–18
    brain changes and, 219–220
    for children, 288
    concentration, 198n3
    contraindications to, 17–18
    EMDR as, 110
    limitations of, with severe trauma, 16–17
    in MBSR, 141
    sweeping, 41
Meditation practices, types of, 15
Meditation skills, client acquisition of, 19
Meditation teachers, qualifications of, 18–19
Memory; see also Traumatic memories
    dissociation of, 227–228
    emotional, of children, 292–293
    retraumatization and, 64

Memory overgenerality; *see* Overgeneralized memory
Mental health, spirituality and, 159
Metacognitive awareness, 19–20, 360
Metta meditation; *see* Loving-kindness *(metta)* meditation
Mind
  habits of, MBSR and, 151–152
  IPNB definition of, 218
  theories of, 126
Mindful Attention Awareness Scale (MAAS), 47
Mindful movements, for children, 288
Mindful self-compassion training, 55
Mindfulness; *see also* Embedded relational mindfulness
  adaptations for children, 287–289
  clinical benefits of, 216
  components of, 305–307
  in DBT, 75
  definitions of, 14–15, 198, 216, 229–230, 275, 285–286, 332–333
  EMDR and, 115
  foundations of, 289–293
  IFS and, 130–132
  impaired integration and, 216–218
  and improvement of mental processes, 218
  in MBSR, 148
  for overcoming dissociation, case example of, 303–305
  overgeneralized memory and, 96
  research on, 217–218
  seeking and, 202
  self-compassion and, 47–48
  in sensorimotor psychotherapy, 229–231, 230f
  stimulus focus in, 235–236, 235f
  and therapeutic skills in embedded relational mindfulness, 232–234
  therapist and, 24–25
  as therapy commonality, 360
  and transformation of suffering, 198–199
  and valued action (*see* Acceptance and commitment therapy (ACT))
Mindfulness groups
  limitations of, with severe trauma, 16–17
  referrals to, 18
  trauma-focused, 18
Mindfulness Intervention for Child Abuse Survivors studies, 143–145
Mindfulness meditation
  versus seated meditation practice, 310
  and transition to exposure, 310–311
  TRD and
    implementing, 310–311
    rationale for using, 308
    structuring sessions of, 308–309
    therapist monitoring of, 309–310
    TRD and, 305–311
Mindfulness practices
  for autonomic reactivity, 262
  for chronic pain, 261–265
  versus compassion, 349–350
  for establishing safety, 265
  for illness anxiety, 262–263

integration of, 15
for pain experience, 263
risks of, 264–265
for self-soothing, 263–264
for unwanted mental contents, 264
Mindfulness programs, for veterans with PTSD, 274–275; *see also* Traumatized veterans
Mindfulness skills, client acquisition of, 19
Mindfulness-augmented trauma therapy, types of, 17–20
Mindfulness-based approaches
  development of, 2
  empirical validation of, 2
  types of, 2
  without ethical/religious contexts, 201n4
Mindfulness-based cognitive therapy (MBCT), 15
  depression and, 47
  trauma-related chronic depression and, 96–98
Mindfulness-based cognitive therapy for children (MBCT-C), 287–289
  home practice and, 296
Mindfulness-based relapse prevention (MBRP), 15
Mindfulness-based stress reduction (MBSR), 15–16, 140–156
  adaptations of, 152–153
  appropriate candidates for, 146–147
  and avoidance of stigma, 246–247
  and avoidance of trauma narrative, 249
  background of, 141
  balancing awareness and compassion in, 151
  body scan sensitivities and, 153–155
  versus CBCT, 349
  characteristics of, 245–249
  client reactivity and, 148–149
  clinical challenges of survivors and, 146
  community building and, 247–248
  confidentiality guidelines and, 148
  contraindications to, 147
  empowerment through, 247
  enrollment interviews and, 152
  exclusionary criteria for, 278
  incorporating trauma sensitivities into, 147–148
  introducing mindfulness into, 148
  mindfulness skills and, 248–249
  naming habits of mind in, 151–152
  nonjudgmental stance of, 247
  nurturing quality of, 251
  participant choices/control in, 148
  participant reactions to, 144–145
  preliminary studies of, 276–278
  providing directions and guidelines for, 150
  and reduced risk of emotional flooding, 251
  research evidence for, 143–145
  safe attachment to instructor of, 250
  safety concerns in, 147–148, 250
  self-compassion and, 54
  and self-efficacy, 250
  self-empowerment and, 251

for sexual abuse survivors, 5
    for low-income minority women, 6
standard curriculum for, 246
teacher/therapist characteristics for, 147–
    148
theoretical considerations in, 142–143
and tools for self-regulation, 251
transcending self-loathing cycle in, 151
trauma-related adaptations of, 249–251
for traumatized veterans (see Traumatized
    veterans)
for underserved trauma populations,
    243–256
    rationale for, 244–245
whole-self approach of, 248
Mindfulness-oriented interventions
hybrid approach to, 16–20
mechanisms of, 62
Multimodal therapies, 12–13
Multiplicity of mind, 125–127

N

Nairn, Rob, 51
Narcissism, versus self-compassion, 49
Narrative, verbal, limitations of, 237–238
National Institute of Mental Health (NIMH),
    Collaborative Depression Study of, 92
Neff, Kristin, 4
Neurobiology; see Interpersonal neurobiology;
    Neuroscience
Neuroception, versus perception, 231–232
Neuroscience
of contemplative practices, 6
loving-kindness meditation and, 35–36
PTSD findings from, 158
of traumatic abuse, 31–32
Neurotransmitter levels, yoga and, 171
Nonjudgmental stance, in DBT, 80–81
North American Vipassana Prison Trust,
    336–337
Nucleus accumbens, in seeking circuitry,
    187–188
Numbing, 13
    chronic pain and, 261

O

Ogden, Pat, 6
One-mindful, defined, 81
Opioids
fear and seeking circuitries and, 196–197
satisfaction circuitry and, 189–190
Opposite action, in DBT, 82–83
Overgeneralized memory
chronic depression and, 95–96
downstream consequences of, 95–96
key variables in, 95
mindfulness and, 96
posttrauma emotional disturbance and,
    94–95
as predictor of depression risk, 96
trauma and, 93–95
war trauma and, 94–95
Ozawa-de Silva, Brendan, 7

P

Pain, 11–30
avoidance of, 260–261
chronic (see Trauma-related chronic pain)
dissociation and, 32, 259
engaging, 14
experimentally produced, 266–267
mindfulness approaches to, 6, 263
versus suffering, 21–22, 289
as trigger for fight-freeze-flight response, 259
unprocessed, 31–32
Pain paradox, 13–14
Panksepp, Jaak, 187
Parker, Robert A., 7
Peritraumatic dissociation, 302
Perpetrators, nonjudgmental descriptions of,
    80–81
Personal Values Questionnaire, 67
Phillips, Jenny, 7
Pleasure, brain opioids and, 189–190
Positive/preferred cognition (PC)
aspiration and, 110–111
in EMDR, 108, 110–111
future ideal state and, 119
Posttraumatic stress disorder (PTSD); see PTSD
Prisoners, traumatized; see Traumatized
    prisoners, vipassana meditation for
Prisons
hypermasculine and violent culture of, 330
lack of trauma treatment in, 331–332
mental health treatment and, 329–330
trauma-informed correctional care and,
    331–332
Psychoanalysis, PTSD and, 12
Psychoeducation, for children, 293
Psychological homeostasis, maintaining, 13–14
Psychological mindfulness, versus EMDR, 115
Psychological trauma, 11
Psychology; see also Buddhist psychology
Western, versus Buddhist psychology, 16
Psychosynthesis, 127
Psychotherapy, sensorimotor; see Embedded
    relational mindfulness; Sensorimotor
    psychotherapy
PTSD
Buddhist practice and, 104–105
childhood trauma and, 214–215
in children, 285 (see also Childhood trauma)
DSM-5 diagnostic criteria for, 142, 212
EMDR and, 102–103
    case example of, 103–104
emphasis on symptoms of, 61
felt sense of, 158–162
interventions for, 1
MBSR and, 142–156
neuroscience findings from, 158
normalizing coping strategies for, 150
overgeneralized memory and, 94
prevalence among veterans, 273
rationale for mindfulness programs for,
    275–276
risk factors for, 215–216
samsara and, 105

PTSD (*continued*)
  symptom clusters in, 45, 46t
  symptoms of, 12

R

Raison, Charles L., 7
Rape
  prevalence of, 243
  of prisoners, prevalence of, 329
Rape survivors, triggering memories and, 63
Reactivity
  MBSR and, 149–150
  in PTSD, 146
Recovery, seeking circuitry and, 193–197, 195f, 197f
Reexperiencing
  client responses to, 171
  in PTSD, 146
Refuge; *see* Inner refuge
Regression, 317
Relationship problems, MBSR and, 142–143
Reward circuitry, seeking circuitry and, 187
Risk factors
  embedded relational mindfulness and, 231–232
  for emotional flooding, with MSBR, 251
  in exposure therapy, 332
  mindfulness practices and, 264–265
  for PTSD, 215–216
  for recurrent depression, 91
  in sensorimotor psychotherapy, 231–232
Rogers, Carl, 136, 160
Rozelle, Deborah, 5

S

Safe place resource, and EMDR, 106–107
Safety
  client's neuroception of, 232
  mindfulness practices for establishing, 265
  MSBR and, 147–148, 250
  in sensorimotor psychotherapy, 231–232
  trauma recovery and, 330
Samsara, PTSD and, 105
Satisfaction circuitry, 189–190
  healing cycle and, 196–197
Schwartz, Richard C., 5
Second-arrow issues, 22
  mindfulness practices and, 263
  and psychological/neurobiological mechanisms of action, 266–267
  separating two arrows meditation and, 268
  urge surfing for pain meditation and, 268–269
  working with, 23–24
Seeking circuitry, 187–189
  and contemplative practices for seeking true goods, 200–205
  and contemplative practices for transforming suffering, 197–199
  and cultivation of love, kindness, compassion, 203–204
  cycles of suffering and, 191, 192f
  healing and, 193–197, 195f, 197f

imaginary rewards and, 188–189
  and love, kindness, compassion, 203
  mindfulness and, 202, 202n5
  misunderstanding of, 201–203
  and other "true goods," 204–205
  pleasure and, 188
  quick fixes and, 188
Self
  access to, 131–132
  in ACT model, 66–67, 71
  as Buddha Nature, 133
  in IFS model, 130
  of therapist, 135–136
Self leadership, 125
Self-acceptance, as therapy commonality, 360
Self-blame, 43
  de-shaming and, 34–35
Self-compassion, 4, 44–50
  in CBCT, 343, 354
  children and, 293
  defining, 44
  hard wiring for, 43–44
  healthy psychological functioning and, 279–280
  as heart of mindfulness, 47–48
  lack of, 45–46
  MBSR and, 54
  mindfulness and, 47–48
  misconceptions about, 48–50
  protective function of, 46
  versus self-pity, 49
  in therapy relationship, 51–52
  trauma and, 45–46
  in trauma treatment, 50–54
Self-compassion break, 53–54
Self-compassion interventions, 53–54
Self-Compassion Scale (SCS), 44, 47
Self-compassion training programs, 54–55
Self-criticism, *versus* self-encouragement, 49
Self-efficacy, MBSR and, 250
Self-empowerment, MSBR and, 251
Self-evaluation, of therapist, 82
Self-kindness, 44; *see also* Loving-kindness *(metta)* meditation
Self-regulation
  mindfulness and, 219
  tools for, MSBR and, 251
  in trauma-sensitive yoga, 178–180
Self-soothing
  chronic pain and, 260
  mindfulness practices for, 263–264
Self-to-Self connectedness, in IFS, 136–137
Semple, Randye J., 7
Sensorimotor psychotherapy; *see also* Embedded relational mindfulness
  case example of, 234–237
  clinical "map" of, 229–231, 230f
  therapeutic relationship in, 231–232
Settling skills, 19
Sex offenders
  adolescent (*see* Focusing-oriented psychotherapy, with adolescent sex offender)
  working with, 317–318

Sexual abuse of children; *see also* Childhood trauma
  MBSR and, 5
"Should-ing," 290
Siegel, Daniel J., 6
Siegel, Ronald D., 6
Sparks, Flint, 5
Spiritual transformation
  life-changing crises and, 159
  seeking circuitry and, 193–197, 195*f*, 197*f*
Spirituality, mental/physical health and, 159
Stewart, Bruce, 336, 337
Stress response
  inward turning of, 45, 46t
  PTSD symptoms and, 45, 46t
Suffering
  avoidance-related, 62
  breaking cycles of, 194–195
  Buddhism and, 21, 42, 104–105, 334
  cycles of, brain circuitry and, 191–193
  dissociation and, 32
  exploring causes of, in CBCT, 346
  versus pain, 21–22, 289
  spirituality and, 159–160
  transforming
    contemplative practices for, 197–200
    seeking circuitry and, 194–195, 195*f*
Suppression, effects of, 63
Survivors
  and appropriateness of meditation, 17–18
  challenges of, 146
  and risk of mental disorders, 140
  self-compassion and, 49
  struggles of, 1
Sweeping meditation, 41
Systems thinking, 125

T

Talk therapy, body wisdom and, 158
Therapeutic interventions, traditional, resistance to, 12
Therapist
  acceptance by, 33–34
  in ACT model, 69–70
  felt sense response of, 161–162, 167
  MBSR and, 147–148
  mindfulness of, 24–25
    in DBT, 81–82
  self of, 135–136
  sufficient experience/training for, 361
Therapist–client relationship, 24–25
  developing, 32–33
  embedded relational mindfulness and, 231–234
  self-compassion in, 51–52
  in sensorimotor psychotherapy, 231–232
Thich Nhat Hanh, 202, 203
Thinking
  depressive, 97–98, 98*f*
  systems, 125
Thoughts
  changing relationship to, *versus* changing content of, 349–350

children's relationship with, 289
intrusive
  mindfulness practice and, 276
  trauma-related chronic pain and, 260–261
  nonfactual nature of, 290–291
Tibetan Buddhism
  CBCT and, 343
  IFS and, 128
Tolstoy, Leo, 159–160
Transcendental meditation, 16
Trauma
  broadened understanding of, 1–2
  and crisis of faith, 159
  definitions of, 31
  developmental, 210–213 (*see also* Interpersonal neurobiology)
  emotional and psychological effects of, 243–244
  felt sense of, 158–162
  groups at risk for, 244 (*see also* Mindfulness-based stress reduction (MBSR), for underserved populations)
  impacts of, 11–12
  memories of, 11–12
  overgeneralized memory and, 93–95
  prevalence of, 243
  self-compassion and, 45–46
  transdisciplinary approaches to, 3–4
  types of, 1–2
  unconscious processes and, 227–228
  Western definition of, 11–12
Trauma Center at the Justice Resource Institute (JRI), 170
Trauma interventions
  evidence-based, symptom focus of, 244
  mindfulness-based, 305–310 (*see also* Mindfulness-based approaches; specific approaches)
  types of, 17–20
Trauma narratives, avoiding reliving of, 249
Trauma processing, in EMDR, 107–109
Trauma recovery, Herman's three-stage model of, 330–331
Trauma-informed correctional care, 331–332
Trauma-related chronic pain, 257–272
  autonomic reactivity and, 258–259
  co-occurrence with PTSD, 274
  fear and, 260
  fear of intrusive thoughts and, 260–261
  illness anxiety and, 259
  and lack of self-soothing, 260
  mechanism of, 257–261
  mindfulness practices for, 261–269
  psychological and neurobiological mechanisms of action in, 266–267
Trauma-related dissociation (TRD), 301–313
  assessment of, 304–305
  differential diagnosis of, 304–305
  mindfulness meditation and, 305–306
    case example of, 303–304
    considerations for using, 306–310
    implementing, 310–311
  symptoms of, 302

Trauma-related dissociation (TRD) (*continued*)
  trauma triggers and, 301, 304
  types of, 302–303
Trauma-sensitive yoga, 170–171
  adding complexity to, 177
  advice and caution for, 180–181
  befriending body and, 177
  case examples of, 173–176, 178–180
  self-regulation in, 178–180
  in treatment context, 171–177
Traumatic abuse, neuroscience of, 31–32
Traumatic memories; *see also* Memory
  characteristics of, 97
  increasing acceptance of, 19
Traumatized prisoners
  contemplative practices and, 332–333
  correctional care and, 331–332
  exposure therapy and, 332
  and lack of trauma treatment, 331–332
  offenses and sentences of, 338
  prison culture and, 330
  and stages of recovery and treatment,
    330–331
  vipassana meditation for, 7, 329–342
    at Donaldson Correctional Facility,
      336–339
    outcome studies of, 337–339
Traumatized veterans
  MBSR and loving-kindness meditation for,
    273–283
  MBSR outcomes and, 278–279
  prevalence of, 273
  with PTSD, 274–280
    exclusion criteria for MBSR and, 278
    future directions for, 278–280
    MBSR studies and, 276–278
    mindfulness programs for, 274–275
    rationale for mindfulness programs for,
      275–276
  reactions to meditation programs, 275
Triggers
  examples of, 104, 304
  fear and seeking, body sensations and,
    190–191
  identification of, 20
  somatic responses to, 171–172
  trauma-sensitive yoga and, 175
  TRD and, 304
True goods
  healing cycle and, 195–197, 197f
  religious/spiritual traditions and, 201
  seeking cycle and, 196
    contemplative practices for, 200–205

Trust, between therapist and client, 32–33
Turcotte, Shirley, 317

U

Uncertainty, developmental trauma and, 219
Unconscious processes, trauma-related,
  227–228
Urge surfing, 20

V

Vajrayana Buddhist practice, 116
Valued Living Questionnaire, 67
Values; *see also* Core values
  in ACT model, 67–68
  connecting to, 4
  conversations about, 67
Values Compass, 67
Verbal narrative, limitations of, 237–238
Veterans; *see* Traumatized veterans
Vietnam veterans, overgeneralized memory and,
  93–94
Violence, in prisons, 330
Vipassana, defined, 334
Vipassana meditation
  Buddhist psychology and, 334–336
  prison-based, 7
    at Donaldson Correctional Facility,
      336–339
    Goenka approach to, 334–336, 334n1
    outcomes of, 333
Visualizations, in loving-kindness meditation,
  36

W

Waelde, Lynn C., 7
War trauma, overgeneralized memory and,
  94–95
Watkins, Helen, 127
Watkins, John, 127
Western psychology, *versus* Buddhist
  psychology, 16
Williams, J. Mark G., 5
Wisdom, Buddhist perspective on, 20–21

Y

Yoga, 18, 170–181; *see also* Trauma-sensitive
  yoga
  in CBCT, 353–356
  for children, 288
  health benefits of, 170
  neurotransmitter levels and, 171